PEDIATRICS RECALL
2nd edition

RECALL SERIES EDITOR

LORNE H. BLACKBOURNE, M.D.
General Surgeon
Fayetteville, North Carolina

PEDIATRICS RECALL
2nd edition

Editors:

EUGENE D. MCGAHREN III MD
Associate Professor of Pediatric Surgery and Pediatrics
Division of Pediatric Surgery
Departments of Surgery and Pediatrics
University of Virginia Health System
Charlottesville, Virginia

WILLIAM G. WILSON MD
Professor of Pediatrics
Department of Pediatrics
University of Virginia Health System
Charlottesville, Virginia

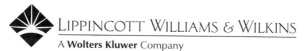
LIPPINCOTT WILLIAMS & WILKINS
A **Wolters Kluwer** Company
Philadelphia · Baltimore · New York · London
Buenos Aires · Hong Kong · Sydney · Tokyo

Editor: Neil Marquardt
Development Editor: Emilie Linkins
Managing Editor: Amy Dinkel

351 West Camden Street
Baltimore, Maryland 21201-2436 USA

530 Walnut Street
Philadelphia, Pennsylvania 19106 USA

The publisher is not responsible (as a matter of product liability, negligence,
or otherwise) for any injury resulting from any material contained herein. This
publication contains information relating to general principles of medical care
which should not be construed as specific instructions for individual patients.
Manufacturers' product information and package inserts should be reviewed
for current information, including contraindications, dosages, and precautions.

Printed in the United States of America

Library of Congress Cataloging-in-Publication Data

Pediatrics recall / editors, Eugene D. McGahren, William G. Wilson.—2nd
ed.
   p. cm. — (Recall series)
  Previous ed. cataloged under: McGahren, Eugene D.
  Includes index.
  ISBN 0-7817-2611-5
   1. Pediatrics—Examinations, questions, etc. 2. Pediatrics—Outlines, syl-
labi, etc. I. McGahren, Eugene D. II. Wilson, William G. (William Grady),
1949– III. Series.

  RJ48.2 .M37 2002
  618.92′00076—dc21   2001038525

*The publishers have made every effort to trace the copyright holders for bor-
rowed material. If they have inadvertently overlooked any, they will be
pleased to make the necessary arrangements at the first opportunity.*

We'd like to hear from you! If you have comments or suggestions regarding
this Lippincott Williams & Wilkins title, please contact us at the appropriate
customer service number listed below, or send correspondence to
book_comments@lww.com. If possible, please remember to include your
mailing address, phone number, and a reference to the book title and author
in your message. To purchase additional copies of this book call our customer
service department at **(800) 638-3030** or fax orders to **(301) 824-7390.** International customers should call **(301) 714-2324.**

02 03 04
1 2 3 4 5 6 7 8 9 10

Dedication

Gene McGahren would like to dedicate the second edition to Catherine, Christopher, and Caroline for their love and humor always.

Bill Wilson dedicates the second edition to Allen and Laura.

Contents

SECTION I
OVERVIEW AND BACKGROUND INFORMATION

SECTION II
NEWBORN CARE

SECTION III
AMBULATORY PEDIATRICS

SECTION IV
PEDIATRIC DISEASES

Contributors

Stephen Borowitz, MD
Professor
Division of Gastroenterology
Department of Pediatrics
University of Virginia Health System
Charlottesville, Virginia

Robert J. Boyle, MD
Professor
Division of Neonatology
Department of Pediatrics
University of Virginia Health System
Charlottesville, Virginia

Marguerite Crawford, MD
Fellow in Cardiology
Department of Pediatrics
University of Virginia Health System
Charlottesville, Virginia

Kimberly Dunsmore, MD
Associate Professor
Division of Hematology and Oncology
Department of Pediatrics
University of Virginia Health System
Charlottesville, Virginia

Nancy L. McDaniel, MD
Associate Professor
Division of Cardiology
Department of Pediatrics
University of Virginia Health System
Charlottesville, Virginia

Eugene D. McGahren III, MD
Associate Professor of Pediatric
Surgery and Pediatrics
Division of Pediatric Surgery
Departments of Surgery and
  Pediatrics
University of Virginia Health System
Charlottesville, Virginia

Victoria Norwood, MD
Associate Professor
Division of Nephrology
Department of Pediatrics
University of Virginia Health System
Charlottesville, Virginia

W. Davis Parker, Jr., MD
Eugene Meyer II Professor of
  Neuroscience
Departments of Neurology and
  Pediatrics
University of Virginia Health System
Charlottesville, Virginia

Vito Perriello, MD
Pediatric Associates
Charlottesville, Virginia

Erick J. Richmond, MD
Fellow in Endocrinology
Department of Pediatrics
University of Virginia Health System
Charlottesville, Virginia

Frank T. Saulsbury, MD
Professor
Department of Pediatrics
University of Virginia Health System
Charlottesville, Virginia

Linda Waggoner-Fountain, MD
Assistant Professor
Department of Pediatrics
University of Virginia Health System
Charlottesville, Virginia

William G. Wilson, MD
Professor of Pediatrics
Department of Pediatrics
University of Virginia Health System
Charlottesville, Virginia

Paul Wisman, MD
Pediatric Associates
Charlottesville, Virginia

William A. Woods, MD
Assistant Professor of Emergency
    Medicine and Pediatrics
Departments of Emergency
    Medicine and Pediatrics
University of Virginia Health System
Charlottesville, Virginia

Preface to the Second Edition

Pediatrics Recall provides information in a concise question-and-answer format, which allows easy access to material that is essential for medical students during their third-year clinical clerkships in pediatrics. The book covers basic issues in neonatal and pediatric fluid management, blood products, nutrition, emergencies, growth, and intensive care. In addition, an entire chapter is devoted to issues relating to the adolescent patient. Disease entities are organized into chapters according to the systems involved. Descriptions of the individual diseases include signs, symptoms, essentials of pathophysiology, treatments, and possible outcomes. Students may use the question-and-answer format to work through each condition from presentation and diagnosis to therapy and outcome.

Pediatrics Recall is not intended to be used as a primary text. Rather, it allows students to review essential information in an efficient format that is designed to facilitate retention.

Changes to the second edition of *Pediatrics Recall* reflect input from students, residents, community physicians, and pediatric generalists and specialists in both the primary writing and review of the text. We have added a chapter devoted to hernias and abdominal wall defects; incorporated new diagrams, tables, and charts; and increased the use of cross-references within the book. We hope that this book will be useful to you and we welcome your suggestions.

Acknowledgments

The editors would like to thank Peg Lascano and Emilie Linkins. Their undying help and enthusiasm made this 2nd Edition of Pediatrics Recall a reality.

The editors would also like to acknowledge the contributors to the first edition. They created the foundation upon which the second edition is built.

Mark A. Brown MD
Pamela Clark MD
William L. Clarke MD
Michael D. Dickens MD
Patricia Hagan MD
Rajesh Malik MD
Robert S. Michel MD
Alan A. Rogol MD, PhD
Jocelyn Schauer MD
Deborah E. Smith MD
Richard D. Stevenson MD
Kathryn Weise MD
Claudia C. Zegans MD
Eugene D. McGahren III MD
William G. Wilson MD
Stephen Borowitz MD
Robert J. Boyle MD
Frank T. Saulsbury MD
Paul Wisman MD
Victoria Norwood MD
W. Davis Parker Jr. MD
Nancy L. McDaniel MD
Kimberly Dunsmore MD
Vito Perriello MD

Section I

Overview and Background Information

1   Introduction

USING THE STUDY GUIDE

This study guide was written to accompany the pediatric clerkship, and we welcome any feedback or suggestions for improvement. The objective of the guide is to provide a rapid overview of common pediatric topics, but keep in mind that this is NOT an all-encompassing source (i.e., you will have to consult major textbooks to round out the information in this guide). The guide is organized in a self-study quiz format. By covering the information and answers on the right side of the page with the bookmark, you can attempt to answer the questions on the left to assess your understanding of the information. Keep the guide with you at all times, and when you have even a few minutes (e.g., between patients), hammer out a page or at least a few questions.

PEDIATRIC NOTES AND PRESENTATIONS

DOCUMENTATION AND COMMUNICATION

In addition to documentation and communication functions, the content of admission and progress notes implies much about the ability of the medical student or resident to gather and analyze data and formulate a treatment plan. Therefore, pertinent negative findings (i.e., the normal findings that the student or resident chooses to include in the written notes) convey the student's problem-solving abilities. In addition, many pediatric, medical, or surgical services expect the medical students to write a detailed discussion of the patient's condition at the end of an admission or progress note. Make certain you understand what is expected of you.

ADMISSION NOTES

The format of an admission note may vary in different institutions, but the note generally contains the following information:

1. Name of patient
2. Age
3. Gender
4. Reason for admission (presenting complaint or diagnosis)
5. Informant (historian)
6. Referring physician or health professional (if referred)

7. History of present illness
8. Past medical history (including, as indicated, prenatal and newborn history)
9. Immunizations
10. Allergies
11. Current medications
12. Hospitalizations
13. Surgeries
14. Developmental history
15. Review of systems
16. Physical measurements (height, weight, head circumference)
17. Vital signs (usually temperature, pulse, respiratory rate, blood pressure)
18. Physical examination
19. Assessment
20. Plan

The organization of the admission note may vary. Because pediatrics encompasses a broad age range, certain elements may be included or excluded, depending on the situation. For example, the elements of the history for a 3-year-old with seizures and developmental delay may not be the same as those for a 16-year-old with an ankle fracture.

PROGRESS NOTES

Progress notes should be concise and convey information about the patient's status, test results, and current treatments and plans. Editorial comments, criticisms of other services or the nursing staff, and humor should all be avoided. Most hospitals use some modification of the **SOAP note** as the standard for progress notes: **S**ubjective (what the patient says he/she feels), **O**bjective (what the physical examination reveals), **A**ssessment (interpretation of the information obtained), **P**lan (treatment plan).

ORAL PRESENTATIONS

The format of an oral presentation depends on the situation. Presentations are usually brief on work and checkout rounds and are more detailed during attending or teaching rounds. You must clearly communicate to your colleagues the important information needed for patient care. Presentations during teaching rounds usually allow more time for discussing differential diagnoses and basic science correlations.

Presentations, like written notes, convey information about the student's ability. A clear, well-organized presentation, with discussion of the patient's differential diagnosis and plans for evaluation and treatment, implies much about the clinical and analytical skills of the student.

COMMON ABBREVIATIONS

Although abbreviations are a part of the medical culture, they may be misinterpreted. A written note that does not use abbreviations is much less likely to be misinterpreted than one that is filled with abbreviations. Be careful in using abbreviations, because many of them have several different interpretations, depending on the context and the patient. For example, the abbreviation CP could mean cerebral palsy, cleft palate, chest pain, or carotid pulse. When in doubt, write out a term. Most hospitals have a list of approved abbreviations. Make certain that you use abbreviations that are approved in your hospital. Remember that the purposes of written notes are documentation and communication.

Δ	Change
ā	Before
ABG	Arterial blood gas
As and Bs	Apnea and bradycardia
AD	Autosomal dominant
ADH	Antidiuretic hormone
ADHD	Attention deficit hyperactivity disorder
AGA	Appropriate for gestational age
AIDS	Acquired immunodeficiency syndrome
ALL	Acute lymphocytic leukemia
	Acute lymphoblastic leukemia
ALTE	Acute life-threatening event
AMA	Against medical advice
AML	Acute myelocytic leukemia
ANC	Absolute neutrophil count
ANLL	Acute nonlymphocytic leukemia
AP	Anterior-posterior
AR	Autosomal recessive
AS	Aortic stenosis
ASD	Atrial septal defect
B	Bilateral
BA	Bone age
BAER	Brainstem auditory evoked response
BE	Barium enema
bid	Twice a day
BM	Bone marrow (aspirate)
	Bowel movement
BP	Blood pressure
BPD	Bronchopulmonary dysplasia
BUN	Blood urea nitrogen
c̄	With
CA	Cancer
	Chronologic age
C & S	Culture and sensitivity
CBC	Complete blood (cell) count
cc	Cubic centimeter
CC	Clinical clerk
CDC	Centers for Disease Control and Prevention
CDH	Congenital diaphragmatic hernia
	Congenital dislocation of the hip

CF	Cystic fibrosis
CHD	Congenital heart disease
CHF	Congestive heart failure
CMV	Cytomegalovirus
CN	Cranial nerve
CNS	Central nervous system
C/O	Complaint of
CP	Cerebral palsy
	Cleft palate
CPAP	Continuous positive airway pressure
CPR	Cardiopulmonary resuscitation
CSF	Cerebrospinal fluid
C-spine	Cervical spine
CT	Computed tomography
CVA	Cerebrovascular accident (stroke)
CVP	Central venous pressure
C/W	Compatible with
	Consistent with
CX	Culture
CXR	Chest radiograph
D/C (or DC)	Discontinue
	Discharge
DDST	Denver Developmental Screening Test
DI	Diabetes insipidus
DIC	Disseminated intravascular coagulation
DM	Diabetes mellitus
DNA	Deoxyribonucleic acid
DNS	Dextrose in normal saline
DTaP	Diphtheria/tetanus/acellular pertussis/ immunization (also known as DTP: diphtheria, tetanus, and pertussis vaccine)
DTRs	deep tendon reflexes
D#W	Dextrose in water (#% glucose in grams/dL [e.g., D5W])
DX	Diagnosis
ECG/EKG	Electrocardiogram
ECMO	Extracorporeal membrane oxygenation
EEG	Electroencephalogram
EGA	Estimated gestational age
EMG	Electromyogram
ESR	Erythrocyte sedimentation rate
ESRD	End-stage renal disease
ETT	Endotracheal tube
FiO$_2$	Fraction of inspired oxygen
FROM	Full range of motion
GBS	Group B streptococcus
G tube	Gastrostomy tube

GU	Genitourinary
HAL	Hyperalimentation
Hct	Hematocrit
HFJV	High-frequency jet ventilation
HFOV	High-frequency oscillatory ventilation
Hgb	Hemoglobin
HiB	Haemophilus influenzae B vaccine
HIE	Hypoxic ischemic encephalopathy
HIV	Human immunodeficiency virus
HPV	Human papillomavirus
HMD	Hyaline membrane disease
HSP	Henoch-Schönlein purpura
HSV	Herpes simplex virus
ICH	Intracranial hemorrhage
ICP	Intracranial pressure
IDDM	Insulin-dependent diabetes mellitus
IM	Intramuscular(ly)
I/O	Intake and output
IPV	Inactivated injectable poliovirus vaccine
IRDS	Infantile respiratory distress syndrome
ITP	Idiopathic thrombocytopenic purpura
IUGR	Intrauterine growth retardation
IV	Intravenous(ly)
IVH	Intraventricular hemorrhage
IVIG	Intravenous immunoglobulin
IVP	Intravenous pyelogram
LA	Left arm
	Left atrium
LE	Lower extremity
LFTs	Liver function tests
LGA	Large for gestational age
LLL	Left lower lobe of lung
LP	Lumbar puncture
LR	Lactated Ringer's (solution)
LUL	Left upper lobe of lung
LUQ	Left upper quadrant
LV	Left ventricle
LVH	Left ventricular hypertrophy
MAP	Mean airway pressure
MD	Medical doctor
	Muscular dystrophy
MMR	Measles, mumps, rubella vaccine
MS	Mitral stenosis
	Morphine sulfate
	Multiple sclerosis
MSPN	Medical student progress note
MVA	Motor vehicle accident
NAD	No acute distress

	No apparent distress
NARD	No apparent respiratory distress
ND	Nasoduodenal
NEC	Necrotizing enterocolitis
NG	Nasogastric
NGT	Nasogastric tube
NJ	Nasojejunal tube
NPO	Nothing by mouth
NPR	Nothing per rectum
NSR	Normal sinus rhythm
OFC	Occipitofrontal circumference
OM	Otitis media
OPV	Oral poliovirus vaccine
PA	Posterior-anterior
	Pulmonary artery
PAC	Premature atrial contraction
PDA	Patent ductus arteriosus
PE	Physical examination
	Pulmonary embolism
PEEP	Positive end-expiratory pressure
PEG	Percutaneous endoscopic gastrostomy
PID	Pelvic inflammatory disease
PIP	Positive inspiratory pressure
PO	By mouth
PPHN	Persistent pulmonary hypertension of the newborn
PR	By rectum
PRN, prn	As needed
qd	Daily
qid	Four times a day
qod	Every other day
RA	Radial artery
	Right atrium
RAM	Rapid alternating movements
RBC	Red blood cell
RDS	Respiratory distress syndrome
RLL	Right lower lobe of lung
RLQ	Right lower quadrant
RML	Right middle lobe of lung
ROM	Range of motion
	Rupture of membranes
RSV	Respiratory syncytial virus
RUL	Right upper lobe of lung
RUQ	Right upper quadrant
RV	Right ventricle
RVH	Right ventricular hypertrophy
Rx	Treatment
s̄	Without

SCT	Sacrococcygeal teratoma
SEM	Systolic ejection murmur
SGA	Small for gestational age
SIADH	Syndrome of inappropriate antidiuretic hormone secretion
SIDS	Sudden infant death syndrome
S/P	Status post
STD	Sexually transmitted disease
SVC	Superior vena cava
SVT	Supraventricular tachycardia
SX	Sign(s) or symptom(s)
TB	Tuberculosis
TBW	Total body water
TEF	Tracheoesophageal fistula
tid	Three times a day
Tmax	Maximum temperature
TOF	Tetralogy of Fallot
TOGV	Transposition of the great vessels (Also known as TOGA; transposition of the great arteries)
TPN	Total parenteral nutrition
TRP	Tubular reabsorption of phosphate
TTN	Transient tachypnea of newborn
UAC	Umbilical artery catheter
UPJ	Ureteropelvic junction
URI	Upper respiratory infection
U/S, US	Ultrasound examination
UTD	Up to date
UTI	Urinary tract infection
UVC	Umbilical vein catheter
VCUG	Vesicocystourethrogram Voiding cystourethrogram
VDRL	Venereal Disease Research Laboratory (test)
VER	Visual evoked response
VSD	Ventricular septal defect
VUR	Vesicoureteral reflux
WBC	White blood cell (count)
WNL	Within normal limits
$\bar{x}$	Except

2

Pediatric Procedures

VENIPUNCTURE/IVS

What are 3 indications for peripheral IVs in infants and children?

1. Administration of resuscitative fluids
2. Administration of maintenance fluids
3. Access for medications and parenteral nutrition

What are appropriate-size IVs for infants?

24 or 22 gauge

For toddlers?

22 gauge

For school-age children?

22 or 20 gauge

For older children and adolescents?

20, 18, or 16 gauge

What are the preferred sites for IVs?

A peripheral location is preferred, usually the foot, the dorsum of the hand, and in infants, the scalp. The saphenous or antecubital veins are next options. In children old enough to walk, hand and arm sites are best. IV sites should be carefully secured (especially for infants). However, excessive wrapping with gauze should be avoided so that the IV can be easily inspected and potentially serious problems (e.g., extensive infiltration) can be avoided.

What is the best technique for placing an IV?

Most health care workers have a technique that works best for them. The extremity is immobilized while placing the IV. (An assistant will be needed for placing IVs in neonates and toddlers.) The skin over the vein is pulled tautly, allowing the IV needle to puncture through the skin without creating redundancy. Once a flash of blood is obtained, the needle is advanced about 1 mm to ensure that the plastic catheter is in the vein. The catheter is then inserted over the needle. Have securing materials, including tape and an extremity board, ready when the IV is placed.

List 3 complications of IVs.

1. Infiltration
2. Thrombophlebitis
3. Necrosis of surrounding soft tissue; usually associated with infiltration of high-concentration calcium solutions or pressors administered through peripheral IVs. Generally, administration of such agents through peripheral IVs should be avoided.

How are these 3 complications treated?

1. Infiltration: remove the IV, elevate the extremity, and apply a warm soak.
2. Thrombophlebitis: same as for infiltration. Occasionally, an associated cellulitis may need to be treated with antibiotics.
3. Necrosis of soft tissue: remove the IV. Treat like a burn by applying antibiotic ointments (e.g., silver sulfadiazine [Silvadene], bacitracin). Any eschar should be removed. In rare cases, skin grafting may be necessary.

How can the pain of IV placement be minimized?

Prilocaine cream (EMLA) can be applied to the IV site before placement. In older, more cooperative children, subcutaneous 1% lidocaine may be an alternative.

LUMBAR PUNCTURE

List 3 indications for lumbar puncture (LP).

1. Suspicion of meningitis (Ch 27)
2. Administration of intrathecal medications
3. Any other need to evaluate CSF

List 3 contraindications to LP.

1. Evidence of increased intracranial pressure (ICP) when positioning the patient

2. When positioning the patient for an LP would risk cardiopulmonary compromise
3. Infection of the skin overlying the site of an LP

Should a contraindication to an LP delay antibiotic treatment or other therapy that may be needed?

No

How is an LP performed?

The patient is in a flexed lateral decubitus position. The skin is sterilized and the L3–L4 or L4–L5 interspace is identified for the LP. Local anesthesia (1% lidocaine) is given subcutaneously at the site of the LP. Usually a 22-gauge 1½-inch spinal needle is used. The needle is advanced slowly until it has entered the CSF space, which usually feels like a small "pop." This sensation may not be felt in a neonate. An opening CSF pressure may be obtained. CSF is then allowed to drip into specimen containers. The needle is withdrawn and pressure is placed on the site.

List 4 studies that should be performed on a CSF specimen.

Culture and sensitivity, cell count, glucose and protein concentration

What is a normal CSF red blood cell (RBC) count?

Normal CSF contains no RBCs. Presence of RBCs suggests a traumatic LP or a subarachnoid hemorrhage.

How may these be differentiated?

RBC count should decline from the first collection sample to the last with a traumatic LP.

What is a normal CSF white blood cell (WBC) count?

0–5 WBC/mm^3. The count may be as high as 15 WBC/mm^3 in newborns. Presence of polymorphonuclear neutrophil leukocytes (PMNs) within this count is **abnormal** although 1–2 PMN/mm^3 may be present in a newborn.

What is a normal CSF protein concentration?

Up to 150 mg/dl in the neonate, but falls to a normal range of 10–25 mg/dl by 6–12 weeks of age. It rises to adult range of 20–45 mg/dl during puberty. CSF protein increases approximately l mg/dl per 1000 RBC/mm^3 in a bloody specimen.

What is a "traumatic" LP (a.k.a. "bloody tap")?

An LP contaminated by blood from a surrounding vessel. Usually this confounds the neutrophil and protein count. It is best to rely on the bacterial culture of this kind of specimen (instead of adjusting the neutrophil or protein counts to account for the traumatic LP) or to obtain another LP sample at a later time.

SUPRAPUBIC PUNCTURE

What is an indication for suprapubic puncture?

Requirement for a sterile urine collection; it is usually performed in infants and toddlers because it is difficult to obtain a midstream urine specimen

What is the technique for suprapubic puncture?

After adequate hydration, a full bladder can be percussed. The suprapubic skin is disinfected. A 22- or 25-gauge needle is placed through the skin and into the bladder at a site about one fingerbreadth above the pubis. One or two milliliters of fluid are obtained for culture.

ARTERIAL PUNCTURE

What are 2 indications for arterial puncture?

1. When measurement of an arterial blood gas (ABG) is required.
2. When a blood sample is needed and a vein cannot be accessed, an artery provides a good site, particularly in an infant.

List 2 arteries that are preferred for drawing blood in infants.

The **radial** or the **dorsalis pedis** arteries. The femoral, brachial, or axillary arteries are less desirable because thrombosis and arterial insufficiency to the respective limb may occur.

List 3 instances in which an arterial cannula should be placed.

1. For constant monitoring of blood pressure (BP)
2. When frequent blood samples are required, especially in an infant or premature baby
3. When frequent ABG measurements are required

What are the best sites for arterial catheters? (List 3)

Radial and dorsalis pedis arteries. In the newborn, an umbilical artery catheter (UAC) can be placed for up to 10–14 days. (Ch 8, p 66)

What is the technique for blood sampling via an artery?

Usually a thin needle (25- or 23-gauge) is used. It is placed into the artery at a 45° angle facing toward the proximal end of the artery. The practitioner should make one clean pass and then pull the needle back until the tip is within the lumen of the artery. (Avoid "searching" for the artery with the needle.) The sample can then be taken.

What are the best techniques for placement of an arterial catheter?

Similar principles hold for placement of a catheter. Sometimes an angle of about 30° is better. After blood is obtained, the catheter should pass easily over the needle. If it does not, a small guidewire may be helpful. The needle is removed, the guidewire is passed through the plastic catheter, and the catheter is advanced over the guidewire. Arterial catheters are secured with tape in neonates and usually with a suture in toddlers and older children.

What are 2 complications of arterial catheters?

Thrombosis with ischemia to the affected extremity (rare when the radial or the dorsalis pedis arteries are used, because there is usually collateral flow to the palmar and plantar arches in the hand and the foot, respectively).

3

Fluids and Electrolytes

MAINTENANCE FLUID REQUIREMENTS

What are 3 primary methods for calculating maintenance fluid requirements?

Basing calculation on: **body weight** (most common); **body surface area;** and **caloric requirements** and **expenditures**

How is Body Surface Area (BSA) calculated?

$$\text{BSA (m}^2) = \sqrt{\frac{\text{Height (cm)} \times \text{weight (kg)}}{3600}}$$

What are approximate maintenance fluid requirements for infants, toddlers and young children?

Fluids

100 ml/kg/24 hr for first 10 kg of body weight
50 ml/kg/24 hr for second 10 kg of body weight
25 ml/kg/24 hr for each subsequent 10 kg of body weight

Electrolytes

Sodium: 3 mEq/100 ml
Chloride: 2 mEq/100 ml
Potassium: 2 mEq/100 ml

What are approximate maintenance fluid requirements for older children (10–14 years of age)?

Water: 1500 ml/m^2/24 hr
Sodium: 30–50 mEq/m^2/24 hr
Potassium: 20–40 mEq/m^2/24 hr

DEHYDRATION

What is it?

Depletion of total body water

List 4 common pediatric causes of dehydration.	Gastrointestinal (GI) losses (e.g., from gastroenteritis, diarrhea), inadequate fluid intake, excess renal losses, increased insensible losses (e.g., fever, sweating)
List 6 findings in mild dehydration.	Loss of 3%–5% of body weight, normal hemodynamic parameters and skin turgor, dry mucous membranes, slight decrease in urine output, and decreased tearing
List 6 findings in moderate dehydration.	Loss of 8%–10% of body weight, decreased skin turgor, dry mucous membranes, relatively normal hemodynamic parameters, decreased urine output, and slight to moderate increase in heart rate
What are the findings in severe dehydration?	Loss of 10%–15% of body weight, abnormal skin turgor and color, dry mucous membranes, rapid heart rate, decreased blood pressure (BP) (although it may still be normal!), poor peripheral perfusion, no urine output or tears
What is important to remember regarding the relationship between BP and dehydration in the infant and child?	Infants and children may maintain a relatively normal BP until a severe degree of dehydration (15%–25%) has occurred! The physician must monitor other parameters (i.e., heart rate, urine output, skin turgor, mucous membranes, mental status, etc.).

ISOTONIC DEHYDRATION

What is it?	Dehydration with maintenance of normal Na^+ concentration; as dehydration worsens, K^+ and blood urea nitrogen (BUN) tend to increase, and bicarbonate (HCO_3^-) tends to decrease.
What will happen to urine specific gravity?	It will increase. However, infants have poor ability to concentrate urine; thus, specific gravity may reach only 1.020, even in cases of severe dehydration.
What is the most common cause of isotonic dehydration?	GI losses secondary to viral or bacterial enteritis

What are the electrolyte concentrations of GI fluids?

Table 3–1. Electrolyte Concentrations of GI Fluids

Fluid	Na^+ (mEq/L)	K^+ (mEq/L)	Cl^- (mEq/L)
Gastric	20–80	5–20	100–150
Pancreatic	120–150	5–15	75–120
Small intestine	100–150	5–15	90–130
Bile	120–170	5–15	80–120
Diarrhea	10–130	10–100	10–100

What is the treatment strategy?

Calculate fluid and electrolyte losses using body weight, electrolyte values, and estimated time of dehydration. Then, rehydrate with appropriate fluids over 24–48 hours. **Note:** Replace K^+ more slowly because K^+ needs time to move intracellularly, where it is the predominant electrolyte. K^+ is added after normal renal function is confirmed.

HYPERNATREMIC DEHYDRATION

What is it?

Loss of more body water than solute, or administration of excess sodium, resulting in elevated serum sodium (> 145 mEq/L)

What are 4 causes of hypernatremic dehydration?

1. **Increased Na^+** (excess Na^+ intake or administration, hyperaldosteronism)
2. **Water loss** (excess respiration and perspiration, diabetes insipidus (DI) [Ch 21, p. 302.])
3. **Water loss that is greater than Na^+ loss** (GI and renal losses)
4. **Abnormal central control of osmotic balance** (essential hypernatremia)

List 5 signs and symptoms.

Lethargy, irritability, muscle weakness, convulsions, coma

Why is hypernatremic dehydration dangerous?

Since losses are more from intracellular than intravascular spaces, the symptoms may be masked until dehydration becomes severe.

How is hypernatremic dehydration treated?

Rehydrate **slowly** with low-sodium fluid to avoid rapid fluid shifts to the intracellular spaces. Usually, the deficit should be replaced over 48 hours.

What may happen if correction is too rapid?

Cerebral edema

HYPONATREMIC DEHYDRATION

What is it?

Relative depletion of sodium compared with total body water loss

What are 4 common etiologic factors?

GI losses, renal losses (including those caused by diuretics), adrenal insufficiency, third-space losses (e.g., ascites, postsurgical, burns)

List 11 signs and symptoms.

Anorexia, nausea, muscle cramps, lethargy, disorientation, agitation, diminished or pathologic reflexes, Cheyne-Stokes respiration, hypothermia, pseudobulbar palsy, seizures

What is the treatment?

Isotonic saline, administered at a rate determined by assessment of fluid and electrolyte losses and adequacy of rehydration. In some cases, judicious administration of hypertonic saline may be beneficial.

4

Blood and Blood Products

What are the uses of "whole blood"?

Sometimes used for volume expansion in emergencies in which there has been acute blood loss. Since the advent of component therapy, whole blood has few uses.

What constitutes a unit of packed red blood cells (RBCs)?

300 ml ($\pm$50 ml) with a hematocrit of 65%–80%

List 2 uses of packed RBCs.

Correct anemia and improve oxygen-carrying capacity of blood

By what percent does a packed–red-cell transfusion of 3 ml/kg raise the hematocrit?

Approximately 3%

What are the indications for irradiated blood products?

Situations in which the recipient might be at risk for engraftment by the donor cells (e.g., premature infants and immuno-compromised patients)

List 4 commonly used products that need to be irradiated for these patients.

RBCs, platelets, whole blood, leukocytes

What are indications for use of cytomegalovirus (CMV)-negative blood for transfusion?

CMV-negative blood is used for premature infants, transplant patients who are CMV-negative, bone marrow transplant recipients, patients with AIDS, and any others who might be at risk for symptomatic infection because they are immunocompromised.

List 2 indications for granulocyte transfusion.

Neutropenia (or defective neutrophil function); serious infection that is not responding to antibiotics

What constitutes a unit of platelets?

About 5×10^{10} platelets in 40–70 ml of plasma if stored at 20°C-24°C or 20–30 ml of plasma if stored at 1°C-6°C

List 2 indications for platelet transfusions.

Thrombocytopenia and **severe platelet dysfunction** (Ch 15, p. 182.)

What volume of a platelet solution, stored at 20°C–24°C, is given to raise the platelet count by 50,000?

10 ml/kg should raise platelet count by about 5.0×10^4/ml.

What is fresh frozen plasma (FFP)?

Plasma from whole blood. About 80% of FFP is made up of plasma proteins.

How much fresh frozen plasma is needed to raise clotting factors by 10%–20%?

10–15 ml/kg

List 3 of the therapeutic uses for immunoglobulin.

Replacement in immunodeficient patients; treatment of Kawasaki disease; to convey passive immunity to susceptible patients exposed to a variety of specific infections, such as tetanus, hepatitis B, rabies, and varicella-zoster (Ch 28, p. 396)

What is cryoprecipitate?

A plasma preparation containing factor VIII, von Willebrand factor, and fibrinogen (Ch 15, p. 181.)

List 4 risks that are associated with the use of blood products.

Risks vary with the type of product, clinical situation, and patient, but include: infection (e.g., HIV, hepatitis B and C, CMV), sensitization, immune response, graft-versus-host reaction.

5

Pediatric Nutrition

Why do nutritional considerations in pediatric patients differ from those in adults?

Growth, maturation, and development are anabolic processes that increase the nutritional needs of children.

What is the caloric content of fat?

9 kcal/g

Of carbohydrates or protein?

4 kcal/g

What are the caloric requirements of a healthy term infant?

On average, 100 kcal/kg/day

What are the fluid requirements if provided by an enteral route?

About 150 ml/kg/day

Recommended protein intake of infants?

Approximately 2.0–2.2 g/kg/day

What is the caloric content of breast milk?

It varies; averages about 20 kcal/30 ml

Of commercial infant formula?

Most contain 20 kcal/30 ml.

List 5 advantages of breast-feeding

Easily available, inexpensive, promotes mother–child bonding, less immunogenic, contains antibodies (which may reduce incidence of infection)

Do breast-fed infants require supplementation?

Yes. Breast-fed infants require **vitamin D, fluoride** (after age 6 months), and **iron** (after age 4–6 months) supplementation.

List 4 contraindications to breast-feeding.

1. Certain medications the mother may be taking (e.g., antimetabolites, chloramphenicol)

2. Certain maternal infections (e.g., HIV, active TB in the mother)
3. Maternal substance abuse
4. Abnormal gag reflex or swallowing in the infant

What is the best regimen for breast-feeding?

On-demand feeding early until the milk supply has been established and feeding is going well. Intervals between feedings can be gradually increased as the length of each feeding increases.

At what age does breast-feeding usually stop?

It varies. Some parents wean the child around 9 months of age, as the child learns to drink from a cup. Usually breast-feeding does not extend beyond 18 months of age.

What are essential amino acids?

Amino acids that cannot be synthesized and must be acquired through the diet

List 7 essential amino acids.

Isoleucine, leucine, lysine, phenylalanine, threonine, tryptophan, and valine

What are essential fatty acids?

Fatty acids that cannot be synthesized and must be obtained from dietary sources

Name 2 essential fatty acids.

Linoleic acid and linolenic acid

List 4 symptoms of essential fatty acid deficiency.

Diarrhea, dermatitis, hair loss, and skin abnormalities (e.g., poor wound healing)

What is MCT oil?

A medium-chain triglyceride preparation which may be used as a calorie supplement.

Name the fat-soluble vitamins.

Vitamins A, D, E, and K

Why is vitamin K given to newborns?

Newborns may be deficient in vitamin K, and administration of the vitamin helps prevent hemorrhagic complications caused by deficiency of vitamin K-dependent coagulation proteins.

What is the primary carbohydrate in breast milk and in cow's-milk–based formulas?

Lactose

List 3 indications for using a lactose-free formula.

Galactosemia; lactose intolerance (either temporary or persistent); formula intolerance

When are "special" formulas used?

A variety are available for specific patients and clinical problems including malabsorption, inborn errors of metabolism, protein allergies and nutritional deficiencies.

When are solid foods introduced?

Usually 4–6 months of age. This varies markedly, depending on the preferences of the parents and physician.

What solid food is introduced first?

Usually an iron-fortified single-grain cereal

Why use single-grain cereals?

A single grain allows easier identification of specific foods or ingredients that may not be tolerated by the infant.

What kinds of foods should be avoided for young children?

Foods that are easily aspirated or need to be chewed by molar teeth

Do older infants need vitamin supplementation?

Children on a well-balanced diet probably do not need vitamin supplements.

Do vitamin supplements have a role in treating children with mental retardation?

There are few studies to support their general use in these children. Children whose diets are inadequate or who have specific nutritional needs (or deficiencies) may benefit from specific supplements.

What is marasmus?

Wasting of muscle and subcutaneous fat from malnutrition

What is kwashiorkor?

Malnutrition in which there is relative protein deficiency; affected children are usually edematous

Are vegetarian diets safe for children?

A well-planned vegetarian diet that contains all the essential amino acids is probably safe for children.

Will a vegetarian diet provide an adequate amount of vitamin B_{12}?

Because vitamin B_{12} comes from animal sources, strict vegetarians may be at risk for vitamin B_{12} deficiency.

INTRAVENOUS AND PARENTERAL ALIMENTATION

Note: Most hospitals have established intravenous alimentation protocols, many using computer templates for calculation of components. Students and house officers should familiarize themselves with these protocols.

What are indications for intravenous alimentation?

Generally, an inability to maintain adequate fluid or nutritional balance by enteric (oral or feeding tube) fluid or nutrient intake

What is TPN?

Total **P**arenteral **N**utrition—implies parenteral administration of sufficient calories and nutrients for growth and weight gain. TPN is administered via a central venous route.

List 6 components of TPN.

Nitrogen source (amino acids), calories (primarily from glucose), electrolytes, vitamins, minerals, water. (Lipids are administered in a separate preparation.)

What are 4 indications for TPN?

Severe GI disease, extensive bowel resection, inflammatory bowel disease, conditions that necessitate bowel rest or prohibit oral or enteric intake for an extended period of time

When should total (central) parenteral nutrition be used?

When a period of greater than 2 weeks of intravenous alimentation is anticipated

When should peripheral hyperalimentation be used?

Usually when a short-term need is anticipated, or when the peripheral alimentation is used as a supplement to enteral nutrition

What is the main limiting factor of peripheral hyper-alimentation?

The highly osmotic content of hyper-alimentation solutions may be irritating to peripheral veins. Generally, 10%–12.5% dextrose is the upper limit for peripheral infusion. Therefore, it is not usually possible to administer total parenteral nutrition via a peripheral vein.

What is "D10"?

10% dextrose (in water or another solution). This means 10 g of dextrose per 100 ml of fluid.

What is the caloric density of dextrose monohydrate?

3.4 kcal/g; for D10, this means 34 kcal/100 ml fluid

What is Intralipid?

A fat emulsion that serves as a source of fatty acids and calories. A 10% solution of Intralipid contains 1.1 kcal/ml.

How is Intralipid administered?

Intralipid cannot be mixed in the hyperalimentation solution and is usually given parenterally via a Y-connector.

What is the source of protein in TPN?

Usually a commercially prepared amino acid or protein solution.

How is centrally administered TPN initiated?

It is usually begun with a 10% dextrose solution (with electrolytes) as maintenance fluid, with incremental increases (by 2.5%/day) as tolerated, up to a 20% dextrose solution. The amino acid mixture is then added, and the infusion rate is increased until the desired intake is achieved. Intralipid is administered in an amount to provide appropriate balance of carbohydrate, protein, and fat calories.

How are vitamins administered?

Usually in a mixture prepared for this purpose and added to the TPN

How are TPN patients monitored?

Each shift:

Glucose and ketones in urine—test each shift until regimen is established, then daily

Daily:

1. Weight
2. Strict intake and output measurements
3. Electrolytes and glucose—daily until regimen is established, then every 3

days (or weekly), depending on the protocol of the institution
4. Lipemia—visual checks

Weekly:

Complete blood count (CBC), total protein, calcium, magnesium, phosphorus, hepatocellular enzymes, bilirubin, and creatinine, serum triglycerides (if using lipids); obtain sample immediately before infusion

Monthly:

Zinc, copper and iron levels

List 12 complications of TPN.

Infection (particularly line infections), hyperglycemia, hypoglycemia (if TPN is stopped too quickly), acidosis, abnormal liver function (particularly from cholestasis), hypocalcemia, hypomagnesemia, trace metal deficiency, hyperlipemia, hyperammonemia, thrombosis, hyperbilirubinemia

6

Pediatric Emergencies

RESUSCITATION IN CHILDREN

What principle should be applied first in all pediatric emergencies?

Remember the ABCs: Airway, Breathing, and Circulation must be confirmed or established before further interventions. This may require placement of an oral airway or endotracheal tube (ETT) and will almost always require an IV or intraosseous catheter.

In what 4 ways does the pediatric airway differ from that of adults?

The pediatric airway diameter is smaller; the larynx is cephalad; the tongue is relatively larger; and the narrowest part of the airway is the subglottic region. In addition, a child's occiput is larger, relative to body size, than that of an adult and thus affects body positioning when the airway is being treated.

Where is the easiest place to palpate a pulse in an infant?

The brachial artery

How does pediatric cardiopulmonary arrest differ from adult cardiopulmonary arrest?

Cardiopulmonary arrest typically begins with respiratory arrest in children and cardiac arrest in adults.

How should a newborn be stimulated to determine responsiveness?

Rub the infant's back or the soles of her feet

What is the minimum resuscitation effort needed for every newborn?

Warm and dry the infant. Consider suctioning the oral and nasal secretions.

What is the most common cause of pathologic brady-cardia in the newborn?	Respiratory insufficiency
What historical information is important in resuscita-tion?	An **AMPLE** history: **A**llergies, **M**edications, **P**ast medical history, **L**ast meal, **E**vents of this illness

RESPIRATORY DISTRESS

What is respiratory distress?	A set of clinical signs observed when increased breathing work is required to compensate for hypoxia, hypercarbia, or airway obstruction
List 6 common clinical signs of early respiratory distress.	Anxiety, irritability, use of accessory muscles of respiration (e.g., nasal flaring, sternocleidomastoid, intercostals, abdominal musculature), tachypnea, tachycardia, hypertension
Are there any absolute laboratory or radiographic findings that define respiratory distress or failure?	NO. Laboratory studies may help determine the cause or show trends, but they must be placed in the context of the physical findings and history.
List 6 common postoper-ative causes of respiratory distress.	Atelectasis, pulmonary edema, pleural effusion, pneumothorax, malpositioned ETT, aspiration
Posttraumatic causes? (List 5)	Pulmonary contusion; pneumothorax, hemothorax, or both; disruption of an airway; injury to the diaphragm
Infectious causes? (List 5)	Pneumonia, pleural effusion, empyema, croup, epiglottitis
Causes from primary lung disease? (List 2)	Asthma, cystic fibrosis (CF)
Other causes? (List 2)	Aspiration of a foreign body, anatomic airway anomaly
What happens if respiratory distress is not treated?	The patient may progress to **respiratory failure.**

List 4 criteria for evaluating the pediatric airway when determining the need for intervention.

Airway patency, airway anatomy, adequacy of respiratory effort, oxygenation

What 3 maneuvers can be done to achieve airway patency?

1. Elevate the child's shoulders (remember the large occiput causes neck flexion).
2. Position the child's jaw (i.e., thrust forward) to eliminate occlusion of the airway by the tongue.
3. Suction any secretions.

What is the most useful medication in pediatric resuscitation?

Oxygen

When should intubation be undertaken?

When child is showing clinical signs of progression toward respiratory failure after simple interventions, **even if laboratory values of arterial blood gas (ABG) are acceptable**. (Ch 8, p 64, intubation in neonates.)

What happens if respiratory failure is not treated?

Untreated respiratory failure leads to cardiac arrest.

Why are young children often pretreated with atropine prior to intubation?

Laryngoscopy can cause bradycardia in an infant or toddler.

How does the practitioner estimate the appropriate size (mm inner diameter) for an ETT?

1. Use the following formula:

$$\frac{\text{Child's age in years} + 16}{4}$$

2. Estimate the tube size based on the size (width) of the child's fifth finger

List 7 options for airway control.

Nasopharyngeal airway, oropharyngeal airway, orotracheal intubation, nasotracheal intubation, cricothyroidotomy, tracheostomy, percutaneous transtracheal ventilation

Name 3 syndromes that would make a child difficult to intubate.

Down syndrome, Pierre Robin malformation complex, Treacher Collins syndrome

Why is intubating a child with Down syndrome difficult?	A child with Down syndrome has macroglossia, a small trachea, and may have C1-C2 ligamentous instability.

HYPOTHERMIA

What is hypothermia?	Core body temperature below 36°C
List 2 reasons for infants being at higher risk for hypothermia than adults.	1. Their ratio of body surface area to weight is higher than that of adults. 2. Infants do not have the motor control to cover themselves.
List 3 common early signs.	Shivering, vasoconstriction, elevated blood pressure
List 9 late signs.	Lethargy, dysarthria, decreased deep tendon reflexes, sluggish pupillary reactions, anisocoria, decreased heart rate and cardiac output (but elevated blood pressure), ECG abnormalities, dysrhythmias, respiratory depression
List 3 physiologic results of moderate hypothermia.	Increased metabolic rate, increased cardiac output and oxygen consumption, increased respiratory effort
List 5 physiologic results of severe hypothermia.	Decreased cerebral metabolic rate, decreased cardiac output, respiratory acidosis, loss of protective airway reflexes, hypoglycemia (in infants)
List 3 common causes of hypothermia.	Induced hypothermia (e.g., intraoperative heat loss, infusion of large volumes of cold fluid), exposure (especially after trauma), near drowning
How is hypothermia diagnosed?	By rectal or other core temperature measurement {e.g., esophageal probe}
List 2 ways it is treated	1. Eliminate ongoing heat loss. 2. Gradually rewarm patient at approximately 1°C/hr.
List 3 methods for rewarming.	1. **Surface rewarming:** blankets, heat lamp 2. **Core rewarming:** warm inhaled gases, warm IV fluids, peritoneal lavage

3. Extracorporeal techniques: cardiopulmonary bypass

What must be carefully monitored during rewarming?	**Electrolytes** and **acid–base** status; acidosis and associated hyperkalemia may worsen during rewarming. **Avoid burning tissue with heat lamps**.
How long should a patient with accidental hypothermia be resuscitated?	This issue is controversial. Neurologic signs are absent at < 25°C—27°C; defibrillation is difficult at temperatures < 30°C. Exercise clinical judgment. A usual rule of thumb: **a patient is not dead until he is warm and dead!**

MAJOR TRAUMA: PEDIATRIC ASPECTS

AIRWAY

What are the 3 major points to remember in any pediatric trauma situation?	The **ABCs: A**irway, **B**reathing, **C**irculation
In what 4 ways does the pediatric airway differ from that of adults?	(See Resuscitation, p. 27)
How is an airway established in an infant or child?	Inline, cervical spine immobilization should be secured. The jaw may be thrust forward to eliminate occlusion from the tongue. An oropharyngeal airway may be placed, or an ETT may be placed if needed.
How is an airway established if a child has severe facial fractures or if an ETT cannot be placed?	A 14-gauge needle is used to pierce the trachea at the cricothyroid membrane. Jet ventilation is then accomplished—up to 60 breaths/minute. This procedure is best performed on the infant or small child. For an adolescent, a surgical cricothyroidotomy may be made.

Circulatory Support

What is the best way to establish access for circulatory resuscitation in the event of trauma?	Establishment of **two large-bore peripheral IV lines**. The size of the IV line should be appropriate for the size of the infant or child. (Ch 2, p 10)

What access route is used if IVs are unsuccessful?

An intraosseous line–a 16-gauge IV needle or bone marrow aspiration needle is placed directly into the bone marrow.

What are the 2 preferred sites for placement of an intraosseous line?

1. **Proximal tibia** (most preferred) approximately 1 finger-breadth below the tibial tuberosity.
2. **Distal femur** (second preferred) approximately 1 finger-breadth above the knee.

How long may intraosseous lines stay in place?

No longer than **6 hours**

What is the circulating blood volume of an infant or toddler?

80 ml/kg

What resuscitative strategy should be used for the infant or child who has experienced trauma?

The first IV bolus should be **20 ml/kg of lactated Ringer's solution.** A second bolus is given if hemodynamic stability is not obtained. If resuscitation is still in doubt, 20 ml/kg of blood is given and sources of ongoing blood loss are sought.

What are the 5 most likely sites of ongoing blood loss after trauma?

Abdomen, chest, retroperitoneum, femur fracture, intracranial bleeding in infants **(Note: In all patients except infants, intracranial bleeding alone does not account for hemodynamic instability.)**

What is characteristic about the child's ability to compensate for intravascular volume loss?

Generally, blood pressure (BP) is maintained until 25%–40% of intravascular volume is lost. Therefore, watch for **tachycardia** and **decreased urine volume. When BP begins falling, the child may be exhibiting circulatory collapse.**

Why can children maintain BP with a greater degree of hemorrhage than adults can?

Pediatric cardiac output is more heart rate-related. Adult cardiac output is more preload-dependent.

List the 3 best signs of adequate circulatory resuscitation.

Adequate **urine output,** pulse, and blood pressure

Why do children have pulmonary contusions more frequently than adults do?	Relatively softer ribs do not absorb the energy of impact.
Give 2 reasons that children have spleen and liver injuries more commonly than adults do.	1. Small iliac crests; automobile lapbelts restrain the abdomen and not the pelvis. 2. Large spleens and livers, relative to their body size, protected by soft ribs and relatively thin abdominal muscles.
How can many of these injuries be prevented?	Education about proper use of car seats and boosters can decrease the risk of severe injury.

HEAD TRAUMA

What kind of injury is most responsible for childhood deaths beyond 1 year of age?	Head trauma
What percent of children with head trauma have a skull fracture?	Approximately 35%
What percent of children with skull fractures have an intracranial hemorrhage (ICH)?	Approximately 30%
How should a child with a severe head injury be approached?	**ABCs—A**irway, **B**reathing, and **C**irculation—are the top three priorities. **Cervical spine immobilization** must be maintained.
What percent of children who die of brain injury have NO evidence of a skull fracture?	50%
What percent of children with epidural hematoma do NOT have a skull fracture?	50%
What is the most common cause of head trauma in children?	Motor vehicle accidents

List 4 other causes.

Bicycle accidents, motorcycle accidents, falls, child abuse

What is a concussion?

A brief, variable, reversible alteration in consciousness with amnesia of the events immediately surrounding the injury (Ch 13, p 141)

List 7 indications for hospitalization after a concussion.

(In many health centers, any child who suffers a concussion is observed in the hospital overnight.) Specific indications are: Deterioration in level of consciousness, persistent confusion and lethargy, excessive vomiting, lack of accurate history of the trauma, focal neurologic signs, presence of skull fracture, seizures (Ch 25, p 345)

What is the grading scale for concussions?

Grade 1: transient confusion for less than 15 minutes without loss of consciousness
Grade 2: transient confusion or signs for longer than 15 minutes without loss of consciousness
Grade 3: any loss of consciousness

How soon after a first concussion may a child resume contact sports?

Grade 1 concussions: child may resume as soon as the same day if she remains asymptomatic (a normal neurologic exam) after stress (sprints, push-ups).
Grade 2 concussions: child must remain asymptomatic for 1 week.
Grade 3 concussions: child must be asymptomatic for 2 weeks.

List 2 complications of concussions.

1. Second impact syndrome (e.g., from ischemia or hypoxia) leading to death from cerebral edema
2. Permanent decrease in cognitive function after a first concussion in a child with some cognitive impairment or after a second concussion in a cognitively normal child.

What is a subdural hematoma?

A collection of blood between the dura and cerebral mantle

List 7 typical signs and symptoms.

Poor feeding, failure to thrive, irritability, lethargy, vomiting, fever, and "setting sun" position of the eyes because of increased intracranial pressure (ICP). These signs may vary with age of the child.

What can an eye exam show?

Retinal or subhyaloid hemorrhage—present in 50% of children with subdural hematoma.

How is the diagnosis made?

With CT or MRI

What is an epidural hematoma?

A collection of blood in the extradural space, usually caused by a rupture of the middle meningeal artery or tears in the dural vein; therefore, **blood usually collects rapidly.**

What is a typical course of symptoms?

A child will suffer a **brief concussion**. Often there is a **lucid interval** before the onset of vomiting, headache, and focal neurologic signs.

What is the treatment for a subdural or an epidural hematoma?

Decompression of the hematoma

What is the prognosis?

Usually good, unless there is underlying brain injury or the hematoma was not recognized in a timely fashion

List 5 types of insults that can lead to potential severe brain dysfunction.

Penetrating injury, contusion, ICH, shear injuries, and the subsequent cerebral edema that can result from these injuries

Can intracranial blood loss cause hypotension?

In the infant it can. In an older child, another source of blood loss must be sought.

Why is cerebral edema bad?

It causes an increase in ICP, thus compromising cerebral blood flow.

What is the formula for cerebral perfusion pressure?

Cerebral perfusion pressure = mean arterial pressure–ICP

List 4 causes of elevation in ICP.

Cerebral edema, hypoxia, hypercarbia, acidosis

List 6 specific interventions to treat cerebral edema.

(These interventions must be individualized to the needs of the patient.) Oxygenation, elevation of the head of the bed, judicious use of IV fluids, adequate ventilation or hyperventilation, monitoring of ICP, and administration of mannitol

What is the prognosis for seizures that develop within a few minutes or hours of head trauma (i.e., acutely after trauma)?

The seizures are usually brief and do not have long-term sequelae.

What is the prognosis if seizures develop over the first 48 hours after injury?

These are **early posttraumatic seizures.** The child should be treated for the seizures. Most children are treated with phenytoin to prevent further brain injury from secondary seizure.

What is the most important determinant of neurologic outcome following head injury?

Duration of coma

How does the outcome for children compare with that of adults if the brain injuries are similar?

Children generally do better.

How does the outcome for children younger than 2 years compare with that of older children if the brain injuries are similar?

Children younger than 2 years do worse.

SEIZURES

What is a seizure?

Clinical manifestation of synchronized electrical discharges of CNS neurons

What are the signs and symptoms of motor seizures in children?

They are characterized by patterns of movement that relate to the patterns of electrical discharges and are usually, but not always, accompanied by impaired consciousness.

Of nonmotor seizures?

They may be manifested only by loss of responsiveness to the environment and

may be mistaken for coma without
seizures.

How are seizures classified?

Table 6–1. International Classification of Epileptic Seizures

Classification	Subclassification
Partial (focal, local)	
Simple partial seizure	With motor signs
	With somatosensory or special sensory symptoms
	With autonomic signs or symptoms
	With psychic symptoms
Complex partial seizure	Simple partial onset followed by impairment of consciousness
	With impairment of consciousness at onset
Partial seizures evolving to secondarily generalized seizures	Simple partial seizures evolving to generalized seizures
	Complex partial seizures evolving to generalized seizures
	Simple partial seizures evolving to complex partial seizures evolving to generalized seizures
Generalized (convulsive and nonconvulsive)	
Absence seizure	Typical absence
	Atypical absence
Myoclonic seizure	
Clonic seizure	
Tonic seizure	
Tonic-clonic seizure	
Atonic (astatic) seizure	
Unclassified epileptic seizure	

What are the physiologic results of brief seizures (seconds to a few minutes)?

It is believed that brief seizures do not harm brain tissue, but the child may sustain secondary injury (e.g., may aspirate, strike head, drown, become hypothermic) through loss of protective reflexes.

What are the physiologic results of prolonged seizures (> 30 minutes)?

They may cause direct injury to brain tissue through electrolyte shifts, increased cerebral blood flow, and elevated ICP.

What are common physiologic causes of seizures?

A unifying cause is unknown, but most are probably associated with an imbalance between effects of excitatory neurotransmitters (e.g., glutamate) and inhibitory neurotransmitters (e.g., GABA).

What are common pathologic causes?

Table 6–2. Common Pathologic Causes of Seizure

Fever
Infection
    Encephalitis
    Meningitis
    Abscess
Traumatic brain injury
Hypoxic–ischemic injury
Metabolic disorders
    Acute electrolyte abnormalities
    Genetic metabolic disease
Drugs or toxins
Infantile spasms
Brain malformation or tumors
Primary or idiopathic seizure disorders
    Benign neonatal seizure
    Absence epilepsy
    Generalized tonic-clonic seizure
    Myoclonic seizure

List 5 characteristics of a simple febrile seizure.

Generalized tonic-clonic, lasts < 15 minutes, occurs in children 3 months to 5 years of age, occurs on day 1 of illness with high fever, and may be present in family history

List 5 characteristics of a complex febrile seizure.

Lasts ≥ 15 minutes; partial or focal seizures may occur; multiple seizures in 1 day may occur; neurologic deficits or developmental delay may be predispositions; family history may include non-febrile seizures.

List 3 diagnostic studies that are used to evaluate a patient with seizures.

1. **Physical examination** during the episode may be diagnostic of the type of seizure, but not of the cause.
2. **Electroencephalography,** with or without video monitoring, may be useful but should not delay treatment.
3. **Laboratory studies** (such as

electrolytes, glucose, calcium) and evaluation for infection, trauma, toxins, and so forth, may be helpful, depending on the circumstances.

Treatment

What is the main goal of treatment?

Stopping seizure activity rapidly without compromising the patient

List 3 immediate treatment procedures.

1. Evaluate and support airway and breathing.
2. Obtain blood for chemistries (e.g., calcium, sodium, glucose), drug levels, and suspected toxins. Perform bedside glucose screen.
3. Gain venous access; infuse NS or LR. Avoid hypotonic solutions until evaluation of serum electrolytes is performed.

What are the next treatment procedures (10–30 minutes postpresentation)?

Administer anticonvulsants while monitoring cardiorespiratory status:
1. **Rapid-onset, short-acting agents** (e.g., lorazepam). Be prepared to intubate the patient if respiratory depression occurs.
2. **Delayed-onset, long-acting agents** (e.g., phenytoin, phenobarbital)

What are 2 later treatment considerations (30–60 minutes postpresentation)?

1. Consider increasing levels of long-acting anticonvulsant or using additional medications if seizures persist.
2. Pursue diagnostic workup:
Evaluate initial laboratory studies.
Obtain further history.
Consider CT or other imaging studies.
Consider obtaining CSF if no evidence of increased ICP is present.

List 3 possible complications of treatment.

1. Respiratory depression from anticonvulsant drugs
2. Other results of drug toxicity, such as cardiac depression
3. Compromised airway unless appropriately secured initially

What is the outcome?

Brief seizure—good if no iatrogenic complications occur; damage may still occur because of underlying cause

Prolonged seizure—variable, but should be anticipated to be worse than that from a brief seizure

CARDIAC ARREST

What is cardiac arrest?

Pulseless cardiac arrest is a clinical diagnosis based on the absence of a palpable central (femoral, brachial) pulse. It is accompanied by apnea. It may exist in the presence of electrocardiographic complexes.

What are common causes of cardiac arrest in children?

Most pulseless arrests in children are the result of **severe hypoxemia** and **acidosis,** secondary to **respiratory failure or shock** (septic, most commonly).

What are 7 causes of electromechanical dissociation (electrocardiographic complexes without cardiac contractions)?

Hypoxia, blood or fluid loss, tension pneumothorax, cardiac tamponade, electrolyte imbalance, profound hypothermia, drug overdose

What are 4 common causes of primary cardiac failure?

1. **Chronic:** Cardiomyopathy, structural heart disease
2. **Acute:** Myocarditis, endocarditis
   Common causes are associated with poor ventricular function or severe dysrhythmias.

What are the physiologic consequences?

Absent cardiac output causes underperfusion of all organs within minutes. Since cardiopulmonary failure in children usually results from respiratory failure with prolonged, worsening tissue perfusion, organ damage may exist before the cardiac arrest, making full recovery (especially neurologic) unlikely even if spontaneous circulation is rapidly recovered.

What is the initial approach to—and treatment of—cardiopulmonary arrest?

1. Confirm cardiopulmonary arrest and begin CPR. **(Remember, airway is always secured first! Airway, Breathing, Circulation—the ABCs!)**
2. Apply monitoring leads and confirm heart rhythm.

3. Obtain venous or intraosseous access.
4. Identify and treat causes.
5. Perform repeated cardiopulmonary assessments and respond to changes accordingly. **[See Decision Tree in Pediatric Advanced Life Support (PALS) manual.]**

When transport is necessary, what 4 important tasks should be included in the arrangements?

Contact the receiving unit. Copy and retain pertinent records. Obtain permission to transport. Remain with patient while awaiting transport, in order to perform and respond to continuing assessments.

What are possible complications of treatment?

Iatrogenic complications include injury to respiratory, cardiac, and neurologic systems through inappropriate actions or failure to identify further deterioration.

What is the outcome?

Survival with an intact neurologic status after out-of-hospital cardiopulmonary arrest is rare. Organ systems other than the CNS are more resilient and may recover if the brain survives. Witnessed in-hospital arrest has a better, but still poor, prognosis for intact survival.

Why is the outcome of pediatric cardiac arrests so poor?

Children do not die from rapidly treatable cardiac arrhythmias. Children usually go into cardiac arrest as a complication of another end-organ illness, typically respiratory causes.

SHOCK

What is shock?

A clinical state in which delivery of oxygen and metabolic substrates to tissues is inadequate to meet tissues' metabolic demands

What are the 2 stages of shock?

1. **Compensated shock:** BP is maintained within a normal range for age.
2. **Uncompensated shock:** hypotension, with or without low cardiac output, is present.

What is hypovolemic shock?

Shock from loss of blood or body fluid

What are the causes of hypovolemic shock?	Blood loss from trauma or excessive bleeding; body fluid depletion from diarrhea, vomiting, poor fluid or food intake.
What is the earliest sign of hypovolemic shock in children?	Tachycardia
What are the causes of distributive shock?	Total body fluid may be adequate but has left the intravascular space. Distributive shock may result from sepsis, anaphylaxis, or tissue or bowel swelling after surgery.
What is "cardiogenic shock?"	Cardiac pump failure; volume status may be low, adequate, or excessive.

List 4 common causes of cardiac pump failure.

1. **Intrinsic cardiac disease:** including cardiomyopathy, myocarditis, structural heart disease, and dysrhythmia resulting in poor output
2. **Toxin-mediated failure:** including drug-induced state and sepsis-related mediators
3. **Hypoxia**
4. **Acute volume loss in trauma**

What are the clinical signs of compensated shock in children?

Cardiovascular signs? (List 3)

1. BP normal or high (Children maintain BP well until late in shock!)
2. Heart rate usually above normal range for age
3. Decreased peripheral perfusion (peripheral pulses thready or absent; capillary refill time > 2–3 seconds; skin temperature cool)

Respiratory signs? (List 2)

1. Respiratory rate is often increased as compensation for metabolic acidosis.
2. Work of breathing may be increased.

Renal signs?

Decreased urine output

CNS signs?

Child may be agitated, combative, or lethargic

What are the clinical signs of uncompensated shock?

Cardiovascular signs? (List 3)

1. BP below normal range for age
2. Heart rate remains elevated although bradycardia may occur in late shock.
3. Decreased peripheral and central perfusion (peripheral signs of hypoperfusion combined with thready central pulses)

Respiratory signs? (List 2)

1. Respiratory rate may remain elevated or may have fallen despite metabolic acidosis.
2. Work of breathing may be at an elevated, or inappropriately low, rate.

Renal signs?

Decreased urine output

CNS signs?

Child is usually combative or lethargic; may fail to recognize a parent, appear apathetic even with painful stimuli, or be unresponsive or comatose.

What are 2 laboratory signs of shock in children?

1. **Metabolic acidosis,** with or without respiratory compensation; elevated lactate implies poor tissue perfusion.
2. **Hypoglycemia** may be secondary to shock or cause shock.

What are physiologic consequences of shock?

Inadequate tissue perfusion causes end-organ dysfunction and eventually **irreversible organ damage if untreated.**

What is the differential diagnosis of shock in an infant?

Sepsis, meningitis, pneumonia, heart disease (acquired or congenital), metabolic disorder, congenital adrenal hypoplasia, dehydration, posterior urethral valves, malrotation with midgut volvulus.

What is the most common category of symptoms in infants with infections, including meningitis?

Respiratory symptoms

List 3 common symptoms in children with pulmonary edema or cardiogenic shock.

Tachypnea; difficulty or sweating with feeding

What are the 5 cyanotic congenital heart lesions?

1-2-3-4-5 Ts:
Truncus arteriosus (**1** vessel)
Transposition of the (**two**) great vessels
Tricuspid atresia
Tetralogy of Fallot
Total anomalous pulmonary venous return (has **5** words)

What is the initial treatment of shock due to TOGV?

Infusion of prostaglandin E1

What are the 2 primary electrolyte abnormalities seen in congenital adrenal hypoplasia?

Hyperkalemia and hyponatremia

List 3 complications of prostaglandin E1 infusion.

Apnea, agitation, hyperthermia

What is the diagnostic approach for shock?

Identification of shock should be **clinical,** based on interpretation of the physical findings outlined above. Determination of the cause is useful in later treatment but should not delay initial stabilization effort.

What is the reason cardiogenic shock must be differentiated from other forms of shock?

It **requires a different treatment approach** after initial interventions than other forms of shock. Cardiogenic shock should be suspected when symptoms of congestive heart failure (CHF) (e.g., enlarged liver, pulmonary congestion, symptoms of poor cardiac output) are present on initial evaluation or after initial fluid resuscitation.

Treatment

List 2 approaches for definitive treatment of shock.

1. Basic interventions (should be used in all cases of shock)
2. Identification of the cause

What are the 6 basic interventions?

Remember the ABCs!
1. Immediately provide **oxygen** through

an **adequate airway** (native or artificial).

2. If bradycardia and poor perfusion present, proceed as for cardiac arrest.
3. Achieve **vascular access** when shock is recognized.
4. Provide an **initial fluid bolus of 20 ml/kg,** using NS or LR. In infants and children, administer fluid using a large syringe and stopcock, **not** a "wide open" infusion, in order to allow rapid administration while avoiding inadvertent overhydration.
5. Obtain a bedside **glucose** measurement, and treat with 0.5–1.0 g/kg of IV dextrose if patient is hypoglycemic. Consider obtaining other diagnostic studies (e.g., blood studies or radiographs), but ABCs are always first!
6. Reassess **peripheral perfusion**(pulse strength and capillary refill time), **fluid balance** (liver size, urine output), **breath sounds** (work of breathing), and **vital signs.** Repeat fluid boluses with frequent reassessment until patient is no longer in shock or until signs of fluid overload are noted. Colloid may be required as a fluid replacement if colloid (e.g., blood) has been lost.

Remain aware that shock may recur until the predisposing condition has been corrected.

List 2 things the physician should do if the patient displays symptoms of cardiogenic shock during resuscitation.

1. Initiate inotropic support via intra-osseous or central venous access.
   Doses:
   Dopamine: 5–20 mcg/kg/min
   Epinephrine: 0.05–1.00 mcg/kg/min
2. Consult pediatric cardiologist or intensive-care specialist to assist in further management of cardiogenic shock.

List 2 complications of treatment.

1. Failure to correct tissue oxygenation and perfusion deficit before end-organ damage occurs.

2. Overzealous treatment causing fluid overload with resulting pulmonary compromise or, rarely, CHF.

What are the outcomes?

Outcomes depend on the underlying cause and on the phase of shock at which intervention begins. Outcomes are improved by rapid recognition of shock and correction of tissue underperfusion.

UNEXPLAINED COMA

What is coma?

A state of unconsciousness from which one cannot be aroused by stimulation of any magnitude

What is the differential diagnosis of coma in an infant or child?

Structural lesions resulting in increased ICP or seizures, including:
1. Trauma, resulting in shear injury, generalized edema, or an expanding mass lesion
2. Tumor
3. Abscess
4. Hemorrhage
5. Infarction

Functional disorders resulting in bilateral hemispheric dysfunction, including:
1. Hypoxic-ischemic injury
2. Ingestion or poisoning
3. Remote or CNS infection
4. Metabolic derangements, such as hypoglycemia, hyponatremia (usually < 120 mEq/L), severe hypernatremia (cerebral edema), uremia, hyperammonemia, extreme hypercalcemia, or severe hyperglycemia
5. Seizures: postictal state; ongoing electrographic (nonconvulsive) status epilepticus

What are 4 important elements of the physical examination of the coma-tose infant or child?

1. **Rapid evaluation of the ABCs!**
2. **Rapid neurologic examination,** looking for symptoms of trauma, increased ICP, or specific toxidromes
3. If elements of **ABCs** appear acceptable and maintainable,

proceeding with examination for localized lesions, signs of infection, and associated conditions (e.g., cervical spine injury).

4. Assigning a **Glasgow Coma Score** as possible aid in serial evaluations and determining prognosis

List 7 appropriate initial interventions.

Remember the ABCs!

1. Stabilize airway and breathing. The comatose patient usually needs intubation due to diminished or absent airway protective reflexes or poor pharyngeal muscle tone. Consider mild hyperventilation ($Paco_2$ 30–35 mm Hg), administration of mannitol (0.25–0.50 g/kg IV), or both, if increased ICP is suspected clinically.

2. Obtain IV access, and a rapid bedside glucose level. Consider administering dextrose (0.5–1.0 g/kg) and naloxone (0.10 mg/kg, up to 2.00 mg/kg) as a therapeutic and diagnostic trial, as indicated by findings.

3. Continue with more detailed physical examination and delegate someone to obtain a rapid and pertinent history from the best available source.

4. Initiate appropriate consultations (e.g., neurosurgery, neurology, pediatrics, trauma surgery), laboratory evaluations, and imaging studies.

5. Avoid non-essential procedures (e.g., an immediate lumbar puncture [LP]) until the patient is stable.

6. Evaluate for signs of associated shock and treat if present; **brain perfusion must be maintained while avoiding fluid overload if increased ICP exists.**

7. The approach to long-term care is dictated by the patient's underlying cause of coma.

What initial laboratory and imaging studies are appropriate?

The choice of laboratory studies and imaging studies should be guided by the findings of the physical examination and by the patient's history.

First priority of metabolic/ toxin evaluation?

Immediate bedside **glucose** determination and **electrolyte** panel, including **calcium**

Second priority of metabolic/toxin evaluation?

Consider ammonia level; urine toxicology screen or specific toxin levels if history or physical examination findings are suggestive; consider studies for inborn errors of metabolism if suggested by history, in consultation with a medical geneticist.

First priority of imaging studies (CT, MRI)?

Rule out rapidly progressive CNS mass lesion.

Second priority of imaging studies?

Define subtle lesions(s) or repeat initial studies to define progression of an identified lesion.

After initial stabilization and evaluation, what are the monitoring and intervention procedures? (List 5)

These are determined by initial findings and the patient's evolving status.

1. Consider ICP monitoring in consultation with a neurosurgeon if evidence of increased ICP exists or there is a likelihood of development of elevated ICP.
2. If hyperventilation is pursued, an arterial line or end-tidal carbon dioxide monitor is advisable.
3. The nature and frequency of laboratory studies are determined by initial evaluations and patient's responses to interventions. **Hypoglycemia should be corrected immediately, whereas severe hyperglycemia and hypernatremia should be corrected slowly.** Correct severe hyponatremia rapidly to a level of approximately 120 mEq/L; then proceed slowly. Electrolyte corrections must be monitored frequently to avoid complications of therapy.
4. Consider obtaining an EEG if nonconvulsive status epilepticus is a possible cause of coma.
5. If toxic exposure or ingestion is determined, specific therapy (if available) should be initiated in consultation with a toxicologist.

What are the outcomes?
Outcomes depend on the underlying cause of the coma, any associated condition (e.g., secondary hypoxic-ischemic injury, progression of increased ICP), and the ability to reverse the progression of disease.

NEAR DROWNING

What is near drowning?
A submersion incident followed by survival for at least 24 hours, regardless of the ultimate outcome

What is drowning?
A submersion incident that results in death within the first 24 hours

List 4 epidemiologic characteristics of near drowning in children and infants.

1. Near drowning is more common in males than in females.
2. High-risk groups: toddlers, adolescent males, and children with seizure disorders.
3. Most drowning or near drowning in small children occurs during brief periods (< 5 minutes) without supervision, not as a result of neglect.
4. Most near-drowning incidents occur in residential swimming pools, but can occur in any available body of water, including lakes, rivers, 5-gallon buckets (often used for storing liquids), bathtubs, toilet bowls, hot tubs, and standing water on pool covers.

List 3 factors that determine outcome after a near-drowning incident.

1. Duration of the hypoxic insult during submersion
2. Associated conditions (e.g., aspiration injury, electrolyte abnormalities)
3. Complications of therapy.

What is the pathophysiology of submersion injury?
The initial response to unexpected submersion is thought to involve **aspiration** of small amounts of water, which triggers **laryngospasm**. As **hypoxia** and **panic** ensue, **reflex swallowing** of water into the stomach occurs. When hypoxia becomes severe, most victims have **resolution of laryngospasm,** followed by active or passive **aspiration of water.**

During resuscitative efforts, **emesis and aspiration of swallowed water** and gastric contents may occur.

Hypoxic injury to the brain and other organ systems occurs, the extent depending on the length of submersion and the water temperature. Multiple organ system failure may result from prolonged hypoxia or **shock.**

Lung injury may be related to contents of the aspirated water.

Electrolyte disturbances may occur but are rarely observed in patients who survive until arrival at a hospital, unless the patients have aspirated extremely hypertonic solutions.

Infection may ensue, although not commonly from direct aspiration. More likely, hypoxic injury to the gut may be followed by translocation of bowel flora into the bloodstream, resulting in sepsis and associated hematogenous spread of infection.

List 3 appropriate initial interventions (before child is at the emergency department)

1. **On-site basic life support, including ABCs with stabilization of the cervical spine,** is initially appropriate for all cold-water (temperature $< 5°C$) submersion victims—and arguably for all warm-water submersion victims—unless the submersion is known to be exceptionally prolonged.
2. Avoid excessive airway manipulation or pressure on the abdomen to avoid emesis and aspiration.
3. Escalate intervention to advanced life-support measures if needed, with continuation until the patient is evaluated in the emergency department. Many clinicians recommend continuing resuscitative efforts until the patient's core temperature exceeds $32°C$, because

existence or maintenance of a spontaneous cardiac rhythm may not occur below this temperature.

What are appropriate interventions at the emergency department?

Decisions about level of further care are based on level of **neurologic function** and presence or absence of **lung abnormalities.** Patients with normal mental status and lung examination may develop pulmonary edema up to 12 hours after submersion; therefore, observation for at least 4–8 hours is recommended before discharge. All patients with altered mental or pulmonary status should be admitted, because the natural history of either is to worsen before resolution can be anticipated.

How long should cardio-pulmonary resuscitation be continued in a submersion victim who arrives in the emergency department without spontaneous circulation?

This issue is controversial. Many clinicians recommend discontinuing efforts if advanced life-support measures fail to restore spontaneous circulation once the patient has reached a core temperature of 28°C; others suggest using 32°C as a temperature goal.

What management approaches should be taken for the submersion patient who is admitted to the hospital?

Patients will have different treatment and monitoring needs, depending on the degree of hypoxic-ischemic insult and other conditions.

Respiratory care? (List 4 features)

1. Oxygen is given to maintain saturations > 90%.
2. If intubation is required, positive end–expiratory pressure (PEEP) may be necessary to minimize intrapulmonary shunt.
3. ABG monitoring is indicated for the intubated patient.
4. Antibiotic coverage is indicated if the patient has clear signs of pulmonary infection.

Neurologic care? (List 3 features)

1. If the patient is obtunded or has a declining mental status, intubate the trachea to protect the airway.
2. Although increased ICP may occur

secondary to the hypoxic-ischemic insult, ICP monitoring has not been shown to alter ultimate neurologic outcome in this patient group. Efforts to avoid further CNS damage from fluid overload, hypoperfusion, hypoxemia, and seizure activity should be maximized.

3. Other rescue therapies that have been commonly used are prolonged hypothermia, barbiturate coma, and steroids. However, these have not been proven to improve outcome.

Cardiovascular care?

After stabilization of initial cardiac dysfunction associated with hypoxia and acidosis, further impairment of cardiac function is associated with hypoxic cardiomyopathy or sepsis. Management of the depressed myocardium requires arterial and central venous pressure (CVP) monitoring and may require cardiac-output monitoring using thermo-dilution in severe cases. Catecholamine support may be needed.

Infection management?

Infection is managed symptomatically. Infection may be secondary to trans-location of gut flora through an ischemic bowel or caused by aspiration of grossly contaminated water.

What are 3 common cate-gories of complications of therapy?

1. **Respiratory complications**—usually due to barotrauma from high ventilatory needs and may include acute pneumothoraces or fibrosis.
2. **Neurologic complications**—largely due to progressive cerebral edema secondary to the initial hypoxic insult but may be exacerbated by shock, fluid overload, and prolonged seizures.
3. **Nosocomial infection**—a possibility during prolonged invasive monitoring or prolonged intubation.

List 4 indicators of poor outcome after near drowning.

1. Documented submersion > 5 minutes
2. The need for CPR in the emergency setting

3. A serum pH < 7 or fixed and dilated pupils in the emergency setting
4. Need for cardiotonic drugs during resuscitation.

However, the only factor consistently predicting poor outcome is the need for continued CPR in the emergency department for nonhypothermic patients.

What is the role of prevention?

Since near-drowning outcomes are largely determined by the degree of the initial hypoxic insult, prevention is of paramount importance. Current areas of focus include improved legislation for barrier requirements around pools, education of the public about drowning risks in the home and around natural bodies of water, and encouragement of CPR training for pool owners.

7

Growth and Development

GROWTH

What is the most important feature to remember about growth?	Growth is a **dynamic,** not a static, process.
What is the best way to evaluate growth?	Longitudinally along a time line, either by direct observation or by evaluation of accurate historical data
Why are growth charts important?	They facilitate growth data analysis and they are a record of data points, allowing easy comparisons with previous points and standard growth patterns. (Samples of selected growth charts, as published by the NCHS, in collaboration with the National Center for Chronic Disease and Health Promotion [Centers for Disease Control and Prevention—CDC] are shown in Figures 7–1 and 7–2.)
What is growth rate?	Change in a growth parameter over time. When evaluating growth abnormalities, the growth rate is frequently more important than an isolated data point.
When is growth most rapid?	Relative growth is most rapid during fetal development. Adolescence is the time of greatest postnatal growth.
What is the normal rate of weight gain for infants?	After the initial postnatal water loss (about 5%–10% of birth weight) during the first few days after birth, an infant should gain about 1 oz (30 g) per day.
At what age does an infant double his birth weight?	Usually at 6 months of age

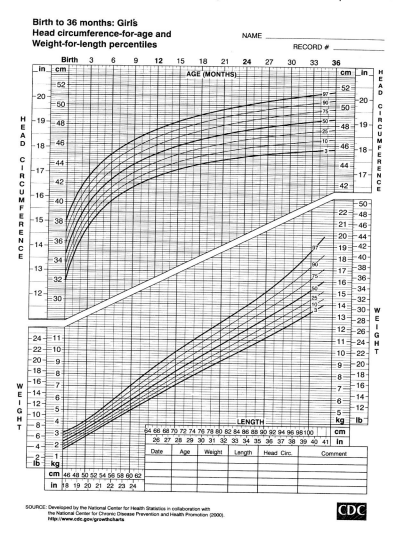

Fig 7–1. Growth chart for girls from birth to 36 months: Head circumference-for-age and weight-for-length percentiles. (Source: National Center for Health Statistics in Collaboration with the National Center for Chronic Disease Prevention and Health Promotion. Revised November 21, 2000. http://www.cdc.gov/growthcharts.)

What height and weight should a normal child be at 4 years of age?

About 40 inches tall and 40 pounds

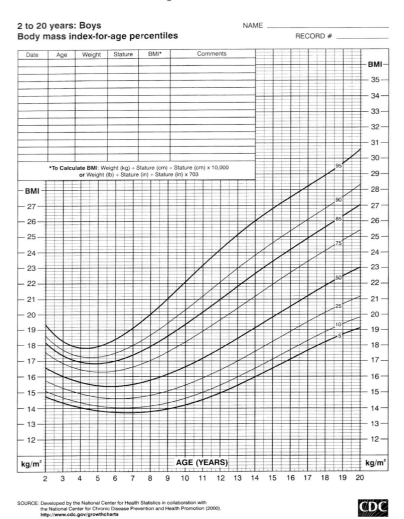

Figure 7–2. Growth chart for boys 2 to 20 years of age: Body mass index-for-age percentiles. (Source: National Center for Health Statistics in Collaboration with the National Center for Chronic Disease Prevention and Health Promotion, 2000. http://www.cdc.gov/growthcharts.)

What is meant by the "upper:lower segment ratio"?

The ratio of the length of the upper segment (i.e., distance from top of the pubis to top of the head) to the length of the lower segment (i.e., distance from the top of the pubis to the bottom of the feet).

How do upper:lower segment ratios vary with age?	Infants and young children have relatively short lower limbs, so the upper:lower ratio is higher in young children than in adults.
What is the normal upper: lower segment ratio at birth?	1.7 : 1
What is the normal upper: lower segment ratio at 10 years of age?	1 : 1
What other variables are important in interpreting upper:lower segment ratios?	Normal values for upper:lower segment ratios can vary with gender and with race or ethnicity.
At what age do first teeth usually erupt?	About 5–8 months; central mandibular incisors usually appear first.
Which permanent teeth usually appear first and when?	First molars ("6-year molars") around 5–7 years.

DEVELOPMENT

Why is development an important pediatrics issue?	It reflects neurologic maturation and social and sensory development in the child. Abnormal development may reflect a neurologic, medical, or social problem.
How does sensory impairment affect development?	Children with undetected hearing or visual deficits may not develop certain skills at the appropriate age.
What areas of development are monitored?	Gross motor, fine motor, social, and language development (should be included in the routine physical examination)
What are representative gross motor milestones at the following ages:	
1 month?	Lifts head from prone position
2 months?	Holds head upright without wobble

3 months?	Regards hand
4 months?	Purposeful grasp; rolls front to back
6 months?	Beginning to sit without support; rolls back to front
9 months?	Sits well without support; up on all fours; crawls
8–10 months?	Pulls to standing; walks with support
13–15 months?	Walks independently
18 months?	Walks up and down stairs; begins to run
24 months?	Jumps in air

What are representative fine motor milestones at age:

2 months?	Follows visually past midline
3–4 months?	Grasps objects and brings to mouth
6 months?	Places objects carefully rather than dropping them, transfers hand-to-hand
9 months?	Clasps hands
9–10 months?	Demonstrates pincer grasp
15 months?	Scribbles; stacks 2 cubes
18 months?	Stacks 4 cubes
24 months?	Stacks 8 cubes

What are representative social milestones at age:

6–8 weeks?	Smiles responsively
2 months?	Smiles when seeing mother
4 months?	Smiles spontaneously

6 months?	Copies facial expressions
9 months?	Fears strangers; shows separation anxiety; plays interactively (peekaboo, patty-cake)
12 months?	Drinks from cup and finger-feeds self
15 months?	Uses spoon; imitates adult actions
18 months?	Removes clothing; uses cup
24 months?	Begins toilet training; puts on clothing

What are representative language milestones at age:

2 months?	Coos responsively
4 months?	Social laughter
6 months?	Makes nonspecific vowel sounds
9 months?	"Dada" and "Mama" (nonspecific)
12 months?	"Dada" and "Mama" plus 2 other words
15 months?	Several more words
18 months?	Combines 2 words into phrases
24 months?	Combines 3 or more words
36 months?	Most speech clear to strangers
48 months?	Toddler stuttering subsiding

What is the Denver Developmental Screening Test?	A screening test developed for the quick assessment of developmental milestones
Does developmental delay imply later mental retardation?	No. Mental retardation usually refers to cognitive and problem-solving deficits, whereas developmental delay includes a wide range of skills that may be adversely affected by medical or neurologic problems that may not affect cognition. Mental retardation implies a permanent

deficit while aspects of developmental delay may be temporary or permanent depending on the causes.

PUBERTY

(Also see Chapter 14, Adolescent Medicine)

What is puberty?	The development of secondary sexual characteristics and the maturation of gonadal function
When does puberty usually begin in boys and what is the usual progression?	Around 11.5 years of age; begins with enlargement of the testes, followed by appearance of pubic hair and linear growth spurt.
What is the normal age range of onset of puberty in boys?	Approximately 9.5–13.5 years
When does puberty usually begin in girls and what is the usual progression?	Around 10.5 years of age; usually begins with breast buds (thelarche), followed by appearance of pubic hair, growth spurt, then menarche.
What is the normal age range of onset in girls?	8–13 years
When does the maximum growth velocity occur?	Usually 1.5 years after the beginning of puberty
When does menarche occur?	Usually 2 years after appearance of breast buds
What is precocious puberty?	Onset of puberty before age 8 (females) or 9 (males).
Is precocious puberty more common in boys or girls?	Girls
What is the most common cause of precocious puberty in girls?	Idiopathic precocious puberty (Ch 24, p. 329.)
What is delayed puberty?	If there has been no development of secondary sexual characteristics by age 13 (girls) or 14 (boys). (Ch 24, p. 331.)

Section II

Newborn Care

8

Perinatal Care and Evaluation of the Newborn

APGAR SCORES

What is the Apgar score?

A method of evaluating a newborn introduced in 1953 by Dr. Virginia Apgar. Five physical signs are identified and a score of 0, 1, or 2 is given to each sign at 1 minute and 5 minutes after birth.

What are the 5 signs evaluated, and what constitutes a score of 0, 1, and 2 for each sign?

See Table 8–1 for the signs and Apgar evaluation scoring.

What is the APGAR mnemonic?

Appearance, **P**ulse, **G**rimace, **A**ctivity, and **R**espirations

What do the 1- and 5-minute scores imply?

The 1-minute score indicates the infant's initial condition. The 5-minute score indicates the infant's improvement, continued well-being or subsequent decline (depending on the initial score).

Should additional Apgar assessments be made beyond 5 minutes?

If the Apgar score is < 7 at 5 minutes, checking of Apgar scores every 5 minutes for the subsequent 20 minutes is helpful to assess resuscitation efforts.

NEWBORN RESUSCITATION

INITIAL ASSESSMENT

List 3 components of initial assessment and management of a newborn.

1. Gentle suction of the mouth, nose, and pharynx with a bulb syringe or suction catheter

Table 8–1.
The Apgar Evaluation Scoring

	Scores		
Sign	*0*	*1*	*2*
Color	Central cyanosis	Peripheral cyanosis	Completely pink
Heart rate	Absent	< 100 beats/min	> 100 beats/min
Reflex irritability	No response	Grimace	Cough or sneeze
Muscle tone	None	With some flexion	Well flexed or spontaneous movement
Respiratory effort	Absent	Irregular or weak cry	Regular or strong cry

2. Drying of the infant to minimize evaporative heat loss with warming via radiant heat
3. Evaluation of the infant's color, respiratory effort, and heart rate

What are the potential risks of suctioning?

Deep suctioning should be avoided in the initial resuscitation because this may induce laryngeal spasm, increase vagal tone resulting in apnea and bradycardia, or result in trauma to the pharynx or esophagus.

How should the infant be positioned as he is transferred from the mother to the resuscitation table and while on the resuscitation table?

The head should be placed in the dependent position (approximately 20°–30° below horizontal) to facilitate drainage of secretions from the pharynx.

INTUBATION

What is the primary indication for intubation?

Inability to oxygenate and ventilate an infant adequately via bag-and-mask ventilation

List 5 signs of inadequate oxygenation and ventilation.

1. Poor color
2. Poor (or lack of) responsiveness
3. Lack of movement of chest with bag-and-mask ventilation
4. Falling oxygen saturation
5. Falling heart rate

What is appropriate positioning for bag-and-mask ventilation?	Placement of the mask over the mouth and nose with the head and neck slightly extended
What sizes of endotracheal tubes (ETTs) are appropriate for infants?	**Uncuffed tubes** with internal diameters of 2.5, 3.0, or 3.5 mm, depending on the infant's size (see Ch 6).

List 6 important anatomic and position considerations during intubation.

1. The infant's head and neck should be slightly extended.
2. The larynx is more anterior and caudad in the neonate than in the older child or adult.
3. The epiglottis tends to hang over the vocal cords.
4. A straight-blade laryngoscope with a Miller 0 or 1 blade is usually most useful for visualizing the airway.
5. The ETT should be placed only 1.0–1.5 cm beyond the cords to avoid main-stem (usually right-sided) intubation. A weight-to-distance correlation of 1-2-3 kg : 7-8-9 cm (i.e., tube marking at infant's lip) is extremely useful for determining the appropriate distance for tube placement.
6. The chest should be auscultated for symmetrical breath sounds over both lung fields and absence of sounds over the stomach. There should be symmetrical chest rise, and ideally the infant's heart rate and color will improve. Chest x-ray confirms the appropriate placement of the tube.

UMBILICAL VESSEL CATHETERIZATION

When are umbilical-vein catheters (UVC) used?	Primarily in premature and acutely ill infants.
List 3 purposes of a UVC.	1. Central venous pressure monitoring 2. Administering intravenous fluids, hyperalimentation, and medications 3. Sampling blood when needed
Where should the tip of the UVC lie?	The junction of the right atrium and inferior vena cava (level of T10–T11)

List 7 potential complications of a UVC.	Vascular embolization, vascular spasm, vascular perforation, infection, hemorrhage, venous congestion of the lower extremities, thrombosis (e.g., thrombosis of the portal vein, resulting in portal hypertension)
List 3 uses for an umbilical artery catheter (UAC).	1. Monitoring pulse and blood pressure (BP) 2. Access for blood samples and arterial blood gas (ABG) 3. Administering of fluids, medications, and hyperalimentation
Where should the tip of a UAC be placed?	Either just above the bifurcation of aorta (level of L3–L5) or above the celiac axis (level of T6–T10)
List 9 complications of a UAC.	Vascular embolization, thrombosis, vascular spasm, vascular perforation, ischemic or chemical necrosis of abdominal viscera, infection, hemorrhage, impaired circulation to the leg, renovascular hypertension
How long may umbilical vein or artery catheters remain in place?	UVCs should be removed within 7 days and UACs within 10–14 days.

EVALUATION OF THE NEWBORN

How are newborns classified?	By **gestational age** and **size**
List the 3 gestational ages and the span each includes.	**Preterm:** less than 37 weeks gestation **Term:** 37 weeks to less than 42 weeks **Postterm:** 42 weeks and beyond.
What is SGA?	**S**mall for **G**estational **A**ge
List 5 concerns about SGA.	Increased caloric needs (relative to their weight), a higher mortality rate, increased risk of malformations, hypoglycemia, and congenital infections.
What is symmetric growth retardation?	Growth retardation of length, weight, and head circumference

List 3 implications of symmetric growth retardation.	1. An insult early in the pregnancy (e.g., teratogen) 2. A malformation syndrome (including chromosome abnormalities) 3. Early infection Alternatively, the parents may be small in stature.
Implications of asymmetric growth retardation?	If weight is disproportionately low (relative to length and head circumference), it implies an insult later in pregnancy (e.g., maternal hypertension, placental insufficiency).
Do all cases of SGA have an identifiable cause?	No. As many as 40% of cases will have **no** identifiable etiologic factors.
What is LGA?	**L**arge for **G**estational **A**ge
List 3 causes of LGA.	1. Maternal diabetes (including gestational diabetes) 2. Beckwith-Wiedemann syndrome 3. Twin–twin transfusion (recipient twin LGA)
Do all cases of LGA have an identifiable cause?	No
List 3 complications of LGA.	1. Hypoglycemia 2. Increased incidence of injury at birth 3. Complications related to underlying cause
What is an IDM?	**I**nfant of a **D**iabetic **M**other
List 6 risks of IDM.	Hypoglycemia, hypocalcemia, polycythemia, respiratory distress, renal vein thrombosis, and malformations—particularly congenital heart disease (CHD) and variants of caudal regression syndrome
What 2 tests assess gestational age?	New Ballard Score and Dubowitz exam
What is the significance of meconium staining?	It may reflect in utero stress and places the infant at risk for meconium aspiration (Ch 10, p 92).

What is the normal new-born heart rate?

> 100 beats/min (usually 120–160 beats/min)

When should a newborn be examined?

In the delivery room. A complete physical examination should be done within 12 hours of birth.

List 4 purposes of the delivery room assessment.

1. Determine if the infant will need resuscitation
2. Assess for obvious malformations or abnormalities
3. Estimate gestational age
4. Assess the infant's cardiopulmonary transition from the intrauterine environment to the outside world

List 3 purposes of the later, more complete examination.

1. Evaluate infant for malformations
2. Establish normalcy of growth and function
3. Document physical findings

What 3 physical measurements are routinely taken?

1. Head circumference (using greatest occipital-to-frontal diameter)
2. Weight
3. Crown-to-heel length

All measurements should be analyzed, using standard curves, for appropriateness for gestational age.

What is the normal new-born respiratory rate?

40–60 breaths/min

How should the complete physical examination of the newborn proceed?

The examiner should note the vital signs and general appearance, and take advantage of the infant's current state. If the infant is sleeping or is quiet, auscultation of the heart and lungs, and palpation and auscultation of the abdomen are done first followed by a head-to-toe inspection and palpation. Unique aspects of the physical examination of a newborn include evaluation of patency of the nasal passages, palpation of the kidneys, and evaluation of the hips for dislocation or laxity. Ophthalmologic exam, including evaluation of the red reflex, and otoscopic exam are performed later in the exam. The formal part of the neurologic exam completes the physical examination.

What is vernix caseosa?

A white greasy coating on the skin of newborns; more common in preterm infants.

What is lanugo?

Fine hair that covers the body of infants; more common in premature infants.

What are mongolian spots?

Bluish discoloration of the skin, usually over the buttocks and lower back; more common in racial groups with darker skin pigment.

What are milia?

Tiny white papules that form over the surface of sebaceous glands; they are often present over the nose.

What are milaria?

Clear (crystallina) or inflamed-appearing (rubra) vesicles that form over obstructed sweat glands; they are often seen with overheating.

What is erythema toxicum?

A benign, splotchy pattern of erythema and pustules filled with eosinophils. Typically appears on face, trunk, and extremities. **Must be distinguished from staphylococcal rashes or herpes**.

List 3 characteristics of staphylococcal rashes.

1. Pustules
2. Generalized erythema
3. Bullous eruptions (referred to as staphylococcal scalded skin syndrome, toxic epidermal necrosis, or Ritter disease)

What is a characteristic of herpes simplex rashes?

Vesiculobullous eruptions (may be only a few) on an erythematous base

What is a "blueberry muffin" rash?

Macular, raised, purple lesions—indicates congenital rubella (Ch 27, p. 391)

Is palpable breast tissue normal in newborns?

Yes. About 1 cm of palpable breast tissue may be present in males or females due to maternal estrogens.

Are heart murmurs common in newborns?

Soft, short systolic murmurs are common. Loud or harsh murmurs should arouse suspicion.

Name 5 heart defects associated with cyanosis.

The "5 Ts":
1. Tetralogy of Fallot
2. Total anomalous pulmonary venous return
3. Truncus arteriosus
4. Transposition of the great vessels (TOGV)
5. Tricuspid atresia (Ch 16, p. 186)

What condition is associated with diminished or absent femoral pulses?

Coarctation of the aorta (Ch 16, p. 198)

How is the fontanel measured?

Anteroposterior and side-to-side dimensions (largest measurement of each).

List 4 disorders that are associated with an enlarged anterior fontanel.

Hydrocephalus, hypothyroidism, hypophosphatasia, skeletal dysplasias (e.g., osteogenesis imperfecta)

List 3 kinds of disorders that are associated with a small fontanel.

Microcephaly, craniostenosis, craniosynostosis syndromes

What is molding?

Temporary misshaping of the cranium, usually related to infant's position during the latter part of pregnancy and labor

What is a cephalohematoma?

A hematoma beneath the periosteum of the cranium

What is caput succedaneum?

Edema of the soft tissues of the scalp

How can cephalohematoma and caput succedaneum be differentiated?

Cephalohematomas do not cross suture lines.

What is ocular hypertelorism?

True ocular hypertelorism is an increased distance between the orbits.

What is the red reflex?

The red reflection of the retina through the lens of the eye; a normal red reflex implies that there are neither large lens opacities nor large retinal tumors.

Why is a catheter passed through both sides of the nose?

To rule out choanal atresia or stenosis

Why not do this immediately after birth?	It may cause a vagal response with bradycardia.
Why is it important to have patent choanae?	Infants are obligate nose breathers, so choanal atresia can cause respiratory distress.
What are "Epstein pearls"?	Small, white, epithelial inclusion cysts seen in the midline of the roof of the mouth. Similar lesions may be seen in the gums. They resolve spontaneously.
What is the most common fracture during delivery?	Fracture of the clavicle
How large is the newborn liver?	The liver may be palpable 1–2 cm below the right costal margin.
What is the normal number of vessels in the umbilical cord?	Three vessels (two arteries and one vein)
When does the umbilical cord usually dry and fall off?	Usually before 3 weeks of age
What is acrocyanosis?	Bluish discoloration of the hands and feet; not rare in newborns but may be abnormal in older infants
What is harlequin color change?	Reddening of one side of the infant, with a sharp line of demarcation at the midline; may be related to autonomic factors; usually benign and self-limited
What is cutis marmorata?	Reticulated mottling of the skin; may be seen transiently in infants who are cold; also seen as a more persistent finding in infants with Down syndrome or other specific disorders
What is the normal penis length for a term male infant?	About 3–4 cm shaft length
What is hypospadias?	Abnormal location of penile urethral meatus along the ventral aspect of the shaft

What is chordee?

Bowing or bending of the penile shaft

How do the labia minora vary with gestational age?

The labia minora are prominent in preterm females, usually protruding beyond the labia majora. They regress as the infant enlarges.

What is the significance of hair, swelling or reddish discoloration in the lumbosacral area?

This is sometimes associated with spina bifida.

What is the significance of a dimple at the base of the spine?

Dimples located **below the gluteal crease** are usually insignificant. Dimples **higher along the spine** require investigation for occult spina bifida or tethered cord.

What is syndactyly?

Cutaneous fusion of the digits

What is polydactyly?

Extra digits

What is developmental dysplasia of the hip?

This term is sometimes used synonymously with congenital dysplasia of the hip; however, it is also a broader term that includes hip dislocation that may not be evident immediately at birth.

List 2 ways to screen for it.

1. Observation for asymmetry of fat folds and discrepancy in leg length
2. Passively abducting the hips (i.e., Ortolani maneuver) or adducting and rotating each hip (i.e., Barlow test)

Which gender is affected more often?

Females

What if the neonate's feet or legs turn in?

Newborns may exhibit a variety of findings related to in utero positioning. If the foot or leg can be easily brought to a neutral or beyond-neutral position, the finding should resolve over several weeks. Otherwise, orthopedic consultation may be required for forefoot, hindfoot, tibia, or hips.

List 4 key components of the neurologic examination of a newborn.

Mental status, cranial nerve function, motor function, reflexes

How can mental status be examined?

Generally, awake infants are in a state of "quiet alertness." Abnormalities of mental status may manifest as unusual irritability or lethargy.

List 10 components of the examination of the CNS.

Examine for:
1. Blinking when light is shone in eyes (II, VII)
2. Fixation on and tracking of objects (II, III, IV, VI)
3. Pupillary reaction (II, III)
4. Extraocular movements (III, IV, VI)
5. Corneal reflex and withdrawal on pinprick to face (V)
6. Facial movement and symmetry (VII)
7. Hearing (e.g., response to hand clap) (VIII)
8. Sucking (V, VII, XII)
9. Swallowing (IX, X)
10. Strength and integrity of sternocleidomastoid (XI) and tongue (XII)

What are 2 things to look for when examining motor function?

1. Spontaneous movement
2. Muscle tone, both active and passive (e.g., posture, resistance to passive motion)

What are primary (primitive) reflexes?

Inherent reflexes present during the first few months of life.

Why are they important?

Absence of primary reflexes suggests CNS depression.

List 4 commonly tested primary (primitive) reflexes.

1. Moro reflex: Rapid abduction and extension of arms in response to sense of falling (examiner lifts infant slightly off bed and releases).
2. Finger grasp: Infant flexes fingers to grasp when examiner's index finger is placed in hand and slight traction is applied.
3. Automatic walking: Infant tries to support with feet when held upright; moves feet to "walk" when tilted forward.
4. Suck-swallow reflex: Infant sucks and swallows when an examiner's finger (clean) is placed in the infant's mouth.

Why give a newborn vitamin K?	Newborns may be deficient in vitamin K; the vitamin prevents hemorrhagic disease due to deficiency of vitamin-K–dependent coagulation factors.
Why put prophylactic antibiotics in the infant's eyes?	To prevent gonococcal eye infection (ophthalmia neonatorum)
What antibiotic is used?	0.5% erythromycin or 1% tetracycline ophthalmic ointments or 1% silver nitrate solution
Is circumcision of males routine?	No. The indications for circumcision are primarily cultural and religious. Parents should be appropriately informed about the pros and cons of the procedure.
What percentage of males are circumcised?	60%–70%
Should local anesthesia be used for circumcision?	Yes (usually 1% lidocaine)
Is nonretractile foreskin a cause for concern?	Most foreskins will not retract completely in the newborn, but this condition usually improves with age.
Are there benefits of circumcision?	Some studies suggest that the incidence of penile inflammation, penile cancer, urinary tract infections (UTIs), and sexually transmitted diseases (STDs) (including HIV disease) is lower among circumcised males.
List 5 contraindications for circumcision.	Hypospadias (Ch 22, p. 307), chordee, micropenis, ambiguous genitalia (Ch 24, p. 341), and bleeding disorder (or family history of a bleeding disorder)—a contraindication until the child has been tested and either is found to be unaffected or is successfully treated (Ch 15, p. 178)
When can feedings begin for a newborn?	**Breast:** breast feed immediately after delivery and q 3–4 hours or on demand. **Formula by bottle:** begin when respiratory status is stable, and q 4 hours or ad lib.

What laboratory studies should typically be obtained in the newborn?

1. Capillary Hct and bilirubin at 4 hours when Rh sensitization is known or newborn is pale in color, twin gestation, IDM, or SGA. Investigate if Hct < 40 or > 70 and bilirubin > 4 mg/dl.
2. Glucose screen within 1 hour and prn if weight < 2500 g or > 90th percentile for gestational age (LGA); or if newborn is jittery, has unstable temperature, or has apnea. Investigate if value < 60 mg/dl.
3. At discharge, Hct and state-required blood screens. [These vary from state to state and may include screens for hypothyroidism, tyrosinemia, phenylketonuria, galactosemia, maple syrup urine disease, homocystinuria, biotinidase deficiency, adrenal hyperplasia, hemoglobinopathies, and cystic fibrosis (CF), among others.]
4. Hearing screen prior to discharge
5. Home visit or physician's office visit within 48 hours after discharge for infants discharged prior to 48 hours of age

Is a car seat required for all infants for discharge home?

Yes; seat insert is needed for infant weighing < 3000 g

9 ___

Common Clinical Problems

JAUNDICE

What is it?

Accumulation of bilirubin in the epidermal tissues of the body, resulting in a yellowish tinge to the skin, sclera, and mucosa

At what bilirubin level is jaundice usually evident?

Serum levels > 5.0 mg/dl

What type of bilirubin is most commonly elevated in the neonate?

Unconjugated bilirubin

What is the physiology of elevated bilirubin?

Unconjugated (indirect) hyperbilirubinemia is secondary to increased production of bilirubin (e.g., excess red blood cell (RBC) destruction), decreased hepatic conjugation of bilirubin, increased absorption of bilirubin from the intestine (enterohepatic circulation) and/or decreased hepatic uptake of bilirubin. **Conjugated** (direct) hyperbilirubinemia is caused by hepatobiliary dysfunction or extrahepatic biliary obstruction.

What are the complications of hyperbilirubinemia?

Persistent and pathologic elevation of bilirubin in the newborn may cause an excess of free bilirubin (unconjugated bilirubin not bound to albumin or other serum proteins). This potential neurotoxin may cause **kernicterus,** an often-irreversible phenomenon characterized by jaundice, alteration of neurobehavioral status, and injury to the brain. Long-term sequelae of kernicterus may include deafness, cerebral palsy, or death.

What level of bilirubin is excessive in neonatal jaundice?

Controversial. In healthy term infants, an unconjugated bilirubin concentration > 20 mg/dl is potentially a cause for concern. Prematurity, acidosis, and other conditions may lower the threshold at which hyperbilirubinemia may cause damage.

What is the differential diagnosis?

Unconjugated hyperbilirubinemia may be physiologic (i.e., caused by immature hepatic enzyme pathways in the newborn) or may be associated with breast feeding. More pathologic causes include:
1. Rh, ABO, or other RBC isoimmunization complications
2. RBC membrane defects (e.g., congenital spherocytosis)
3. RBC biochemical defects (e.g., G-6-PD deficiency)
4. Deficiency in glucuronyl transferase (e.g., Crigler-Najjar syndrome)
5. Hypothyroidism
6. Bruising
7. Bacterial or viral sepsis
8. Resolving cephalohematoma or caput succedaneum with subgaleal hemorrhage.

Conjugated hyperbilirubinemia may be caused by direct hepatic insult from asphyxia, sepsis, congenital metabolic toxins, or by intrahepatic or extrahepatic biliary obstruction.

List 5 important components of the clinical evaluation.

1. Pertinent history should identify maternal complications with pregnancy or delivery; maternal and neonatal blood types, and direct Coombs' results; feeding history; time of onset and duration of jaundice.
2. Clinical examination should be thorough and should include a neurobehavioral exam and evaluation for signs of sepsis.
3. Pertinent studies include fractionated bilirubin level, Hct, and evaluation of a blood smear for evidence of hemolysis; evaluation of liver function

and hepatocellular integrity is
necessary with conjugated
hyperbilirubinemia.
4. With conjugated hyperbilirubinemia,
ultrasound of the liver and biliary tree
or nuclear medicine excretion studies
may be needed to rule out anatomic
abnormalities (e.g., biliary atresia).
5. Liver biopsy may be needed in certain
cases.

What is the treatment?

Unconjugated hyperbilirubinemia:
prophylactic or therapeutic phototherapy;
infants at high risk of kernicterus may
need exchange transfusions of whole
blood.
Conjugated hyperbilirubinemia: treat
the underlying liver disease or other
disease process

NEONATAL SEIZURES (SEE CH 6, P. 36, AND CH 25, P. 345)

**What is the incidence of
seizures in neonates?**

0.8%–1.0% of all live births; more
common in preterm infants

What do seizures reflect?

Seizures may indicate underlying illness
or metabolic derangement. All seizures
require prompt evaluation!

**What are common mani-
festations of seizures in a
neonate?**

Seizure activity in the newborn may be
focal, clonic, multifocal clonic, tonic, or
myoclonic movements.
Subtle seizures may manifest with sudden
onset of apnea; intermittent vasomotor
phenomena; oromotor, ocular, or facial
tics; or repetitive motion of facial muscle
groups.

**List 2 complications of
seizures.**

1. Respiratory compromise or apnea.
2. Prolonged seizure activity may cause
permanent brain injury.

**What is the most common
cause of seizures?**

Hypoxic-ischemic encephalopathy, which
is caused by intrauterine or birth-related
insult

**List 7 other common causes
of seizures.**

1. Infection: bacterial or viral infection or
toxoplasmosis

2. Imbalances in the blood concentrations of glucose, Na^+, Ca^{2+}, and Mg^{2+}
3. Intracranial hemorrhage (ICH)
4. CNS malformation
5. Drug withdrawal
6. Inborn errors of metabolism
7. Benign familial neonatal seizures

List 4 important factors in the history when evaluating a seizure.

1. Complications during pregnancy or delivery
2. Maternal drug use
3. Family history of seizures
4. Risk factors for sepsis

What 4 diagnostic studies should be performed?

1. Blood chemistries (e.g., electrolytes, calcium, magnesium, glucose, arterial blood gas [ABG])
2. Evaluation for sepsis, including lumbar puncture (LP)
3. CT or MRI to evaluate for hemorrhage, ischemia, or CNS malformation
4. Electroencephalogram (EEG) for detecting subtle seizures

What do skin vesicles or mucosal lesions suggest?

Herpes simplex encephalitis may present after the first week of age with seizures, lethargy, irritability, or a sepsis-like syndrome.

What is the treatment for neonatal seizures?

Treat the underlying cause.
Also:
1. Attention to airway and respiratory support
2. Electrolyte replacement as needed
3. Antibiotics and acyclovir therapy as clinically indicated
4. Anticonvulsant therapy (e.g., phenobarbital and phenytoin) titrated for effect
5. Surgical procedures for certain malformations or hemorrhages

What is the prognosis?

The prognosis depends on the etiologic factors.

List 3 signs of poor prognosis.

1. Seizures caused by hypoxic-ischemic encephalopathy or CNS malformation

2. Seizures initially occurring less than 12 hours after birth
3. Refractory seizures persisting beyond 24 hours after birth

What percentage of infants with seizures will have neurodevelopmental problems?

25%

NEONATAL ANURIA AND OLIGURIA

What is neonatal oliguria?

Urine output of < 15–20 ml/kg/day in the first 24–48 hours after birth. Many infants may only void once in the first 24 hours after birth. (See Ch 21, p. 293.)

What is neonatal anuria?

Failure to void within the first 48 hours after birth

What percentage of newborns void within 24 hours?

92%. Voiding in the delivery room "counts."

Within 48 hours?

99%

What is normal urine output for an infant after 24–48 hours?

~2 ml/kg/hr

What are causes of oliguria?

Prerenal in origin until proven otherwise! Oliguria is usually secondary to hemodynamic compromise caused by sepsis, CHD, dehydration, hypoxia, or (rarely) renovascular accident.

What are 2 causes of oliguria due to urinary retention?

1. Renal malformation
2. Obstruction of urinary outflow tract (e.g., posterior urethral valves)

List 6 causes of intrauterine anuria.

Bilateral renal agenesis, severe congenital polycystic kidney disease, posterior urethral valves, maternal or neonatal drug exposure, CNS disease (e.g., meningitis), spinal cord malformation (e.g., myelomeningocele)

List 2 complications of intrauterine anuria.

Oligohydramnios, pulmonary hypoplasia

What is the incidence of renal malformations, and what is the most common one?

5–6 per 1000 live births; horseshoe kidney is most common.

List 5 primary renal causes of anuria.

Bilateral renal agenesis, multicystic renal disease, congenital polycystic kidney disease, nephritis, exposure to nephrotoxins

List 4 important obstructive lesions.

1. Ureteropelvic junction obstruction
2. Posterior urethral valves
3. Duplication of the calyces, renal pelvis, or ureters
4. Urethral atresia

Why is family history important?

Some congenital renal disorders are inherited.

What are 2 important aspects of prenatal and intrapartum history?

1. Maternal history of oligohydramnios
2. History consistent with a hypoxic-ischemic event.

Many urinary anomalies are now diagnosed antenatally by ultrasound.

List 2 ways of evaluating prerenal compromise in the neonate.

1. Fluid bolus challenge of 10–20 ml/kg
2. Single-dose furosemide therapy (1.0 mg/kg) following a bolus dose of isotonic fluids may help rule out more severe pathology.

List 2 important components of the clinical evaluation of oliguria or anuria.

1. Evaluation of perfusion and blood pressure (BP)
2. Abdominal exam with careful palpation of kidneys; inability to palpate may suggest agenesis or absence of kidney; palpation of mass may suggest polycystic kidney or hydronephrosis due to urinary obstruction.

List 3 important laboratory values in evaluating a neonate with oliguria or anuria.

1. Blood chemistries
2. Blood urea nitrogen (BUN) and creatinine concentrations (IMPORTANT: neonatal electrolytes and chemistry values typically reflect the mother's values in the first 24 hours of the newborn's life)
3. Urinalysis

**What are the 2 most help-
ful imaging studies?**

1. Renal ultrasound—the kidneys should
   be evaluated in any infant with
   multiple congenital anomalies.
2. Nuclear medicine excretion studies
   may help assess the relative function
   of each kidney.

**List 4 treatments that may
be included in the management of neonatal oliguria
or anuria.**

1. Judicious use of IV fluids to maintain
   adequate urine output
2. Maintenance of normal BP; renovascular accidents, renal dysplasia, and
   postobstructive disorders are associated with severe hypertension
3. Peritoneal or arteriovenous dialysis if
   renal failure ensues
4. Transplantation of kidneys;
   transplantation in the neonate has
   been successfully performed

What is the outcome?

Varies, depending on the cause. Prompt
diagnosis and treatment of oliguria and
anuria prevent continued renal
deterioration.

FAILURE TO PASS MECONIUM

**When is meconium
normally passed?**

95%–97% of healthy term newborns pass
meconium in the first 24 hours. Sick term
infants and healthy preterm infants may
not pass meconium for 3–5 days.

**List 3 signs of failure to
pass meconium.**

Abdominal distention, feeding
intolerance, emesis. Any bilious emesis
requires prompt evaluation and should be
considered volvulus until proven
otherwise.

**What is the differential
diagnosis?**

1. Hirschsprung disease (Ch 19, p. 265)
2. Meconium ileus
3. Meconium plug
4. Anorectal malformation or atresia (i.e.,
   imperforate anus)(Ch 19, p. 251)
5. Malrotation of the bowel (Ch 19, p. 266)
6. Small-left-colon syndrome in the
   infant of a diabetic mother
7. Maternal medication, especially
   magnesium sulfate

8. Atresia of the duodenum, jejunum, ileum, or colon (Ch 19, p. 269)
9. Intestinal duplication

In any of these conditions except meconium ileus or imperforate anus, meconium may still pass appropriately!

List 4 important aspects of the clinical evaluation.

1. Confirm patency of rectum with digital exam or passage of soft catheter
2. Water-soluble contrast study of lower and upper gastrointestinal tract to determine if obstruction is present
3. Rectal biopsy if Hirschsprung disease is suspected
4. Assessment for cystic fibrosis (CF)

List 2 possibilities for treatment.

1. Water contrast enema may alleviate meconium plug or meconium ileus. (Examiner must consider Hirsch-sprung disease or CF in infants with meconium plug.)
2. Surgical exploration and repair may be necessary when an obstructing pathology exists. Maintenance of fluid and electrolyte homeostasis and hemodynamic status is imperative in these cases.

NEONATAL CYANOSIS

What is it?

Bluish tint of the skin: reflects the presence of 3–5 g/dl of reduced Hgb in the blood

What must the O_2 saturation be for an infant with polycythemia to demonstrate cyanosis?

< 88%

An anemic infant?

< 70%

List 5 common causes of cyanosis.

Primary lung disease, poor cardiac output, congenital cyanotic heart disease, pulmonary hypertension in the newborn, methemoglobinemia

Many healthy newborn infants may have cyanosis of the extremities (acrocyanosis)

with a normal pink color centrally, due to cooling, immature regulation of skin blood flow, or both.

Why are prenatal and peri-natal histories important?

Intrauterine or birth-related complications may indicate sepsis, asphyxia, or pulmonary insult as causes of cyanosis.

List 3 significant findings on clinical examination.

Heart murmurs, absent distal pulses, respiratory distress

Why is a chest radiograph important? (List 2 reasons)

1. Evaluation of the lung fields for evidence of primary lung disease
2. Evaluation of cardiac size and shape for evidence of CHD.

What are 2 significant findings for ABG?

1. PaO_2 level > 60 mm Hg on room air virtually excludes cyanotic heart disease.
2. Failure to demonstrate a rise of PaO_2 > 100 mm Hg in response to oxygen suggests a cardiac rather than pulmonary etiologic factor.

What is the significance of chocolate-colored blood?

It may indicate methemoglobinemia.

What condition may cause a 5%–10% difference in O_2 saturation between the arms and legs?

Pulmonary hypertension

Why?

Pulmonary hypertension may cause shunting through a patent ductus arteriosus (PDA). Blood supply to the right arm is preductal and to the legs is postductal.

What is the treatment for cyanosis?

Treat the underlying disease. Antibiotics are useful in fighting infection. Oxygen and ventilatory support may be required for noncyanotic heart disease and primary lung disease. Nitric oxide or extracorporeal membrane oxygenation (ECMO) therapy, or both, may be needed for refractory pulmonary disease, sepsis, and persistent pulmonary hypertension.

NEONATAL RESPIRATORY DISTRESS

What is the most common reason for admitting a newborn to a level II or III neonatal intensive care unit?	Respiratory distress
List 4 features of respiratory distress.	Tachypnea (i.e., > 60 breaths/min in any infant); use of accessory muscles of respiration (e.g., nasal flaring, intercostal retractions, grunting); hypoxia; hypercapnia
What is the most common cause of neonatal respiratory distress?	Primary lung disease
List 3 types of restrictive (poor lung compliance) conditions.	Pneumonia, surfactant deficiency (respiratory distress syndrome [RDS]) (Ch 10, p. 89), malformation of the lung or chest wall
Give an example of a type of obstructive (normal compliance) condition.	Aspiration syndromes—for example, aspiration of blood, amniotic fluid, meconium (Ch 10, p. 92), or gastric contents
List 12 other common causes of respiratory distress.	CNS injury; obstruction of upper airway by nasopharyngeal tissues (as in choanal stenosis or atresia) or the tongue (as in severe micrognathia); primary malformations of lung tissue; pulmonary edema; retained fetal lung fluid following precipitous vaginal delivery or cesarean section; pleural effusion; excessive incursion of abdominal contents; diaphragmatic hernia; hypoplastic lungs (caused by renal dysfunction or other causes of oligohydramnios); infection; polycythemia; transient tachypnea of the newborn (TTN) (Ch 10, p. 91)
List 6 important factors in evaluation.	Clinical history and examination, chest radiograph, ABG, hematocrit, assessment for cardiac disease, evaluation for sepsis

NEONATAL HYPOTONIA

What is the normal resting position for a newborn?	Elbows and knees flexed; hands most often in the fisted position
For a premature newborn?	Flexed and fisted less frequently
List 5 characteristics of hypotonia	1. Extension of extremities 2. Open hands 3. Occasionally exaggerated "frog-leg" position when supine 4. Child not withdrawing into flexion with noxious stimuli 5. Diminished primitive reflexes because of poor truncal tone
What causes hypotonia?	Conditions that are **genetic** or **acquired** in the intrauterine environment or during the birth process
List 5 causes of hypotonia without weakness.	Maternal disease or medication; placental insufficiency; sepsis; direct CNS injury; severe respiratory disease
List 6 causes of hypotonia with weakness.	Nervous system impairment—specific disorders in the neonate include: 1. Direct CNS or spinal cord injury 2. Anterior horn cell degeneration (e.g., infantile spinal muscular atrophy) 3. Variants of congenital myasthenia gravis 4. Myotonic dystrophy and other muscular dystrophies 5. Myotubular myopathy 6. Congenital metabolic disorder should be suspected in any infant with sudden onset of lethargy, hypotonia, or seizures.
Why is family history important?	Because of possible genetic etiologic factors. In addition, infants with congenital myotonic dystrophy may show no clinical or electrical signs of myotonia; however, often the mother will.
List 5 important laboratory studies.	Blood chemistries, sepsis evaluation, acid-base status, plasma ammonia concentration, creatinine phosphokinase (CPK) levels

What imaging studies are helpful?	Cranial and spinal MRI or CT
Why are the electro-encephalogram and electromyogram important?	They can help rule out seizures and abnormalities of skeletal muscle innervation.
What is another important test?	Muscle biopsy
What can rule out myasthenia gravis?	Neostigmine and atropine challenges
What consultants are commonly needed?	Neurologists and genetic consultants provide workups of specific congenital metabolic disorders.
What is the treatment?	Treatment must be tailored to underlying etiologic factors.
What is the prognosis?	The outcome depends on specific disease present; genetic counseling may be helpful in certain cases.

10

Diseases of the Newborn

PERIVENTRICULAR–INTRAVENTRICULAR HEMORRHAGE

What is it?

Intracranial bleeding that most commonly arises from the capillary network of the subependymal germinal matrix layer; arises less frequently from the choroid plexus or the roof of the fourth ventricle (Ch 25)

List the 4 grades (classifications) of these hemorrhages.

Grade I: isolated germinal matrix hemorrhage
Grade II: IVH with normal ventricular size
Grade III: IVH with acute ventricular dilatation
Grade IV: IVH with associated parenchymal hemorrhagic infarct

What is the incidence?

Approximately 40%–50% of infants who weigh < 1500 g and are < 35 weeks gestation have some degree of hemorrhage. Most hemorrhages occur within the first week of life, usually within the first 2 days. Although essentially a condition of premature neonates, it is seen occasionally in full-term infants.

What is the physiology of this condition?

The germinal matrix is a periventricular structure, containing a rich vascular network of primitive vessels most prominent 26–34 weeks from conception. Bleeding from the matrix ruptures into the lateral ventricles.

List 9 predisposing conditions and events.

Most common:

Prematurity, acute respiratory failure requiring mechanical ventilation

Others:	Pneumothorax, hypotension, acidosis, coagulopathy, volume expansion, bicarbonate infusion, birth trauma
List 4 signs.	Hypotension, apnea, metabolic acidosis, bulging of the anterior fontanel in severe cases **At least 50% of infants with hemorrhage have no clinical symptoms.**
List 2 methods that are used for diagnosis.	Ultrasound (usually preferred) or CT scan
What is the treatment?	Supportive care. Anticonvulsants may be required for seizures or seizure prophylaxis. If **posthemorrhagic hydrocephalus** ensues, treatment options include: 1. LPs 2. Drugs (e.g., acetazolamide, furosemide) that induce hyperosmolarity to decrease production of CSF 3. Ventriculostomy 4. Placement of ventriculoperitoneal shunt

RESPIRATORY DISTRESS SYNDROME (RDS)

What is it?	Pulmonary disease associated with prematurity and surfactant deficiency; previously called hyaline membrane disease
What is the incidence?	Age dependent: 60% at 29 weeks gestation. Decreases to less than 1% by 39 weeks gestation
List 5 characteristics of infants who are commonly affected.	1. Infants who have diabetic mothers 2. Infants who have siblings who had RDS 3. Males 4. Infants born by cesarean section without labor 5. Infants who experience perinatal asphyxia Note: Infants who had prolonged ROM

or IUGR, or whose mothers experienced physiologic stress, are relatively spared.

What are the classic features?

Onset of grunting respirations, chest retractions, and increased oxygen requirements. Characteristic radiographic changes occur within 6 hours of onset of symptoms.

List 4 acute and 3 long-term complications.

Acute:

Alveolar rupture (leading to pneumo-thorax, pneumomediastinum, pneumo-pericardium, or interstitial emphysema), infections, intracranial hemorrhage, PDA

Long-term:

Bronchopulmonary dysplasia (BPD), retrolental fibroplasia (also called retinopathy of prematurity), possible neurologic impairment

How is pulmonary imma-turity detected prenatally?

Because fetal lung fluid enters the amniotic cavity, **amniocentesis** provides a means for assessing pulmonary maturity via analysis of phospholipids in the amniotic fluid. Lecithin : sphingomyelin (L:S) ratio of $< 2:1$ and a saturated phosphatidylcholine (SPD) concentration of < 500 are associated with insufficient surfactant and, therefore, with potential RDS.

List 6 components of treatment.

Stabilization of the premature infant, including:
1. Administration of oxygen to keep PaO_2 at 50–80 mm Hg
2. Early surfactant with additional dosing (up to 3–4 doses) as required
3. Lung expansion, using continuous positive airway pressure or intubation and mechanical ventilation with PEEP
4. Thermal neutrality, usually a skin temperature of 36.5°C
5. Cardiovascular support
6. Acid–base and electrolyte therapy as indicated

What is BPD?

A condition characterized by inflammation or scarring of immature lung tissue exposed to high-pressure ventilation, oxygen, or infection.

List 3 preventive measures against BPD.

Administration of prenatal glucocorticoids to mother; surfactant therapy to infant with immature lungs at birth; minimization of ventilator injury from pressure and oxygen

List 5 components of treatment for BPD.

Treatment is mainly supportive. Therapies include judicious fluid–diuretic management, prevention of infection, bronchodilators, glucocorticoids, and nutrition

What is the long-term outcome?

Some children may experience chronic respiratory insufficiency, but many outgrow their BPD and have the potential for normal lives from a respiratory standpoint.

TRANSIENT TACHYPNEA OF THE NEWBORN (TTN)

What is it?

Early onset of mild respiratory distress

What causes TTN?

Any circumstance delaying the clearance of lung liquid by the lymphatics, including elevation of central venous pressure by late clamping of the cord, or cesarean section with limited or no labor.

List 7 features of the classic clinical presentation.

Tachypneic infant with 60–120 shallow respirations per minute; mild cyanosis; mild grunting; nasal flaring; chest retractions; mild respiratory acidosis; mild-to-moderate hypoxemia

List 4 radiographic findings.

Hyperaeration of the lungs, fluid in the interlobar fissures, prominent pulmonary vascular markings, and mild cardiomegaly. These signs usually resolve within 24–48 hours.

What is the treatment?

Supportive care with supplemental oxygen. Diuretics are not helpful. TTN is self–limited

MECONIUM ASPIRATION SYNDROME

What is meconium?	A thick, blackish-green material that accumulates in the fetal intestines beginning at the end of the first trimester. It is the accumulation of debris from the developing gastrointestinal tract.
What 2 conditions can be caused by meconium aspiration?	Significant **pneumonia** and **pneumonitis**
What 2 groups of infants are particularly at risk?	Small-for-gestational-age (SGA) infants and postterm infants. (Meconium-stained fluid is seen in 8%–20% of all deliveries.) Meconium staining rarely occurs before 34 weeks gestation.
How can this syndrome be prevented?	**Maternal management:** amnioinfusion of normal saline to relieve cord compression if fetal distress is evident and to wash out the uterine cavity **Infant management:** suction of the mouth and nose of the infant before delivery of the thorax. The infant's caregiver immediately intubates and suctions the trachea before the initiation of spontaneous respirations if the infant is depressed or has respiratory distress.
What are key components of treatment?	1. When all meconium cannot be removed from the airway and respiratory distress develops, supportive care, especially directed at oxygenation, is established. Infants may require intubation, mechanical ventilation, sedation, and neuromuscular blockade. Inhaled nitric oxide or ECMO may be needed in most severe cases. 2. Antibiotics are given after bacterial cultures are obtained, because meconium may promote bacterial growth, and sepsis may have contributed to the initial passage of meconium.
What are the outcomes?	Historically, meconium aspiration

syndrome has had a high mortality rate—up to 30% of infants who require mechanical ventilation. ECMO saves 85%–95% of infants who would probably otherwise die. Morbidity is more related to the hypoxic insult than to the pulmonary complications.

PERSISTENT PULMONARY HYPERTENSION OF THE NEWBORN (PPHN)

What is it?	PPHN, or persistent fetal circulation, implies pulmonary hypertension, right-to-left shunting at the level of the PDA and patent foramen ovale (PFO), and a structurally normal heart, often with depressed myocardial function and systemic hypotension. The constellation causes **severe hypoxemia**.
List 8 etiologic factors.	Primary (idiopathic) or secondary to: meconium aspiration or other aspiration syndromes; hyperviscosity of blood; neonatal sepsis (see below); intrauterine or perinatal asphyxia; myocardial dysfunction; CDH; neonatal pulmonary disease
List 5 symptoms.	Respiratory distress; cyanosis; gallop rhythm with a blowing murmur of tricuspid regurgitation; shock (Ch 6); heart failure
What does the chest radiograph show?	May reveal underlying lung disease; may show diminished pulmonary markings; or may be normal.
Differential diagnosis?	1. Cyanotic CHD, including transposition of the great vessels (TOGV) (Ch 16), total anomalous pulmonary venous return, pulmonic stenosis or atresia, and Ebstein anomaly 2. Severe pulmonary disease including CDH, pulmonary hypoplasia, and pneumonia
What is the treatment?	Goal is to decrease pulmonary vascular resistance and right-to-left shunting. 1. Supportive management is directed at

correcting acidosis and hypoxemia. Liberal use of oxygen is recommended.

2. If conservative therapy fails, intubation, mechanical ventilation, and sedation, with or without neuromuscular blockade with 100% oxygen, are initiated. Alkalosis (either metabolic or respiratory) aids in pulmonary vasodilation. Some clinicians hyperventilate the infant to Pco_2 20–30 mm Hg and pH 7.45–7.55.

3. Inhaled nitric oxide is an effective pulmonary vasodilator in some infants.

4. Pressors and inotropic agents may be required for systemic hypotension.

5. ECMO may be indicated if conventional therapy fails.

What are the outcomes?

Mortality rate ranges from 20%-40%. The incidence of neurologic sequelae is 12%–25% for survivors. Neurosensory hearing loss has been reported in up to 20% of survivors.

NEONATAL PNEUMONIA

What is the incidence?

Up to 0.5% of live births.

What are the etiologic factors?

Bacterial or viral; may be acquired transplacentally, through the birth canal, or post-delivery.

What is the most common bacterial agent?

Group B *streptococcus,* affecting 1–4 in 1000 live births

List 8 other common bacterial agents.

Escherichia coli (*E. coli*), *Klebsiella* species, Group D *streptococcus, Listeria* species, Pneumococci, *Staphylococcus* and *Pseudomonas* species can cause slightly later-onset disease, and *Chlamydia trachomatis* can cause pneumonia as late as 3–4 weeks after birth.

What are common viral agents?

Prenatally or postnatally acquired CMV, as well as postnatally acquired influenza, RSV, and adenovirus. The latter are

associated with significant morbidity and
mortality rates in infants.

List 4 predisposing factors.

Premature labor; rupture of membranes
before onset of labor, or prolonged
rupture of membranes; prolonged active
labor with cervical dilatation; frequent
obstetric digital exams

**List 8 signs and symptoms
of neonatal pneumonia.**

Nonpulmonary symptoms: Lethargy,
thermal instability, apnea, abdominal
distention, jaundice
Pulmonary symptoms: tachypnea,
cyanosis, respiratory distress

**What are the lung field
findings on chest radio-
graph?**

Vary from streaky density, to diffuse
opacification, to a granular appearance.

**List 4 important studies to
be conducted during
evaluation.**

Blood and CSF cultures; complete blood
count with differential; nasopharyngeal
culture for chlamydia or viruses; tracheal
aspirate for Gram stain and culture if
intubated

What is the treatment?

Initial treatment includes a penicillin
(usually ampicillin) and an aminoglycoside because broad-spectrum
coverage is indicated for early-onset
condition. Treatment for later-onset
pneumonia should also include coverage
for *staphylococcus* organisms. When the
causative organism is identified, treatment may be narrowed and continued for
a minimum of 10 days.

NEONATAL SEPSIS

What is it?

A generalized bacterial infection in a
clinically ill infant with a positive blood
culture during the first month of life

What is the incidence?

It occurs in 1 in 500 to 1 in 600 live births
and is influenced by maternal factors,
including active infection at delivery and
neonatal (especially prematurity) and
environmental factors.

When can infection occur?

1. Before labor, it can occur transplacentally or through the amniotic fluid with or without intact membranes
2. During delivery, as the infant passes through the birth canal
3. Post-delivery

List the 7 most common bacterial agents.

Group B *streptococcus; E. coli; Listeria monocytogenes;* Group A *streptococcus;* Group D *streptococcus; Streptococcus viridans; Staphylococcus* species

List some potential symptoms of neonatal sepsis.

Lethargy, irritability, poor feeding, temperature instability, possible fever if fulminant, tachypnea, hypotension, cyanosis, apnea, tachycardia, seizures, vomiting, diarrhea, hepatomegaly, jaundice, petechiae, and bleeding

Differential diagnosis?

Differential diagnosis includes hemolytic anemia, hypovolemic shock, intracranial hemorrhage, RDS, pneumonia, gastrointestinal anomalies, heart disease, hypoglycemia, or inborn errors of metabolism.

Which blood test is a helpful indicator for sepsis?

WBC with differential. Best indicator is an abnormal ratio of bands to neutrophils (i.e., > 20%) on differential. (Normal WBC for an infant is 8,000–20,000 WBC/mm^3.)

List 3 possible components of treatment.

1. After cultures (blood and CSF) have been obtained, broad-spectrum coverage is initiated with ampicillin and an aminoglycoside, usually gentamicin. When an organism has been identified, coverage is narrowed based on sensitivities and a 7- to 10-day course can be completed.
2. Granulocyte colony-stimulating factor or granulocyte transfusions may be required for desperately ill newborns with neutropenia.
3. ECMO may be employed for infants suffering pulmonary failure secondary to neonatal sepsis.

Immunoglobulin transfusions are still being studied for this population.

What is the outcome?	Mortality rate can be as high as 13%–50%.

NEONATAL BACTERIAL MENINGITIS

(See also Ch 28 for discussion of meningitis, including bacterial meningitis.)

What is the incidence?	Approximately 2–10 of 10,000 live births and is responsible for 1–4 of 100 neonatal deaths.
List 5 of the most common infecting agents.	Same as those discussed in neonatal sepsis (see above); most common are: Group B *streptococcus; E. coli; Listeria monocytogenes; Flavobacterium meningosepticum*—associated with epidemic disease; and *Citrobacter* species—associated with CNS abscess formation.
What are the risk factors?	They are the same as those associated with neonatal sepsis (see above). Meningitis is associated with up to 33% of cases. Local infections of the skin, respiratory tract, and urinary tract can cause bacteremia and thus meningitis. Premature infants and infants with meningomyelocele are at increased risk. Certain strains of bacteria are associated with increased risk—specifically, *E. coli* containing capsular polysaccharide K1, group B *streptococcus* serotype III, and *L. monocytogenes* type IV.
What are the signs and symptoms?	Same as those for sepsis (see above). In addition: Seizures, paralysis of CNS, abnormal cry, focal neurologic signs, bulging fontanel (may be a late sign). Stiff neck and positive Kernig or Brudzinski signs are rarely seen in this age group.
List 2 important factors in evaluation.	1. Every infant with subtle signs of sepsis requires an **LP** with Gram stain, cell count, protein and glucose analysis, and culture of the CSF. 2. **Blood and urine cultures** should also be obtained.

What is the treatment?	**Broad-spectrum antibiotic therapy** (ampicillin and an aminoglycoside) is initiated and tailored to an identified organism and sensitivity. **Gram-positive** meningitis is treated for a minimum of 14 days, whereas **gram-negative** meningitis is treated for 2 weeks after the infection is cleared or 3 weeks minimum, whichever is longer.
What are the outcomes?	Mortality rate ranges from 20%-50%. Morbidity is substantial and includes hydrocephalus, subdural effusions, ventriculitis, deafness, and blindness. Neurologic impairment is evident in 40%–50% of survivors. All survivors require audiologic and neurologic follow-up.

APNEA OF INFANCY AND SIDS

What is apnea of infancy?	Pause in breathing, usually ranging from 5 to > 20 seconds in duration, which arises from a central event, an obstructive event, or a combination of both.
What is the normal physiology of infantile breathing?	While the respiratory system matures, an infant < 6 months of age may experience periodic breathing or isolated, asymptomatic apnea of 5–15 seconds in duration.
When are apneic periods of clinical importance?	When unexplained apnea lasts > 20 seconds or is symptomatic
What is an acute life-threatening event (ALTE)?	Prolonged apnea, resulting in bradycardia and color change, that requires vigorous stimulation or positive pressure ventilation (it was previously also called a near-SIDS event)
List 10 causes of ALTE.	Apnea, gastroesophageal reflux, inborn errors of metabolism, seizures, sepsis, heart disease, apnea of prematurity, breath holding, poisoning, and Munchausen syndrome by proxy or child abuse
What are the treatment options?	1. Up to 30% of cases may be resolved by treating the primary cause.

2. For remaining cases, **apnea monitoring** and **CPR training** of the parents may be recommended.

What is SIDS?

Sudden **I**nfant **D**eath **S**yndrome

What is the incidence?

2 in 1000 live births; results in 6000–10,000 deaths yearly, with a peak incidence at 2–4 months of age

What are the risk factors?

1. Infants who have had an ALTE—these infants are at increased risk for dying from SIDS. However, 93% of infants who die of SIDS have never had such an event.
2. Infants of substance-abusing mothers
3. Infants put to sleep on their abdomens
4. Infants who are stressed (e.g., with an upper respiratory tract infection)

List 6 rules for parents to prevent SIDS.

1. Placing infants **"back to sleep"** (i.e., in a supine sleeping position) is recommended nationally.
2. Have infants on **firm** rather than soft bedding.
3. Avoid overly warm sleeping quarters.
4. Avoid over bundling.
5. Avoid placing objects such as stuffed toys in the cradle or crib.
6. Refrain from smoking around infants.

NEONATAL DIARRHEA

What is it?

Abnormally frequent, loose stools in an infant; may be associated with dehydration, failure to thrive, or systemic illness.

List 2 complications.

Profound dehydration; nutritional deprivation (dangerous for the developing nervous system)

List 7 common causes.

1. Infections (the most common causes), especially **rotavirus** (after 4 months), but also *Salmonella, Campylobacter,* and *E. coli* (during the first 2 months)
2. Primary or secondary carbohydrate malabsorption
3. Fat malabsorption

4. Congenital malformations of the intestines
5. Acquired defects of the bowel (e.g., short-gut syndrome— Ch 19)
6. Hormonal abnormalities (e.g., thyrotoxicosis, congenital adrenal hyperplasia)
7. Allergic conditions (e.g., intolerance to cow's milk protein)

List 3 ways neonatal diarrhea should be evaluated.

1. **History:** should include family history, birth history, and a chronology of the illness.
2. **Physical exam** should be detailed— after an initial assessment of hemodynamic stability and hydration status.
3. **Laboratory tests:** serum electrolytes, BUN, and creatinine; CBC to assess for an associated anemia; and stool studies for culture, rotavirus antigen, WBC and occult blood, and reducing substances.

What is the treatment?

Following fluid and electrolyte stabilization, therapy is determined by underlying condition. Antimotility agents are **NOT** used in infants and have a significant morbidity rate in this age group.

UMBILICAL ABNORMALITIES

OMPHALITIS

What is it?

Infection of and around the umbilicus and the retained umbilical remnant in the infant

What are the signs and symptoms?

Fever and possibly signs of sepsis

What is the appearance of the umbilicus with omphalitis?

Erythema around umbilicus, often extending in a streak up the abdomen along the umbilical vein—infection may spread within hours to become a frank **fasciitis** with **crepitus** and tissue **necrosis**.

List 3 components of treatment.	1. Broad-spectrum antibiotics 2. Umbilical remnant may need to be removed. 3. Aggressive surgical debridement if fasciitis is present.
List 2 ways it can be prevented.	Hand washing, asepsis in handling of fresh cord
What may be a significant associated condition?	Possible link between delayed separation of the cord, omphalitis, and defective neutrophil motility.

UMBILICAL HERNIA (SEE CH. 23, PAGE 320)

UMBILICAL GRANULOMA

What is it?	Persistent granulation tissue on umbilicus after separation of umbilical cord
What are the signs and symptoms?	Persistent discharge or oozing at site of granuloma. Cellulitis may develop around the site, leading to omphalitis.
List 3 components of treatment.	1. Mild cases respond to 1–2 applications of silver nitrate. 2. Some granulomas require surgical excision. 3. If cellulitis begins, infant should be treated with intravenous antibiotics and observed for any progression of infection.

PERSISTENT URACHAL REMNANT

It is a remnant of what structure?	The embryologic connection of the umbilicus to the bladder (allantois); it may take various forms: urachal cyst, urachal sinus, or urachal fistula.
What are the signs and symptoms?	1. Persistent discharge of mucus, pus, or frank urine from umbilicus 2. Cellulitis or sepsis if remnant becomes infected 3. Possible mass (may be tender) in infraumbilical midline position
How is it diagnosed?	Usually by physical exam. Sinogram

(contrast study through the draining umbilical site) or cystogram may reveal sinus or fistula.

What is the treatment?   Surgical excision, usually through infraumbilical midline or curvilinear incision. Remnant must be removed down to level of bladder.

11

Newborn Intensive Care: General Considerations

RESPIRATORS

List 4 basic modalities of oxygen therapy.

1. Nasal cannula with oxygen flow
2. Head box with humidified, heated oxygen to prevent excessive heat loss in the infant, with continuous monitoring of FiO_2
3. **CPAP: C**ontinuous **p**ositive **a**irway **p**ressure administered through nasal cannulae or endotracheal tube
4. Endotracheal intubation with mechanical ventilatory support

List 2 commonly used types of respirators.

1. **Conventional:** oxygen is delivered 20–40 cycles/min and may be pressure-limited, time-cycled, or volume-limited
2. **High-frequency:** facilitated diffusion of gases in lung at 600–900 cycles/min; may be a jet ventilator or oscillator

MONITORS

List 5 ways infants are monitored in the intensive care setting.

1. **Cardiorespiratory (CR) monitor:** detects apnea
2. **Arterial catheters:** catheters placed in an umbilical or peripheral artery for blood gas or chemistry sampling and for continuous BP monitoring
3. **Pulse oximetry:** continuous transcutaneous monitoring of arterial oxygen saturation
4. **Transcutaneous oxygen** (Tco_2): electrode applied to skin measures oxygen crossing skin membrane;

continuous measurement; correlation with arterial PO_2 varies with infant; good for monitoring trends; unreliable with poor perfusion

5. **Transcutaneous carbon dioxide:** same issues as TcO_2

NUTRITION

What IV fluids are appropriate for the newborn infant?

$D_{10}W$ in first 24 hours, except for the very low birth-weight infant who may require only D_5W; add "1/4 normal" saline after 24 hours

At what rate?

80–100 ml/kg/day

When is hyperalimentation used?

For the low birth-weight infant or ill term infant

What are the goals of hyperalimentation?

Goal: ~ 80–120 kcal/kg/day, including 3 g/kg amino acids, 3–4 g/kg fat; calcium, phosphorus, and other electrolytes and vitamins are added

List 2 administration routes for hyperalimentation.

Peripheral IV (limited to 12.5% dextrose) and central venous catheter (up to 25% dextrose)

List 3 routes of enteral feeding.

1. Gavage: feedings through NGT every 2–4 hours or by continuous infusion
2. Nasoduodenal: continuous feeding through transpyloric duodenal tube
3. Gastrostomy: g-tube may be placed when an infant undergoes abdominal surgery and a quick return to oral feeding is not anticipated, or when infant's feeding skills are poor

List 3 basic categories of formula.

1. **Standard formula:** 20 kcal/oz iron-fortified for term infants (same caloric concentration as breast milk)
2. **Premature formula:** 24 kcal/oz (increased sodium, calcium, phosphate and vitamins for improved growth and bone mineralization)
3. **Elemental formula:** blend of hydrolyzed protein and modified fat for improved absorption in infants

with malabsorption or feeding intolerance
Formulas may be milk- or soy-based.

ENVIRONMENT

What is a "closed" unit?	Once an infant leaves a "closed" neonatal intensive care unit (NICU) or newborn nursery (NBN) for the outside world, he/she cannot return to that unit. Subsequent admissions must be to a ward or pediatric intensive care unit (PICU). The bacterial flora of newborns are different from those acquired outside the hospital. Visitors must wear gowns to protect the infants in a NICU or NBN.
Why must a premature baby be kept in an incubator or a bed with an overhead warmer (i.e., a controlled environment)?	The infant's body surface area is large relative to body mass, and she/he cannot regulate body temperature adequately.
When can a premature infant regulate her own body temperature effectively?	Usually when a weight of 1600–2000g is attained.
What is the most likely cause when a premature infant's body temperature is too high or too low?	The temperature of the infant's environment. If appropriate, other reasons for the infant's altered temperature (especially **sepsis**) must be sought.

COMMON QUESTIONS PARENTS ASK

What are survival rates among premature babies?	For infants with birth weights Less than 750 g: < 40% 750–1250 g: 90% More than 1250 g: 95%–98% Congenital malformations and chromosomal anomalies affect these data.
List 7 common complications of prematurity.	Cerebral palsy, developmental delay, visual impairment, hearing impairment, learning disability, chronic lung disease, and mental retardation

What is the incidence of complications among premature infants?

For infants with birth weights
Less than 1000 g: 25%–30%
More than 1000 g: 15%–20%

When can an otherwise healthy premature baby be discharged?

Without major complications, a premature infant is expected to be discharged shortly before its term due date.

Can a mother still provide breast milk for a premature baby?

Yes. Although the infant may not be able to directly breast feed initially, the mother should pump her breasts at least every 3 hours beginning shortly after delivery.

Section III

Ambulatory
Pediatrics

12
The Pediatric Physical Examination

THE WELL-CHILD VISIT

What is the purpose of the well-child visit?

To identify physical, psychosocial, and developmental problems; prevent disease; provide guidance and advice to parents.

List 7 components of the well-child visit.

1. Identifying and responding to parental concerns
2. Historical assessment of physical and psychosocial growth and development
3. History of family-child interactions and problems
4. Age-specific physical examination to look for previously undiagnosed problems, assess previously identified problem areas, and assess normal neurologic development
5. Screening laboratory tests
6. Immunizations
7. Anticipatory guidance

At what ages should visits be scheduled?

1 month, 2 months, 4 months, 6 months, 9 months, 1 year, 15 months, 18 months, 2 years, 3 years, 4 years, 5 years, and every other year thereafter.
These are recommendations of the American Academy of Pediatrics (AAP).

List 2 instances when a visit may be needed for a newborn.

1. A baby who is discharged before 36 hours of age should be seen within 48 hours of discharge.
2. If the mother is breast-feeding for the first time or had a problem feeding a previous child, the infant should be seen at 2 weeks of age.

How long should the well-child visit last?

20–30 minutes

List some common parental concerns for an infant:

Newborn to 2 months of age?

Sleep schedules, feeding, crying

2–3 months of age?

Sleep, interpreting cries, initiation of solid foods, effect of mother going to work

4–6 months of age?

Sleep, scheduling naps, initiation of solid foods, effects of day care

6–9 months of age?

Motor development, child's tolerance of solid foods, patterns of discipline

9–12 months of age?

Motor development, temper tantrums, fear of strangers

12–18 months of age?

Temper, limit setting, night walking

18–24 months of age?

Temper and violence toward other children, limit setting, language abilities

24 months of age?

Toilet training, playing with others

36 months of age?

Social skills

List 4 physical measurements that should be recorded and give the frequency.

1. **Weight:** at every visit (unclothed)
2. **Length:** at every visit until the child can stand cooperatively; then height is recorded
3. **Head circumference** at each visit. Record maximum occipitofrontal circumference.
4. **Blood pressure** (BP): in all 4 extremities at 1 month of age to assess for coarctation of the aorta; routine single extremity BP at every visit beginning at 3 years of age

How are growth parameters tracked?

Using standardized growth curves expressed in percentiles

When is physical growth considered abnormal?

If the child's growth pattern deviates by more than 1 standard deviation from its previous percentile or is more than 2 standard deviations from the mean

What 4 areas of develop-ment are monitored?

Gross motor, fine motor, social, and language development. (See Ch 7, p. 57, for the milestones, by age, for these areas of development.)

What is the most commonly used developmental screening test?

The Denver Developmental Screening Test

At what age should malformations of fetal development or stigmata of syndromes be looked for?

At birth

At what ages should intra-abdominal masses be looked for?

Birth to school age

At what age should retinoblastoma be looked for?

Throughout the first 3 years

At what age should cardiac murmurs be looked for?

At each well-child visit

At what age should visual function be assessed?

By 3–4 months

At what age should congenital hip dysplasia be looked for?

At each visit, until child is walking

When does normal tooth eruption begin?

At 6 months; normal range is up to 15 months

List 2 early milestones of normal hearing.

Responds to sound by 2 months; orients to sound by 4 months

List 3 types of office screening for hearing.

1. Play audiometry at 3 years
2. Pure tone audiometry at 4 years
3. Brain–stem-evoked audiometry by age 6 months if child is in a high-risk group or if a newborn screen is abnormal

When does normal development of secondary sexual characteristics begin?

Girls: between 8 and 12 years of age
Boys: between 10 and 14 years

When does scoliosis commonly become apparent?	Beginning with the onset of puberty through Tanner Stage IV

SCREENING LABORATORY TESTS

List 6 common screening laboratory tests, and when they are performed.

1. Screening for a variety of **metabolic diseases** (e.g., PKU, hypothyroidism, sickle cell disease, biotinidase deficiency, galactosemia) is performed at birth on a state-by-state basis; these tests may need to be repeated if the child is discharged from the nursery early.
2. Screening for **sickle cell disease** (based on ethnicity) at 9 months of age, if not done at birth
3. Screening for **anemia** between 9 and 12 months of age, at entry to school, once in midchildhood, and once in adolescence. Earlier testing may be indicated if there are neonatal problems.
4. Screening for elevated **lead levels** as per current AAP and Centers for Disease Control and Prevention (CDC) protocols
5. **Urinalysis** is controversial, but children are often screened once in infancy and again at school entry.
6. Screening for **tuberculosis**—most children are screened at 12 or 15 months of age and again at school entry. Frequency of screening depends on the area of the country and the child's background (see Ch 28, p. 429, for the Mantoux tuberculin skin test and childhood tuberculosis in general)

IMMUNIZATIONS

List 11 diseases against which children are routinely immunized.	Diphtheria, pertussis, tetanus, polio, measles, mumps, rubella, influenza type B, varicella, hepatitis B, and *Streptococcus pneumoniae*
What source is the authority on immunization schedules?	The AAP's *Redbook;* it is updated every 3 years.

List 3 other vaccines that may be administered.

Influenza types A and B and *Neisseria meningitidis*

ANTICIPATORY GUIDANCE

List 6 topics on which anticipatory guidance may be given to parents.

Injury prevention, poison prevention, development stimulation, nutrition, behavioral development, child's adjustment to family disruptions (e.g., new siblings, moves, illness)

What guidance about injury and poison prevention should be given? (List 7 topics)

1. Use of a proper **infant car seat** from birth to 4 years of age (or 40 pounds), followed by **seat belt** use thereafter (a lift for the seat is helpful for children of young school-age years)
2. **Poison prevention**—beginning at 6 months with reinforcement thereafter; advice should include distribution of ipecac; parents should be advised to conduct a formal safety check of the home before 6 months; discuss drugs, household chemicals, and plants
3. **Firearm safety** in the home beginning at birth
4. **Swimming lessons** beginning by 3 years of age
5. **Bike helmet** use beginning with first tricycle
6. **Burn prevention** throughout childhood; advise parents to adjust water-heater temperature to maximum of 125°F at birth of first child.
7. **Avoid the use of walkers**

Guidance about child's development? (List 3)

Discuss milestones achieved and those to be achieved in the interval before next checkup. Discuss ways to help the child achieve the next milestone in a fun way.

Guidance and advice about nutrition? (List 8)

1. Breast-feed until 1 year; use formula if breast milk is unavailable. (Ch 5, p. 21)
2. Start solid foods about 4–6 months of age (preferably 6 months).
3. Review the principles of a balanced diet regularly.
4. Review the elements of a heart-healthy diet.

5. Review proper elements of food preparation and storage to avoid food poisoning.
6. Avoid constant overfeeding
7. Discuss fluoride supplementation when necessary
8. Monitor for nutritional practices that lead to iron deficiency

Advice about smoking and tobacco products?

Begin discouraging parental smoking at the prenatal visit and every visit thereafter. Offer to prescribe nicotine patch withdrawal systems for the parents.

List 7 major family stresses that the primary pediatrician should be alert for.

Divorce; separation; absence of a parent (e.g., at work) for prolonged periods; parental or sibling illness or disability; a move from one house to another; death of a family member, close friend, or pet; natural disasters affecting the family, such as fire, flood, or hurricane

THE SCHOOL PHYSICAL

What is a "school physical"?

The formal assessment of a child entering kindergarten

When is it performed?

Usually within 6 months of school entry (children are usually $4\frac{1}{2}$–6 years of age); individual state laws vary.

List 3 ways the school physical is different from the well-child visit.

1. Focuses on health and development as it relates to school readiness
2. Seeks to identify problems that may impair educational functioning of the child
3. May be considered (by some parents) as the last of the mandatory well-child examinations; therefore, special care should be taken to identify problem areas

List 8 general components of the school physical.

1. Immunization record review and completion
2. Developmental history and assessment
3. Screening hearing test
4. Screening vision test
5. Screening laboratory tests

6. Complete physical examination
7. Discussion of school placement and the child's potential strengths and weaknesses with the parents
8. Completion of the school form giving direction and advice to the school system about the child's unique needs, if any

List 4 immunizations that are given at the school physical.

1. Final dose of **polio** vaccine
2. Final dose of **diphtheria-pertussis-tetanus** (DTP) vaccine, either regular DTP or DTaP vaccine
3. Second dose of measles-mumps-rubella (**MMR**) vaccine
4. Completed vaccination against **influenza type B**

Note: State laws vary and dictate which immunizations are required for school entry.

What certification must the physician sign?

Usually the physician must certify that the child has received all appropriate immunizations, the child has a medical or religious contraindication, or (if the child is not fully immunized) a plan is in place to complete the required vaccines by an identified date.

List 4 screening laboratory tests that may be performed.

Usually **hemoglobin** (Hgb), **urinalysis,** and a tuberculosis (**TB**) **skin test;** in addition, **lead level** should be tested if there is any history of lead exposure, developmental delay, or anemia

What hearing test is used?

A pure tone audiometry test in a quiet place.

Describe this test.

Each ear is tested individually over a frequency range of 500–4000 Hz, with a minimal threshold of 15–20 decibels for the child to "pass" the test.

List 3 components of the vision test.

1. Visual **acuity** is tested in each eye separately and in both eyes together using a Titmus vision testing machine or a method of equal accuracy.
2. **Color vision** should be tested.

3. An assessment of **strabismus,** including a cover test, is also important.

What are key components of speech evaluation?

The child should **speak clearly** (i.e., physician readily understands) with little hesitation, using **complete sentences**. Occasional **stutter** may be normal, particularly if the child is excited, but facial grimacing, explosive speech, or frustration associated with the stammering is not. The **vocabulary** should excede several hundred words, and the child should know colors and body parts and identify most objects to which the tester points.

What are the standards for math readiness?

1. Should understand the concept of "more" versus "less" and "above" versus "below."
2. Should be able to count and correctly identify the number of raised fingers (up to 5).
3. Should be able to recite back to the examiner **3**-number sequences presented orally.

List 12 questions the physician should ask the parents about the child's social, behavioral, and developmental history.

1. Does the child play regularly with other children and does he/she look forward to these activities?
2. Does the child get frustrated and cry easily? Is the child prone to violent outbursts of temper?
3. How does the child handle conflict resolution in the family?
4. Does the child have trouble separating from the parents?
5. Is the child incontinent when napping during the day?
6. Is the child clumsy or physically awkward?
7. Is the child overly quiet and shy around strangers?
8. Does the child have older siblings in the school?
9. Does the child already like to read and does he/she have the ability to sustain concentration over a given task long enough to complete it?

10. Were the parents worried about this child's development either in the past or presently?
11. Has the child ever attended preschool and, if so, were the teachers there at all concerned about the child?
12. Does the child speak English fluently?

What should the physician do if concerned about the child based on the school physical?

Medical problems should be addressed, and the physician should alert the school to the potential problem so the school can perform an evaluation at the earliest possible date.

List 3 areas of consideration related to the child's size.

1. A child who is unusually small or large may be subject to extra emotional stress from classmates.
2. A child who is unusually small may be underestimated and treated like a younger child.
3. If there has been a recent change in growth pattern greater than one standard deviation, or if the child's size deviates more than 2 standard deviations from the mean, then the child should be assessed for comorbid illnesses associated with growth delay or with overgrowth.

How should the school be informed about any medications the child is taking?

A note is given to the school indicating the medication the child is taking, its therapeutic usefulness, possible side effects, and dosage schedule. The note should also indicate the primary illness that requires medication, whether it is contagious, and what effect it may have on the child's school performance.

List 7 causes of fatigue in a school-age child.

Late bedtime, getting up too early, an overly long bus ride, skipping meals, lack of time to rest or nap at school when the body is tired, frequent mild respiratory viral illnesses contracted in the school setting, and over-involvement in after-school organized activities.

List 4 ways the physician can address a child's physical disabilities with the school.

1. A child with a physical disability needs special communication with the school to ensure appropriate treatment. The school should receive an honest but upbeat appraisal of the child's abilities.
2. Point out activities that may put the child at risk and consult with the teacher for alternative strategies.
3. The teacher's fears about the child's needs in the classroom should be addressed.
4. Any special help the child may need, such as adaptive physical education and time for trips to a physical therapist, should be described in detail.

Advice to parents with a physically disabled child?

Stay involved in your child's classroom activities. Don't be shy and assume that everything will turn out well. If the child is not doing well academically, is fearful of school, doesn't want to discuss school, or seems to have undergone negative personality changes, then the parent should contact both the teacher and physician immediately.

List 2 common specific reasons for school physical examinations.

1. The preparticipation sports physical (Ch 13, p. 130)
2. The physical examination required every 3 years for children receiving special educational assistance.

List 2 purposes of the every-3-years physical examination.

1. To assess any new or changed physical or developmental limitations, including changes in physical functioning (e.g., vision and hearing)
2. To evaluate new information about a child's chronic illness (e.g., new medications or complications) that affects the child's school performance.

COMMON CLINICAL PROBLEMS

WHEEZING

List 8 common causes of wheezing in infants.

Tracheal malformations, vascular rings, tracheoesophageal fistula (TEF)(Ch 19, p. 271), mediastinal masses, aspiration, reflux, cystic fibrosis (CF) (Ch 17, p. 220), and infections (Ch 28, p. 396)

In toddlers? (List 5)	Infection (especially respiratory syncytial virus [RSV] and adenovirus) (Ch 28, p. 210); asthma; CF; foreign body aspiration; tumor (Ch 26, p. 210) (See Ch 17, p. 210, for discussion of asthma, CF, and foreign body aspiration.)
In older children? (List 4)	Infection (especially viral) (Ch 28, p. 217); asthma (Ch 17, p 220); CF (Ch 17, p. 220); tumor (especially lymphoma in the mediastinum) (Ch 26, p. 359)

FEVER

What body temperature classifies as a fever?	Generally, a rectal temperature of > 37.8°C is considered a fever, but some authors use a higher figure (38.0°C–38.2°C). Interpretation of fever may vary with the patient's age.
Does fever equal infection?	No, but the concern about infection depends on the patient's age and clinical status. **Infants with fever should be carefully evaluated for meningitis or septicemia.** (See Ch 28, p. 396, for a discussion of meningitis.)

RESPIRATORY DISTRESS

List 8 causes of respiratory distress in children.	1. **Upper airway obstruction,** including **epiglottitis** (Ch 18, p. 228), peritonsillar or retropharyngeal abscess, foreign body in airway (Ch 17, p. 220), edema, malformations (Ch 17, p. 227), intrinsic or extrinsic masses 2. Lower airway obstruction, including foreign body, bronchiolitis, and reactive airway disease 3. Pneumonia (Ch 17, p. 215) 4. Congestive heart failure or pulmonary edema 5. Trauma 6. Spontaneous pneumothorax (especially thin, adolescent males) (Ch 17, p. 222)

7. Metabolic diseases
8. Muscle diseases

ABDOMINAL PAIN

List possible causes to be considered in the differential diagnosis of abdominal pain in children and adolescents.

Viral gastroenteritis, appendicitis, mesenteric lymphadenitis, bacterial enterocolitis, Meckel diverticulitis, inflammatory bowel disease, hernia with incarcerated bowel, food poisoning, intussusception, abdominal adhesions, pneumonia, acute intermittent porphyria, trauma, volvulus, functional. In girls who have begun menstruating, dysmenorrhea and pregnancy must also be considered as a cause for abdominal pain.

DIARRHEA

List 3 causes of acute diarrhea.

Bacterial infections, such as *Salmonella, Shigella, E. coli, Campylobacter,* and *Yersinia;* viral gastroenteritis; food poisoning

List 9 causes of chronic diarrhea.

Fat malabsorption, CF, dietary allergy, lactose intolerance, bacterial infection, celiac disease, malnutrition, antibiotic use, inflammatory bowel disease

VOMITING

List 13 causes of vomiting.

Viral gastroenteritis, food poisoning, upper gastrointestinal (GI) obstruction, inborn error of metabolism, CNS tumor, motion sickness, sepsis, paralytic ileus, adhesive obstruction (if child has had a prior operation), incarcerated hernia (Ch 23, p. 317), malrotation, appendicitis, intussusception (Ch 19, p. 249)

ACNE

What is it?

A skin condition commonly affecting adolescents, consisting of 4 basic types of lesions: Open and closed comedones, papules, pustules, and nodular-cystic lesions.

List 2 causal factors.

1. During adolescence, **androgens** stimulate the growth of sebaceous glands as well as the production of sebum. Some of these materials are hydrolyzed to free fatty acids, which can cause inflammation.
2. Characteristic abnormal **keratinization** of skin cells at this time also contributes to the lesions.

List 2 features of open comedones ("blackheads").

The orifice of the follicular duct is open and the involved sebum has been oxidized to the black color, usually without a surrounding inflammatory reaction.

List 2 features of closed comedones ("whiteheads").

The follicular duct is occluded, with a surrounding inflammatory reaction.

List 2 ways the development of acne can be minimized.

Cleansing the face 2–3 times daily with a mild soap, and avoiding oil-based skin preparations and makeup

List 3 ways acne is treated.

Topical agents—the most common are benzoyl peroxide and retinoic acid; systemic antibiotics—such as tetracycline or erythromycin, may be needed in more severe cases; 13-cis-Retinoic acid is used for the most severe cases of acne (cystic acne or acne conglobata). **Females of childbearing age being treated for acne should avoid pregnancy (consider birth control) since some treatments may have adverse effects on a developing fetus.**

List 3 potential side effects of retinoic acid preparations.

1. There may be **carcinogenic effects** from the combination of light and retinoids. Therefore, avoidance of sun or, alternatively, the use of sunscreen is recommended for patients using retinoic acid.
2. Retinoic acid also may cause hyperpigmentation in patients with darkly pigmented skin.
3. Retinoic acid and some related compounds are **teratogens**.

INGESTION OF POISONOUS AGENTS

How important are ingestions of poisonous agents in pediatrics?	They are the **4th most common cause of death** in children.
What is the peak age for poison ingestions?	2 years of age; however, teens also are prone to ingesting caustic substances as suicide attempts or gestures
List 3 categories of commonly ingested household materials.	Cleansers (e.g., sodium hydroxide); batteries (potassium hydroxide); miscellaneous acidic agents (e.g., sulfuric acid)
What should be done if a child ingests a poisonous agent?	The poison control center should be called. Instructions will depend upon the agent ingested. Ipecac should be kept in the household in case inducement of emesis is appropriate.
List 2 ways that a child who has ingested a caustic agent is evaluated.	**Esophagoscopy** within 24 hours and **barium swallow** within 48 hours to assess degree of injury, stricture, and esophageal motility
List 2 components of treatment of ingestion of a caustic agent.	1. Ampicillin and gentamicin with hydration should be started when ingestion is suspected. 2. Esophageal strictures may require dilation, placement of a feeding tube (nasogastic or gastrostomy), or anatomic replacement.
List the 2 best methods of prevention.	"Childproofing" the home and educating children and parents

DEVELOPMENTAL DELAY

What is it?	Delay in attaining developmental milestones at the appropriate age (Ch 7, p. 57)
Does developmental delay equal mental retardation?	No. There may be reasons for developmental delay that are unrelated to cognitive skills.
List 3 ways for the physician to screen for developmental delays.	Careful history; thorough physical examination; use of a screening test (e.g., the Denver Developmental Screening Test)

What laboratory, radiographic, or other tests are indicated for developmental delay?	This part of the evaluation should be individualized, using the history and physical examination and the developmental evaluation as starting points. (Ch 7, p. 571)

SHORT STATURE

What is it?	Height less than the second percentile for age (**Note:** definitions may vary)
List the 2 most common causes.	Normal variation, constitutional delay
List 7 other causes.	Endocrine abnormalities (Ch 24, p. 324), metabolic diseases, genetic syndromes, skeletal dysplasias, chromosome abnormalities, chronic diseases, pyschosocial short stature
List 5 ways in which it is evaluated.	History (including family history), review of growth data, physical examination, appropriate radiographic and laboratory studies as indicated
Why are previous measurements so important?	Growth is a dynamic process; evaluation of change over time gives more information than isolated growth points.

OBESITY

What causes obesity?	Caloric intake exceeds caloric expenditures.
What is the most common cause of childhood obesity?	Exogenous obesity (excessive intake)
What is the relationship of obesity to height?	Children with exogenous obesity tend to be taller than average. Most endocrine disorders and syndromes in which obesity is seen are associated with stature that is shorter than average.
List 4 syndromes associated with obesity.	Prader-Willi syndrome, Cushing syndrome (Ch 24, p. 340), pseudohypoparathyroidism type I, growth hormone deficiency (Ch 24, p. 333)

FAILURE TO THRIVE

What is it?	Usually the term refers to failure to gain or maintain weight adequately
List 7 causes.	GI disorders, immune disorders, chronic diseases (consider CF!), inborn errors of metabolism, inadequate nutritional intake, CNS abnormalities, psychosocial problems
List 6 ways it is evaluated.	Careful history, physical examination, weight measurements, review of growth data, and laboratory and radiographic studies as indicated

ENCOPRESIS (SEE CH 19, P. 264)

What is it?	Fecal incontinence due to overretention of stool
List 5 causes.	Psychological problems, Hirschsprung disease (Ch 19, p. 265), chronic stool retention, neurologic abnormalities, hypothyroidism
List 5 ways it is evaluated.	Careful history, physical examination, review of growth data, and laboratory and radiographic studies as indicated. Evaluation should be done to rule out Hirschsprung disease. (Ch 19, p. 265)
List 3 components of treatment.	Treatment depends on the etiologic factors. 1. Educating and supporting the parents and child are key. 2. A "clean-out" regimen, followed by a program to maintain regularity (if not caused by Hirschsprung). 3. Attention to emotional and behavioral issues.

ENURESIS

What is it?	Urinary incontinence in child 5 years of age or older
What is the differential diagnosis?	Urologic abnormalities, neurologic abnormalities (including seizures),

	diabetes mellitus, diabetes insipidus, psychosocial stress
List 5 ways it is evaluated.	Careful history, physical examination, review of growth data, laboratory evaluation (including urinalysis, regardless of suspected cause), and radiographic studies as indicated
What is the treatment?	Depends on the etiologic factors
List 3 components of therapies of nonorganic enuresis.	Medications, alarms, behavioral modification

SCHOOL PHOBIA

What is it?	Fear of school or refusal to attend school
List 3 of the common potential causes.	Real fear of the school environment (e.g., bullies, violence); fear of a teacher; fear of separation from the parent or family
List 3 components of evaluation when somatic complaints are present.	History; physical examination as indicated; detailed interview with the parents and child.
What is the treatment goal?	The goal is to normalize the child's school experience, which usually involves returning the child to the classroom as soon as possible. Parental education is important, as well as additional counseling if the school phobia is a manifestation of more serious emotional problems.

ATTENTION DEFICIT HYPERACTIVITY DISORDER (ADHD)

What is it?	A disorder characterized by limited capacity for attention, overactivity, and impulsivity. It is distinct from abnormal conduct behavior and specific learning disabilities.
What are the etiologic factors?	These are still not fully known.
What is the prevalence?	1.5%–4.0% of children; some studies suggest a higher prevalence

Is it more common in boys or girls?	Boys, by a 5:1 ratio
What is the age of onset?	Usually before 4 years of age
Is family history important?	Yes. ADHD is more common in children who have had family members with ADHD.
List 5 typical characteristics of the history of a child with ADHD.	A history of behavior in specific situations is important, as are birth and neonatal histories. There is often a history of difficult birth, colicky behavior as an infant, sleep difficulties and feeding difficulties as an infant, and excessive temper tantrums as a toddler.
List 4 typical clinical manifestations.	A child (especially in school) may be uncontrollable, refuse to sit still, intrude upon other children, and refuse to follow instructions. During formal examination, symptoms may be difficult to detect because these children can behave well in significantly structured situations.
On what basis is the diagnosis made?	Usually on a clinical basis.
List 7 other causes of difficult behavior for which children with symptoms of ADHD should be tested.	Specific learning disabilities, hearing impairment, petit mal epilepsy, side effects of medication, anxiety or depressive disorders, or poor living situations
List 3 potential components of treatment.	1. Behavioral and psychosocial therapy with a confirmed structure to the child's environment 2. Stimulants, including methylphenidate (Ritalin), dextroamphetamine, pemoline, and clonidine are sometimes used in conjunction with these therapies. 3. Tricyclic antidepressants may also be efficacious.
What is the prognosis?	Prognosis appears to be better if a child with this condition does not exhibit aggression. There are concerns that children with ADHD may be more prone

to alcoholism, sociopathy, and hysteria in adulthood. Steady gainful employment seems to be helpful.

LIMP

List 10 causes of limp.	Foot problems (e.g., calluses, foreign bodies, warts, shoe problems), sprains, strains (Ch 13, p. 136, re sprains and strains), fractures, dislocated hip, toxic synovitis, osteomyelitis, soft tissue trauma, arthritis (septic, inflammatory), and cancer (e.g., osteosarcoma, leukemia, neuroblastoma) (Ch 26, p. 355)
List 4 ways limp is evaluated.	History and physical examination, laboratory and radiographic studies as indicated

HEADACHE

Are headaches a sign of dangerous disease?	Rarely
What are 4 signs that a headache may be serious?	Excruciating pain, stiff neck, accompanying neurologic findings, impairment of consciousness
List 6 characteristics of migraine.	Rapid onset; pain is often hemicranial and behind the eye; visual changes (e.g., seeing flashing lights, black spots); pain is intense and pounding; photophobia; child sleeps and then awakens without headache
Is a family history of migraine common?	Yes
What are possible treatments?	Sleep is often the best treatment. Other therapies include ergot derivatives, isometheptene, and analgesics. Some patients may require chronic treatment with β-blockers, tricyclic antidepressants, or calcium channel blockers. Biofeedback or relaxation therapy may be helpful.
List 7 characteristics of tension headaches.	1. Slow onset of pain 2. Bifrontal distribution 3. Pain is not really debilitating

4. Pain is squeezing in quality and may have a throbbing component
5. No visual changes or photophobia
6. Gradual remission of pain
7. May be associated with definable psychological stress

List 3 treatments of tension headaches.

Analgesics, biofeedback therapy, relaxation therapy

13

Pediatric Sports Medicine

GENERAL ISSUES IN SPORTS MEDICINE

What is the role of a primary care physician in sports medicine?

Roles range from being a team physician to providing medical care dealing with an individual player's specific illness. The primary care physician should be comfortable addressing injuries to bone and joints, nutrition, fitness, and health issues as they relate to sports.

List 4 characteristics of a good sports medicine or team physician.

1. Knowledge of young people and how to deal with them
2. A significant interest in sports
3. Awareness of the demands of a specific sport
4. Appreciation and understanding of the "athletic mentality"

What is the difference between "weight lifting" and "weight training?"

"Weight lifting" is the process of pressing and jerking maximum amounts of weight for a one-snatch opportunity. **"Resistance strength training"** ("weight training") involves selecting a weight that can be lifted or moved in a series of repetitions to attain increased strength and flexibility. Usually 3 sets of 10 repetitions is safe and effective.

Is there a role for "weight lifting" in sports?

Except for weight lifting competition, no.

What is the role of weight training for prepubertal boys and girls (Tanner stage 1 or 2). (Ch 14, p. 152)

1. There is disagreement about the effects of weight training by prepubertal children.
2. Weight training will not result in any significant increase in muscle mass

until testosterone comes aboard later in puberty.

3. Specific muscle training relevant to a certain sport under the supervision of a knowledgeable trainer may increase strength and flexibility to some degree. There is no evidence that this correlates with improved athletic performance.

4. Concern exists about abuse of weight training causing damage to growth plates. (**Pain** is a good indicator that muscle is being abused.)

At what age should a child be allowed to begin participation in competitive sports? Collision sports?

The American Academy of Pediatrics guidelines suggest:
1. Competitive sports: no child under 6 years old
2. Collision sports: no child under 10 years old

List 2 criteria for allowing a child to participate in a sport.

1. The main criterion is that the child states a sincere interest in participating.
2. The physician must feel the child is able to participate safely, based on the physical assessment of the child and the physician's knowledge of the sport and the program the child will be joining.

PREPARTICIPATION SPORTS ASSESSMENT

What are the 3 primary goals of a sports physical examination (PE)?

1. Identify boys and girls at high risk for injury because of disqualifying factors or predisposing conditions.
2. Recommend rehabilitative measures to correct or minimize the risk factor or condition.
3. If rehabilitation is not possible, redirect the boy or girl to another sport in which the risk is lessened.

List 4 skills and strategies for the physician to use in dealing with the injured athlete.

1. Good communication skills to establish rapport and effective dialogue with athletes
2. A knowledge of and interest in the athlete's sport

3. Awareness that return to action as soon as possible is everyone's goal
4. Empowering the patient to participate in his or her healing

What 2 secondary goals or benefits are derived from a sports physical examination (PE)?

1. Educates the athlete about nutrition and fitness and their connection to sports
2. Introduces many participants to health care; the sports PE is frequently the only contact adolescents have with a physician

Is there a standard form or set of requirements for sports PE?

No. Although the American Academy of Pediatrics and American Academy of Family Practice have made recommendations on this issue, state requirements vary.

List 3 reasons the sports PE should be comprehensive.

1. This may be the only physical examination he or she receives.
2. To identify important historical information
3. To determine appropriate level of participation in a suitable sport

What 5 particular factors are important during a comprehensive sports PE?

In addition to the components of a standard physical examination, a sports PE should focus on:

1. **History**—provides highest yield of factors that might affect an athlete's participation. History of any previous injury, individual or family cardiovascular conditions, and previous concussions and head injury should be obtained.
2. **Assessment of physical maturity**— may reveal factors for disqualifying a girl or boy from participating in a collision sport
3. **Musculoskeletal examination**—the most common source of physical findings that predispose to recurrent injury
4. **Measure of fitness and state of nutrition**—especially important for sports in which weight loss is common (gymnastics and wrestling) or in which

obesity might predispose the athlete to heat injury (e.g., football practice in August)

5. **Analysis of history and physical examination and knowledge of the nature of sports**—necessary for making an appropriate recommendation for specific sports participation

List 2 ways in which physical maturity is measured.

1. Tanner stage of pubertal development (Ch 14, p. 152).
2. Measure handgrip strength with a hand ergometer.

Boys and girls should reach what Tanner stages before participating in vigorous competition?

Boys at less than Tanner stage 4 should not participate in collision sports (e.g., football, lacrosse, ice hockey) with fully mature boys because of increased risk for injury, especially to epiphyseal plates. Physical maturity is much more relevant to injury risk than weight or size.

Girls who reach 15 years of age and are still at Tanner stage 2 or less should receive close scrutiny and evaluation before participation in "weight conscious" sports, such as gymnastics, dance, or cross-country running.

As a nonorthopedist, how does a physician conduct a musculoskeletal examination?

Evaluate all joints and muscle groups, including the neck, for level and symmetry of strength, muscle mass, bony structure, and range of motion. Pay special attention to any areas of previous injury.

List 3 areas of fitness that should be determined at the time of the sports PE.

Cardiovascular, pulmonary, and general health and fitness (including nutrition)

List 3 ways cardiovascular fitness is measured.

1. Blood pressure (BP)
2. Cardiac examination for murmur and rhythm, especially after exercise with the heart rate increased.
3. Exercise. One practical method: the athlete performs a 2-minute jumping-jack task at 1 jump/sec. The physician measures resting pulse, pulse

immediately after exercise, and pulse after a 1-minute recovery period. A rise in pulse to > 95 beats/min during exercise, or a drop to $< 2/3$ of the resting level on recovery is grounds for slow and cautious advancement to full practice and activity.

List 2 ways to measure general health, fitness, and nutrition.

1. **Height:weight proportio:** use standard growth chart
2. **Body fat:** the appropriate range in girls and women is 10%–25%; in boys and men, 7%–20%. Body fat lower than these ranges may indicate **malnutrition** or **eating disorders**. Higher body fat indicates obesity and could be a problem in acclimatization to heat.

In what 2 ways is the body fat percentage determined?

1. Determining body density by water immersion (most accurate).
2. Measuring skin fold with calipers.

How is pulmonary fitness measured?

Some sports medicine specialists recommend a pre- and post-exercise FEV_1 test (forced expiratory volume in 1 second) to identify exercise-induced bronchospasm. As much as 10% of the athlete population experiences this condition enough to affect performance.

When should a sports PE be performed?

Ideally, 2–4 weeks before practice begins. If a mild abnormality is noted (e.g., loss of full range of motion of a joint, poor cardiac fitness, or obesity), there is time for appropriate conditioning or rehabilitation.

List 2 formats that are typical for sports PEs.

1. The one-on-one, physician–athlete examination in the physician's office (preferably, the young person's own physician). The young person's own physician knows the athlete well, including history and family, and may be more likely to uncover undue family pressure to participate or to know of history that the young person might choose not to report.

2. A mass-screening format—usually held at a school.

List 2 desirable features of a mass-screening format.

1. Stations where different health care providers perform different aspects of the examination.
2. The last station provides a physician to complete the examination for each child

List 4 duties of the physician at the last station of a mass-screening sports PE.

1. Summarize the findings of the evaluation
2. Give recommendation for participation
3. Discuss the recommendation with the athlete
4. Allow the athlete to ask health-related questions

How frequently should a sports PE be performed?

There is no standard recommendation. The current mode is for a yearly examination.

What laboratory tests should be included in a sports PE?

Routine laboratory tests are not needed on all children; tests should be based on the history or PE.

List 2 instances in which it is reasonable to include urinalysis in an asymptomatic patient as part of a sports PE.

1. For baseline data in case of future injury to the kidney
2. If the boy or girl has not had a urinalysis in the past 2 years and is receiving no other health care

In what instance is it reasonable to test hemoglobin (Hgb) and hematocrit (Hct) as part of a sports PE in an asymptomatic patient?

If the athlete is not receiving any other health maintenance

Is testing of free erythrocyte protoporphyrin and ferritin appropriate?

These may be valuable tests but are not practical in mass screening situations. Low iron stores, even with normal Hbg or Hct, may occur in certain sports fairly commonly and are especially problematic in female athletes.

What are the 4 potential recommendations to an athlete following preparticipation evaluation?

1. **Full participation**—history and PE are normal.
2. **Limited participation**—everything is in normal range, but some factor recommends against participation in a certain sport (e.g., a boy in Tanner stage 3 is recommended for all sports except a collision sport).
3. **Conditional participation**—the child is allowed to participate, but some restrictions or precautions are recommended (e.g., an obese, out-of-shape athlete is required to lose a certain amount of weight before putting on football pads)
4. **No participation**—the boy or girl may be required to get clearance before playing—for example, from an orthopedist because of knee surgery or from a cardiologist because of previous syncope.

What recommendation should be made if a boy or girl has only 1 kidney or has experienced 5 or 6 concussions?

Probably **not to participate in collision sports**. If the family insists on participation, precedents have been set so that courts may allow a child to participate over a physician's recommendation.

What are 8 key ingredients to an excellent sports pre-participation evaluation?

1. Thorough sports-specific and medical and family history
2. Thorough physical and neurologic examination
3. Additional examination:
   - Tanner staging
   - Body fat measurements
   - Pulse—resting, exercise, and recovery
   - FEV_1—pre- and post-exercise
4. Some measurement of iron stores and anemia
5. Performed 2–4 weeks before sports practice begins
6. A quiet and private environment convenient for the athlete, conducive to a good examination and an opportunity for conversation
7. Performed by individual(s)

knowledgeable and interested in athletes and in all aspects of sports
8. Summation by a physician and appropriate recommendation and follow-up for the athlete, family, coach, and school

MUSCULOSKELETAL INJURIES

What are the 2 major types of musculoskeletal injuries?

1. **Traumatic injury:** acute and involves an impact or undesired motion.
2. **"Overuse" injury:** may seem acute but usually has an insidious onset over a long period of time (e.g., stress fracture).

List 7 factors that pre-dispose a sports participant to musculoskeletal injury.

1. Re-injury of a previous injury that had not been totally rehabilitated—the most common cause of injury
2. Imbalance or asymmetry in muscle strength or range of motion
3. Overuse of particular joint(s) or muscle(s)
4. Improper warmup and stretching, which limit flexibility
5. Improper equipment
6. Improper technique in an athletic skill
7. Poor conditioning

What is the difference between a strain and a sprain?

Sprain: injury to a ligament
Strain: injury to a tendon or muscle

What is the most common soft tissue injury?

Muscle hematoma or contusion (a.k.a. "Charley horse"). The goal is to **minimize the amount of bleeding** to prevent myositis ossificans (muscle calcification)

MANAGEMENT OF INJURIES

ACUTE MANAGEMENT

List 5 steps in the acute treatment of a traumatic injury.

1. Calm the injured patient and move others away.
2. Assess for life-threatening situations such as compromised airway, major bleeding, or neck or vertebral spine injury.

3. Get history of the nature of injury and whether any "pop," "snap," or other acute feeling or sound was noted.

4. Check for swelling and ask when it first occurred (if physician was not at the scene of the injury). Immediate swelling is generally due to bleeding. Swelling after the first hour or so usually is secondary to inflammation and exudation of tissue fluid.

5. **"PRICEM"** (a variation of the more familiar "RICE")—is always appropriate for any musculoskeletal injury.

   Protection: If appropriate and possible, immobilize the joint above and below the injury until further assessment.

   Rest: Complete rest for a significant injury is usually indicated for a **minimum** of 48 hours.

   Ice: Cold applied for 20 minutes every 2–4 hours minimizes swelling from bleeding or inflammation. This can shorten the recovery time and reduce muscle destruction.

   Compression: Pressure (e.g., hand compression, elastic bandage) can control bleeding and swelling and minimize destruction of tissue and rehabilitation time.

   Elevation: When possible, elevating the injured area will enhance resolution of swelling.

   Medicine: Judicious use of pain and anti-inflammatory medication.

EARLY REHABILITATION

List 3 goals of rehabilitating an injury.	To return the athlete to his or her sport: 1. As quickly as possible 2. With the greatest likelihood of achieving the previous level of performance 3. With no increased risk of further injury or re-injury.
List 4 goals in developing a treatment plan for an injury.	Recognize that most injuries to muscle, ligaments, or tendons generally cannot be "fixed"—they have to be allowed to heal.

1. Minimize damage to the injured areas
2. Prevent injury to other tissues that might occur through compensatory behaviors if participation continues or resumes prematurely
3. Maintain muscle tone and cardiovascular fitness
4. Gradually return to activity as function and pain permit

When should "early rehabilitation" begin?

As soon as the extent of the injury to underlying structures is determined. Usually within 24–48 hours of injury, stretching, isometric contractions, and passive range of motion exercises to point of minimum discomfort can begin.

List 3 signs of readiness for the early stage of rehabilitation.

1. Acute pain is gone
2. Swelling has decreased to stable point
3. Passive range of motion can be accomplished without pain.

List 3 components of "early rehabilitation."

1. Alternate heat and ice: ice for 10–20 minutes, heat for 15 minutes, ice again for 10–20 minutes (2 or 3 times per day)
2. Stretching and passive range of motion exercises to point of minimum discomfort should be done midway through the ice phase of treatment. Active range of motion exercise can begin when no significant pain occurs.
3. Isometric contractions against resistance can begin. **Always let pain be the limiting guide**.

ADVANCED LEVEL REHABILITATION

When does "advanced level" rehabilitation begin?

It begins when all the above levels are accomplished without pain.

List 5 components of "advanced level" rehabilitation.

1. Continue most early rehabilitation activities (use heat to the injured area before exercising and ice after exercising).
2. More intense stretching, especially before and after exercising.
3. Exercising should consist of range of

motion against resistance (e.g., using weight training principles). Isometrics continue to be good.

4. Cross-training is important to keep non-injured muscles and cardiovascular system fit. It also helps the athlete to feel she is active and contributing to self-healing. For example, judicious use of exercise in water or bicycling provides low impact, good aerobic conditioning so long as careful consideration for the injury site is maintained.

5. A protective device for the injured can be helpful during rehabilitative exercise (e.g., knee/ankle braces; elastic wrap for compression of a muscle injury).

How long does "advanced level" rehabilitation continue?	Until the injured area can be used in a normal manner without difficulty; this can last from approximately 14 days to 4 weeks after injury.

RETURN TO ACTION

What time span does this stage encompass?	From the time when all advanced rehabilitation activities can be accomplished without pain until the injured area is back to full strength.
How soon can an injured athlete return to active participation in sports?	2 weeks to 8 weeks or more depending on injury.
What is the best approach to use with athletes during the return-to-action stage?	Explain to an athlete what must happen before she can participate rather than give a specific length of time. **Pain** is the main determining factor.
List 3 components of management in the return–to–action stage.	1. Continue advanced rehabilitation. 2. Begin a period of regimented, easy use of the injured part. Intensity of use can be carefully increased until goal is reached. Cross-training may be helpful. 3. Continued use of ice and protective devices is advisable. If pain or

difficulty occurs, then the athlete
should back down to an earlier level of
activity and advance more slowly.

**How does one approach an
overuse injury?**

Same as for traumatic injury, except that
usually a reduction in activity or cross-
training may be satisfactory instead of
total withdrawal from activity.

**How does the physician
treat a specific injury such
as a sprained ankle or
painful knee?**

Evaluate the injury as discussed above. If
there is no underlying fracture or major
instability suggesting disruptions of
ligaments, tendons, or other supporting
structures, then following the progression
of management as described above is
appropriate. Many exercise-rehabilitation
program outlines are available in books;
one of these can be plugged into the
Early and Advanced Rehabilitation levels,
but the basic outline above applies to the
majority of specific extremity injuries.

**What is the role of "TENS,"
ultrasound, "whirlpool,"
physical therapy, occupa-
tional therapy, and so forth,
in treating these injuries?**

For most mild to moderate injuries (the
vast majority of those that occur) the
above outline of management by a
primary care physician is all that is
needed.
For more severe injuries, referral to an
orthopedist, a sports medicine facility with
an athletic trainer, or other therapist
should be done. Referral may be helpful if
the athlete does not seem likely to follow a
program on his own.
The therapist may choose to use electrical
stimulation or other treatment modalities.
However, data supporting their
effectiveness are fairly limited and
unimpressive.

**How are injuries graded in
severity?**

Injuries are graded by a somewhat
arbitrary method meant to suggest the
amount of damage and the length and
type of management and rehabilitation
necessary.

**List the grades of ankle
sprains, with the charac-
teristics of each.**

Grade I—Mild pain and slight swelling,
stable joint tests, normal range of
motion, pain-free weight bearing.

> **Grade II**—Moderate pain and intermediate swelling, stable joint, decreased range of motion by a few degrees, and painful weight bearing.
>
> **Grade III** – Severe pain, significant swelling that obliterates landmarks, unstable joint, limited range of motion, and inability to bear weight.

HEAD INJURIES

How are concussions graded?

There are many grading methods with loss of consciousness, pain, confusion, and amnesia being important ingredients. There is not a uniformly accepted system, but **any head injury should be considered potentially serious** until proven otherwise. For simplicity in this discussion we will consider 3 grades of head injury:

1. **Mild concussion**—player is "dazed" without amnesia and no loss of consciousness
2. **Moderately severe concussion**—confusion post-event, retrograde amnesia, or both, plus loss of consciousness of less than 1 minute or even without loss of consciousness
3. **Severe concussion**—signs of moderately severe concussion plus significant loss of consciousness and a prolonged period of confusion

How is each type of concussion managed?

Mild—A person can have significant brain injury without losing consciousness! If the athlete is neurologically intact after being removed from the game, did not lose consciousness, has not had a previous concussion, and is checked every 5 minutes for 15–20 minutes, she may return to action if no delayed signs of amnesia, headache, dizziness, nausea, and so forth develop during that period.

Recent studies suggest that asking the player questions relating to their current activity ("What team are you playing?" to "What is the score?") are more relevant to the player's possible confusion than standard orientation questions ("What is your name/address?").

Moderately severe—The physician should remove the athlete from the contest, perform frequent neurological checks, and transport the player to an emergency facility if any deterioration occurs. Return to practice and play **only** after 1 full week **without any** symptoms, even a mild headache.

Severe—Transport to the nearest hospital by ambulance, with appropriate immobilization techniques. No return to action until 2–4 weeks have passed **absolutely symptom-free**.

What is the danger of repeated head injuries?

The **second impact syndrome**. Death can even occur from a relatively minor blow to the head occurring within a few weeks of a previous concussion if brain swelling persists. This is the reasoning for not allowing an injured player to return to action for a period of time and until **all** symptoms are gone.

How many concussions are too many?

Concussions can have a cumulative destructive effect. Cognitive deterioration, parkinsonian-type disorder, and "boxer's syndrome" have all been attributed to repeated concussions. There are no data to show exactly how many concussions should create major concern. However, there is consensus that a player should not return to action in a season **after 2 significant concussions** without clearance from a neurologist or other appropriate physician. Similar precautions about participation in collision sports should be recommended for a player who has experienced several concussions over a few seasons.

What is a "stinger"?

A "stinger" is a burning or stinging of the arm and hand that can be accompanied by weakness and sometimes paralysis. This occurs from a stretching or compression of the neck, injuring the brachial plexus. Recurrent episodes may lead to permanent weakness.

What are components of the management program for "stingers"?

Initial treatment consists of:
Ice, resting the arm in a comfortable position, anti-inflammatory agents
When the pain is gone and strength returns to normal, the athlete can resume parti-cipation. If symptoms persist for more than 24 hours, a more comprehensive evaluation and rehabilitation program should be arranged. Some athletes with long necks are predisposed to stingers, and a neck collar can be somewhat protective.

EYE INJURIES

When should eye injuries be evaluated by an ophthalmologist?

Injuries with trauma to the globe or the periorbital tissues.

List 5 serious sequelae of trauma to the eye.

Hemorrhage, retinal detachment, hyphema, lens dislocation, and orbital floor fracture

How can eye injuries be prevented?

By using protective eye wear—especially children with visual impairment

MEDICAL ISSUES RELATED TO SPORTS PARTICIPATION

INFECTIOUS DISEASE

What 2 factors should be considered when deciding whether an athlete with an upper respiratory infection or other common viral illness should participate in an athletic contest?

1. Risk to the athlete—the athlete is at greater risk for injury if the illness includes a fever, decreased stamina, or other complicating factor
2. Contagiousness—probably not relevant, as risk is usually minimal
Decision to participate should be made on an individual basis.

List 3 skin lesions that may prohibit an athlete from participating in a sport in which physical contact occurs.

Impetigo, tinea, herpes
A boy or girl should not participate unless the lesions are covered or healing. This is a significant concern in wrestling. (Ch 27, p. 382)

List 3 signs in an athlete with infectious mononucleosis that require a delay in returning to sports participation.

Fatigue, splenomegaly, lymphadenopathy. When splenomegaly is present, no activity that involves exertion or collision should occur for a **minimum of 2 weeks after resolution of splenomegaly**.

What sports should an athlete with a blood-borne infectious disease (hepatitis B, AIDS, HIV) be strongly discouraged from playing?

Sports in which close physical contact and exposure to body fluids and blood occur (e.g., wrestling, boxing) pose the greatest concern.

The athlete's health determines whether participation is advisable. There have been no substantiated reports of these diseases being transmitted through athletic participation. The risk of this transmittal is low, but theoretically it is not zero.

A physician can recommend that an athlete not participate in these sports if infected. However, the athlete cannot be forbidden from playing under present legal interpretations. Note: The physician also operates in the doctor–patient confidentiality relationship.

List 3 things sports physicians can do to prevent spread of these diseases in sports.

1. Encourage hepatitis B vaccine for all athletes, trainers, coaches, referees, and others who might be at high risk for exposure to blood and body fluids.
2. Advise all players about judicious participation in sports if they are infected with any transmissible disease.
3. Practice and encourage the use of the "universal precautions" at all athletic events.

List 5 universal precautions as they relate to sports participation.

1. An athlete should cover wounds whenever possible.
2. If a bleeding wound occurs, the individual's participation stops until the wound stops bleeding and is cleansed and covered securely. Any uniform contaminated with blood should be changed.
3. Skin exposed to blood or other body fluids contaminated with blood should

be cleaned as promptly as possible with soap and warm water.

4. Rubber gloves and disposable towels should be used by individuals when cleaning and handling blood and blood-contaminated materials. These items should be placed in a container lined with a plastic bag for disposal.

5. Any surface contaminated with blood should be cleansed with fresh household bleach solution (one part of bleach to 100 parts of water).

CHRONIC DISEASES

In what sports should an athlete with asthma not compete?

With current therapeutic options, most young people with asthma should be able to participate in any sport they desire. Sports that require more prolonged and constant action (long-distance running, soccer, and field hockey) are more likely to cause difficulty than sports with short bursts of activity (football, tennis, and basketball).

List 2 ways athletes with asthma can maximize their safety and effectiveness in sports competition.

1. Use of peak flow meters to monitor asthma status and helping an athlete learn about his or her "refractory period."

2. Pre-exercise medication (cromolyn, beta-2 agonists, or both) can be helpful in minimizing bronchospasm.

What is the refractory period?

There is a period shortly after beginning exercise when reactive airway bronchospasm is particularly severe. Once that period is passed, there is a **refractory period** during which the airway seems to be particularly open. This period can last for a fairly extended time. If an athlete learns where her "bad" period is, she may warm up more vigorously for that prescribed period, so that when the game or practice begins she is already at the refractory period.

What is exercise-induced asthma?

Bronchospasm that occurs only with exercise

In what 3 ways is it recognized?	1. Shortness of breath occurs with exercise 2. Bronchospasm occurs with exercise 3. Hyperactive airway is identified in exercise portion of physical examination As many as 10% of athletes are identified in preparticipation sports PEs as having hyperactive airway. Many are unaware of problems, but in retrospect may report shortness of breath with exercise that they attributed to being out of shape.
List 2 treatments for exercise-induced asthma.	Pre-exercise use of cromolyn, beta-2 agonists
What is exercise-induced anaphylaxis?	Episodes of apparent syncope with characteristics simulating anaphylactic shock at or near the end of participation in an athletic activity. It can be confused with exercise-induced asthma.
List 3 possible causes.	1. Something triggers the release of histamine or some other mediator, often in people without a history of atopic disorders. 2. A combination of heat, stress, and dehydration may trigger the episode. 3. In other instances various foods appear to be the trigger—but only if the food was eaten near the time of the exercise, because the food alone is tolerated well.
List 4 components of management in severe cases.	The "full court press" of management, including **adrenalin (epinephrine), steroids, IV fluids,** and **antihistamines** and any other supportive measurements appropriate for the situation.
What other allergic disorder can create problems for athletes?	Severe generalized systemic reaction to stings from *Hymenoptera* (e.g., bees, yellow jackets, fire ants)(Ch 29, p. 441 for more on allergic reactions to insect stings and bites)
What athletes are at greatest risk from anaphylaxis and severe allergic reactions?	Participants who are outdoors at a distance from trainers and medical care (e.g., cross-country runners)

List 2 measures that athletes at risk for anaphylaxis can take to prevent or treat allergic reaction.

1. Carrying adrenalin (epinephrine) in an easy-to-administer form
2. Consultation concerning the appropriateness of venom desensitization

What are 2 guidelines for participation in sports by young people with seizures?

1. **Non-collision** sports—Usually youngsters can participate in any non-collision sport including swimming and diving, so long as the seizures are **well controlled** with medications.
2. **Collision sports**—controversy surrounds the appropriateness of playing a collision sport in which blows to the head typical of these sports could lower the threshold for seizure. The issue comes down to an individual decision by the participant, the family, and the physician

What sports should a person with diabetes mellitus avoid?

With good control, good knowledge about his disease, and appropriate precautions and accommodations, a person with diabetes should be able to participate in any sport.

List 3 precautions that should be observed in athletes with diabetes.

1. The coach, trainer, and other teammates should be aware of the athlete's disorder.
2. Glucagon and a source of sugar (e.g., juice, candy bar) should be available at all times.
3. The athlete should always carry identification that includes information about his diabetic condition.

What can the young athlete do to maintain control of his diabetes if he chooses to participate in sports?

Learn what adjustments in diet and insulin (with close monitoring) may be necessary to maintain good control with variations in practice and game times.

NUTRITION

Can an athlete be too obese to participate in sports?

Yes. If an obese athlete (> 20% body fat for boys and men, > 25% body fat for girls and women) has any other risk factors such as hypertension or poor cardiovascular conditioning, he or she is at greater risk and should be evaluated fully and monitored closely.

What is the greatest risk for the obese athlete?

If no other risk factors are present, the greatest risk is the problem of **acclimatizing to heat.**

List 4 ways to manage acclimatization to heat.

1. Begin a conditioning program 2–3 weeks before practice begins.
2. Increase physical activity gradually over a 14-day period.
3. Monitor pre- and post-exercise weight.
4. Take frequent breaks for fluids. (Water is best!)

Can a young person be too thin to participate in sports?

If the participant is physically mature (greater than Tanner stage 3), he should not be at greater risk for injury in a collision sport despite a difference in size from the other athletes.

What 2 groups may be at increased risk in sports?

1. Boys and young men with less than 7% body fat
2. Girls and young women with less than 10% body fat

List 5 factors for which they are at risk.

Decreased endurance, alterations in growth patterns, delayed pubertal development, abnormal or absent menstrual cycles (females), eating disorders

List 4 examples of sports in which the greatest risks occur.

Those in which weight loss tends to be encouraged, such as wrestling, gymnastics, dance, and crew.

Are there safe ways to lose weight if it is indicated or desirable?

It is acceptable to burn **excess** fat to lose weight. A rate of **2 pounds a week** is acceptable. Weight loss accomplished by losing fluid (dehydration) or by losing muscle (malnutrition) can be harmful and can lead to poor endurance and reduced strength.

List 6 harmful effects of rapid weight loss.

Dehydration, malnutrition, electrolyte imbalance, negative nitrogen balance, and renal and liver insults.

What are the calorie requirements of an athlete?

Enough calories to meet basic metabolic needs plus calories required for activity and exercise. **Prepubertal athletes** require additional calories for growth. Most growing, active athletes need 2000–3000 calories per day—and more if they are involved in vigorous activity and endurance sports. No athlete, even those trying to lose weight for wrestling or similar sports, should eat fewer than 1500 calories per day.

What are the best foods for an athlete to eat?	A daily diet that offers plenty of water, 60% carbohydrates, 25% proteins, and 15% fat.
List 3 components of pre-game preparation, from a food and rest standpoint.	1. A good night's sleep for the 2 nights preceding a game or contest. 2. The "night-before" meal should be a high-carbohydrate meal such as pasta. 3. The pre-game meal should be about 4 hours before competition and should also be high in carbohydrates such as pasta. Avoid grease and fat.
What kind of vitamin supplements should an athlete take?	An athlete who eats a normal diet does not need additional vitamins.
How can an athlete gain weight if he or she desires?	A good caloric intake and appropriate weight training add "good" muscle weight to an athlete that can be a positive contribution to performance and appearance. (This is only true for athletes who have entered puberty.)
Are high-calorie and high-protein supplements safe for the athlete?	No. These may create potentially harmful renal solute loads and liver toxicity. Also, creatine and androstenedione should be avoided.

STEROIDS, DRUGS, AND OTHER SUBSTANCES

List 3 dangers of steroids.	Abnormal growth in prepubertal boys and girls; liver, skin, and central nervous system (CNS) abnormalities and adrenal gland suppression; many long-term adverse effects

List 3 common types of substance abuse among athletes and the effects of each.

1. **Tobacco** can be detrimental to lung function and performance in sports, with no redeeming values.
2. **Alcohol** can lead to nutritional and hydration problems, and provides a large number of calories that may not be desirable.
3. **Marijuana** and **cocaine** have adverse effects on lung function and heart function.

HEAT INJURY

List, in order of severity, the 5 types of heat injury syndromes.

From mild to severe:
Heat fatigue, heat syncope, heat cramps, heat exhaustion, and heat stroke

List the symptoms of the 5 types of heat injury.

Heat fatigue: weakness, fatigue, light-headedness

Heat syncope: fainting, frequently at the end of a workout

Heat cramps: painful cramping of muscles, especially in the legs. Sometimes called "tired leg" or "dead leg" syndrome, heat cramps result in fatigue, weakness, and difficulty running

Heat exhaustion: prostration, lethargy, hyperventilation, dizziness, inability to concentrate

Heat stroke: hyperpyrexia, shock, disorientation or confused mental status up to level of coma

List 6 ways the athlete can prevent heat injury.

1. Acclimatize
2. Weigh before and after practice and replace weight loss by frequent and generous intake of water.
3. Wear lightweight clothing until acclimatized.
4. Use a sling psychrometer to measure "wet bulb temperature," humidity, and temperature, and regulate sports practice according to readings.
5. Be aware that lost sodium, potassium, and other salts and minerals are replaced in a normal diet.
6. Watch for early signs of heat injury

and allow generous fluid intake and cool-down.

List 5 components of treatment for heat injury.

1. Stop exercise
2. Lie in cool place with legs elevated
3. Drink lots of water if conscious enough to be safe
4. Remove helmets or other restricting clothing items
5. In case of heat stroke or severe heat exhaustion, IV fluids and other more aggressive emergency-room level treatments should be sought immediately

What is the correct dose for salt tablets or potassium supplements?

No salt or potassium supplements are needed, even with leg cramps. Enough of these elements is provided by a normal diet.

What should athletes drink?

Water is the ideal drink to replace lost fluid. Sports drinks can be too hypertonic during activity, and they can delay stomach emptying and suppress the thirst mechanism. Diluted sports drinks (2–3 parts water to 1 part sports drink) are acceptable.

14

Adolescent Medicine

PUBERTY AND GROWTH

What is adolescence?

The period between childhood and adulthood (the Latin *adolescere* means "to grow up"); generally from 10–21 years (exact limits vary)

What are 5 tasks of adolescence?

Identity formation, autonomy, separation from family, exploration of vocation, and establishment of internal moral standards

What is puberty?

Biologic maturation (L. *pubescere* means "to grow hair")

When does puberty occur?

8–13 years of age in girls; 9–14 years of age in boys

When is menarche?

10–15 years of age (average age is 12); ovulation usually occurs within 2 years after menarche

When does sperm production begin?

13–14 years of age

What are Tanner stages?

Stages of external physical (sexual) maturation

What is Tanner stage 1?

Prepubertal

Stage 2?

Onset of any sign of sexual change; in girls: breast buds, sparse pigmented pubic hair; in boys: enlargement of testes, scrotum, and penis, with sparse pigmented pubic hair

Stages 3 and 4?

Increasing pubic hair; other findings in girls include increased breast tissue, raised areola (stage 4); other findings in boys include continuing enlargement of genitalia

Stage 5?	Adult secondary sexual characteristics; areola now continuous with breast tissue in females, pubic hair on the inner thighs
What is precocious puberty?	Onset of puberty before 8 years of age in girls and before 9 years of age in boys (Ch 24, p. 329)
At what age is puberty considered delayed?	If there has been no development of secondary sexual characteristics by 13 (females) or 14 (males) years of age (Ch 24, p. 331)
List 3 categories of causes of precocious puberty.	1. Idiopathic (most common) 2. Endocrine abnormalities (see Ch 24) 3. CNS abnormalities
List 7 causes of delayed puberty.	Idiopathic (most common); Turner syndrome (in girls); Klinefelter syndrome (in boys) (Ch 30, p. 446); chronic illness; weight problems; CNS abnormalities, including secondary abnormalities; psychological or psychosocial problems
List 5 important factors in the evaluation of abnormal timing of puberty.	History, physical examination, plotting of longitudinal growth data, bone age, laboratory tests as clinically indicated (Ch 24, p. 332)
What information does one use to assess growth at puberty?	Longitudinal data
What are normal growth rates?	Prepubertal: about 5 cm/year During puberty: 9 cm/year for girls; 10 cm/year for boys (boys also have a "strength spurt" near the end of puberty)
List 6 causes of a delayed growth spurt or strength spurt.	Idiopathic, stress, chronic illness, nutritional deficiencies, genetic disorders, endocrine disorders

LEGAL ISSUES

What is emancipation?	Fiscal and physical independence
What is the legal age of emancipation?	Usually 18 years of age; may vary with states (check local statutes)

List 6 types of procedures to which minors can legally consent.

In most states, minors can consent to:
1. Emergency care
2. Diagnosis, treatment, and prevention of STDs
3. Contraception—but not sterilization
4. Diagnosis and management of pregnancy
5. Management of rape or sexual abuse
6. Diagnosis and treatment of mental health problems, including substance abuse

Note: State laws vary and may change regarding these issues.

Who is an emancipated minor? (List 4 categories)

A minor who is currently or was married; a teenage parent; a self-supporting minor living away from home; a minor in the armed forces

BASIC ISSUES OF TEEN HYGIENE

When should a woman have her first pelvic examination?

By 18 years of age; before initiation of sexual intercourse; any time there is a gynecologic problem

List 3 immunizations that are given to adolescents.

1. Second measles-mumps-rubella (MMR) vaccine, varicella vaccine, or both (if not received earlier)
2. Tetanus booster (10 years after previous booster)
3. Hepatitis B series (if not already received)

Note: Some physicians also suggest meningococcal vaccine, depending on the school setting.

When is adult dentition present?

By midpuberty

How often is routine dental care needed?

Hygiene every 6 months; check-up yearly

How often are eye examinations needed?

Every 1–2 years during adolescence, more often if indicated

ACNE

See Chapter 12

MENSTRUATION

List 3 characteristics of a normal menstrual period.	Menstrual flow < 8 days; cycle duration of 21–35 days; blood loss of about 50 ml during menstrual flow

OLIGOMENORRHEA

What is oligomenorrhea?	Too little menstrual bleeding; skipping months
List 8 causes.	Anovulatory cycles, stress, pregnancy, weight change (loss or gain), polycystic ovary syndrome, thyroid disease, increased prolactin production, androgen excess
What is the treatment?	Regulate periods with medroxyprogesterone acetate (Depo-Provera) or oral contraceptives, and treat underlying cause.
What are the 2 most common causes of secondary amenorrhea?	Pregnancy and stress. Other causes, as in oligomenorrhea

POLYMENORRHEA

What is polymenorrhea?	Excessive menstrual bleeding
What are the causes?	Anovulatory cycles, pregnancy problems (e.g., ectopic, miscarriage), sexually transmitted diseases (STDs), endocrine causes (similar to oligomenorrhea), diabetes, blood dyscrasias, iron deficiency
List 4 important factors in evaluation.	History, physical and pelvic examination, hematocrit, platelet count
What is the treatment?	Same as for oligomenorrhea

DYSMENORRHEA

What is dysmenorrhea?	Cramping, colicky pain immediately before or during menses
How common is it?	It is the most common cause of school absence for adolescent females.

List 7 associated symptoms.	Headache, irritability, emotional lability, nausea, vomiting, diarrhea, backache
What are 3 important factors in the evaluation?	History, physical and pelvic examinations
List 3 treatments.	Nonprescription analgesics, nonsteroidal anti-inflammatory drugs (NSAIDs), and oral contraceptives

SEXUALLY TRANSMITTED DISEASES (STDS)

(See Chapter 28)

How common is sexual activity among teenagers?	Varies widely with the population—some studies show 50% of teens engage in sexual activity by 16 years of age and 90% by 19 years of age
How common are sexually transmitted diseases (STDs)?	Present in 25% of sexually active teenagers
List 3 infestations that may be transmitted by close contact.	Pubic lice ("crabs"), body lice, and scabies
List 3 genital infections that are not sexually acquired.	*Monilia*, bacterial vaginosis, folliculitis

PREGNANCY AND CONTRACEPTION

How common is teenage pregnancy?	About 1 million/year in the United States; 50% result in spontaneous or elective abortion and 50% result in live birth
List 4 hazards teenagers face with pregnancy.	Dropping out of school, poor development of job skills, short- or long-term welfare dependency, parenting difficulties.
What are the hazards for children of teenage parents?	Increased incidence of low birth weight, prematurity, health or psychosocial problems related to poverty or poor parenting skills, attention deficit hyperactivity disorder (ADHD)

List 3 components of managing teenage pregnancy.	Teen-oriented obstetric care; promoting the involvement of family and community; long-term follow-up and support after birth of child
List 4 ways teenage pregnancy can be prevented.	1. Education 2. Building teens' skills to enhance self-esteem, self-efficacy, and decision making 3. Understanding abstinence and delayed sexual intercourse as appropriate courses 4. Knowledge and availability of birth control
List 9 methods of birth control.	Abstinence, condom (with spermicide), oral contraceptives (birth control pills), diaphragm (with spermicide), rhythm method, progesterone implant (Norplant), female condom, medroxy-progesterone acetate (Depo-Provera), spermicide (alone)

EPIDEMIOLOGY OF ACCIDENTAL AND NON-ACCIDENTAL DEATH

What are the 3 leading causes of death among adolescents?	Accidents (particularly motor vehicle accidents), homicide, suicide
What segment of the adolescent population is at greatest risk for death from homicide?	African-American males
Are suicide attempts (or gestures) more common in males or females?	Females
What adolescents are at greatest risk for death from suicide?	White males
Are suicide attempts considered to be "acting out"?	All attempts or suicide gestures should be taken seriously and patients should be assessed and hospitalized under observation if they are felt to be at risk. Suicide is frequently a sign of depression or other

mental illness and these underlying psychiatric issues should be explored and treated.

Is there a relationship between gun availability and successful suicides?

Yes. Guns are the most commonly used method of successful suicide. While the guns do not "cause" suicidal behavior, their use by a person with suicidal intent is associated with a high chance of death.

IV

Pediatric Diseases

15

Hematologic Disorders

NUTRITIONAL ANEMIAS

IRON DEFICIENCY ANEMIA

What is it?

Hemoglobin (Hgb) below 95% of the normal for age that is caused by lack of iron (Fe); it is the most common anemia

What are 2 causes?

Inadequate iron in diet or chronic blood loss (e.g., from peptic ulcer, inflammatory bowel disease, Meckel diverticulum, polyp or hemangioma)

What is the physiologic effect?

Decreased production of heme proteins involved in oxygen transport (Hgb), electron transport (cytochromes), and oxidative metabolism (NADH)

What are common signs and symptoms?

Pallor, fatigue, shortness of breath, pica (ingestion of nonfood substances, such as ice, paper, dirt, or clay) (Ch 19, p. 277), spoon-shaped nails (koilonychia), enlarged spleen. If not severe, iron deficiency anemia is usually suggested by routine lab screenings.

What are 4 findings of a complete blood count (CBC) in iron deficiency anemia?

Hypochromic, microcytic red blood cells (RBCs); decreased reticulocytes; decreased mean corpuscular volume (MCV); decreased mean corpuscular hemoglobin (MCH)

What are 4 effects on the indices of iron storage and transport?

Decreased iron, ferritin, and transferrin saturation; increased total iron-binding capacity.

Why are free erythrocyte protoporphyrins (FEP) increased?	Low iron concentration limits the production of Hgb. FEP are heme precursors that accumulate as a result.
List 3 investigations that may be helpful to detect occult blood loss.	Stool guaiac test; urinalysis; a careful menstrual history
How may iron deficiency anemia be diagnosed if other tests and investigations are equivocal?	By the child's response to a trial of iron administration

List 2 treatments.

1. Oral therapy with elemental Fe (3 mg/kg/day for 3–4 months); reticulocyte response should be seen in 1–2 weeks
2. Determine and correct the etiologic factors of Fe deficiency

What are potential side effects of oral Fe administration?	Nausea, abdominal pain, constipation, stained teeth.
What is the result if deficiency is not corrected?	Psychomotor and cognitive functions may become impaired.

FOLATE DEFICIENCY ANEMIA

What is it?	Decreased Hgb caused by folate deficiency. Folate deficiency causes a decrease in folate-dependent enzymes with decrease in 1-carbon transfer reactions
What are common causes?	Dietary deficiency is the most common. Others include: increased folate demands (hemolytic anemia, sickle cell disease, pregnancy), thalassemias, HIV, malabsorption, certain drugs (e.g., antiepileptics, trimethoprim-sulfa, alcohol), a disorder of metabolism.
What are common signs and symptoms?	Pallor, fatigue, shortness of breath; infants may fail to gain weight and suffer chronic diarrhea.

List 6 laboratory findings.

1. CBC: decreased Hgb and increased MCV

2. Hypersegmented neutrophils
3. Low reticulocyte count
4. Low serum folate
5. Elevated serum lactate dehydrogenase (LDH)
6. Nucleated RBCs with megaloblastic morphology

What is the treatment?	Oral supplementation with folate. Increased reticulocytes peak at 1 week and Hgb is normal in 6–8 weeks. Duration of therapy is based on the etiologic factors.

VITAMIN B$_{12}$ DEFICIENCY (PERNICIOUS ANEMIA)

What is it?	Decreased Hgb caused by vitamin B$_{12}$ deficiency
What is the physiologic effect?	Deficit of methylcobalamin (coenzyme B$_{12}$), which is a required cofactor in conversion of homocysteine to methionine (via methionine synthetase). Methionine is critical in formulation of tetrahydrofolates.
List 4 causes.	1. Dietary deficiency (e.g., seen in vegans) 2. Decreased absorption in gastrointestinal (GI) tract (e.g., in a child whose terminal ileum has been removed) 3. Defects in B$_{12}$ transport 4. Defects in B$_{12}$ metabolism
List 5 characteristic laboratory findings.	Increased MCV, multilobed neutrophils, decreased serum B$_{12}$, increased serum methylmalonic acid, increased serum homocysteine
What are common signs and symptoms?	Nausea, diarrhea, abdominal pain, glossitis
What are the neurological sequelae of prolonged B$_{12}$ deficiency?	Subacute degeneration of spinal cord, decreased vibratory and position sense, pyramidal signs, and peripheral neuropathy; cerebral symptoms and depression may be present.

What are findings on bone marrow aspiration?   Megaloblastic changes

What is the Schilling test?   The Schilling test uses vitamin B_{12} incorporated with ^{57}Cobalt (^{57}Co) to test for B_{12} absorption. The labeled B_{12} is given orally and is followed by a large IV dose of unlabeled B_{12}. If the labeled B_{12} is absorbed, it will be displaced by the unlabeled B_{12} and excreted in the urine. If this phase suggests that labeled B_{12} was not absorbed, another oral dose of labeled B_{12} is given simultaneously with intrinsic factor (IF). If labeled B_{12} is then later excreted, the insufficient or poorly functioning IF is the cause for B_{12} deficiency. If labeled B_{12} is still not excreted, a primary malabsorption condition exists.

What is the treatment?   For deficiency without malabsorption or an IF defect, oral vitamin B_{12} is sufficient. A malabsorption or IF defect usually requires vitamin B_{12} injections for life.

What are indicators of appropriate response to treatment?   Clinical improvement, increased reticulocytes, decreased MCV, and decreased methylmalonic acid.

List 2 complications.
1. Rapid correction of severely anemic patients can be associated with thrombosis, embolism, and hypokalemia.
2. Neurologic symptoms usually improve slowly and may not completely resolve.

HEMOGLOBINOPATHIES

THALASSEMIA

What is it?   The thalassemias are a group of inherited anemias caused by gene mutations that affect the synthesis of Hgb chains. Clinical syndromes vary in severity.

Who is most commonly affected?   α-Thalassemia is more common in people of Asian and African ancestry.
β-Thalassemia is more common in people of Mediterranean and African ancestry.

What is the pathophysiology?

Decreased or absent synthesis of α or β chains leads to increased amounts of rare Hgb compared with normal Hgb. Severe forms of thalassemia lead to hemolysis and ineffective RBC production in the bone marrow.

How many α-globin genes are normally present?

Normally, there are **4** α-globin genes (2 on each homologous chromosome 16). Therefore, there are different combinations of α-globin gene abnormalities.

List the 4 types of α-thalassemia and their characteristics.

Silent carrier. (1/4 genes affected): hematologically normal; electrophoresis normal

Thal trait. (2/4 genes affected): mild anemia, decreased MCV, presence of target cells, electrophoresis normal

Hgb H disease. (3/4 genes affected): moderate hemolytic anemia, decreased MCV, presence of target cells, splenomegaly, electrophoresis reveals Hgb A and H (β_4)

Hydrops fetalis. (4/4 genes affected): fetal death, electrophoresis reveals Hgb H and Barts (γ_4)

List the 4 types of β-thalassemia and their characteristics.

β-Thalassemia is more heterogeneous. Severity is based on the specific mutation in a gene rather than the number of genes affected.

Silent carrier: hematologically normal, electrophoresis normal

Thal trait: mild anemia, decreased MCV and MCH, presence of target cells, electrophoresis reveals increased Hgb A_2 and F

Thal intermedia: severe anemia without transfusion requirement, decreased MCV and MCH, presence of target cells, electrophoresis reveals increased Hgb A_2 and F.

Thal major: severe anemia with transfusion requirement, decreased MCV and MCH, presence of target cells, growth retardation, bone deformity, hepatosplenomegaly, electrophoresis reveals increased Hgb A_2 and F

List 3 common diagnostic studies for thalassemia.	CBC; Hgb electrophoresis; measurement of α and β chain biosynthesis
What are the treatments?	
Mild syndromes?	Folic acid supplementation, avoidance of oxidant drugs, transfusion if necessary
Severe syndromes?	Folic acid supplementation, transfusion protocol with chelation of Fe, splenectomy if hypersplenism develops, bone marrow transplantation
What are common complications?	Cholelithiasis (Ch 20, p. 280), increased susceptibility to infection, bone marrow hyperplasias with bone deformity, Cooley's facies, "hair-on-end" skull radiograph; liver, endocrine, and cardiac abnormalities associated with Fe overload

SICKLE CELL DISEASE

What is it?	Hemoglobinopathy in which α chains are normal, but β chains are abnormal because valine is substituted for glutamic acid at position 6
Who is most commonly affected?	People of Central African, Mediterranean, and Indian descent, but sickle cell disease can be seen in any population
What is the pathophysiologic effect?	Hgb S forms polymers within red cells, causing sickling of the cells when Hgb is deoxygenated. This sickling causes sludging and obstruction in vessels with subsequent tissue hypoxia.
List 5 common phenotypes associated with hemoglobin S and their characteristics.	**Sickle trait:** Hgb AS; not associated with increased morbidity and mortality rates **Sickle disease:** Hgb SS; clinically variable in severity from mild to debilitating **Sickle SC disease:** Hgb SC; mild chronic hemolytic anemia with variability in complications from vaso-occlusion; splenomegaly

Sickle β-thalassemia: two forms, β^+ (Hgb A is produced) and β° (Hgb A is not produced); sickle β°-thalassemia (i.e., no Hgb A produced) is clinically similar to Hgb SS; splenomegaly

Sickle α-thalassemia: variable clinical picture

What 3 diagnostic studies are used, and what do they show?

1. CBC: decreased Hgb, normal MCV if not thalassemic
2. Blood smear: sickled forms, target cells, Howell-Jolly bodies
3. Hgb electrophoresis:
   Sickle disease: 80%–100% Hgb S, 0%–20% Hgb F
   Sickle SC disease: 50% Hgb S, 50% Hgb C
   Sickle β-thalassemia: 75%–100% Hgb S, 0%–20% Hgb F, 3%–6% Hgb A_2
   Sickle α-thalassemia: 80%–100% Hgb S, 0%–20% Hgb F

List 5 clinical manifestations of sickling hemoglobinopathies.

1. Vaso-occlusion causing pain in bone, hand and foot ("hand–foot syndrome"), abdomen, or chest. Patient may also experience cerebral vascular accident (CVA) or priapism.
2. Splenic sequestration
3. Aplastic crisis
4. Infection caused by decreased opsonins and splenic function. Infection is **the most common cause of death in children with sickle cell disease.** Common organisms include pneumococci, *Haemophilus influenzae*, *Salmonella*, and *Mycoplasma*.
5. Acute chest syndrome

What is acute chest syndrome?

A serious complication of sickle cell disease. It is one of the most common causes of death in these patients.

List 3 causes.

Infection, pulmonary fat emboli, and pulmonary infarction. However, many episodes do not have an identifiable cause.

List 6 symptoms.

The symptoms may include cough, wheezing, fever, chest pain, extremity pain, and dyspnea.

What are the treatments?   Prophylaxis (vaccines against influenza virus, *H. influenzae, S. pneumoniae*)

For clinical cases: Hospitalization for antibiotics, bronchodilators, transfusions

Bronchoscopy should be considered if there is no clinical response to initial therapy.

What are the treatments for the following clinical manifestations?

For vaso-occlusive crisis?   Hydration and pain medications

For CVA?   Exchange transfusion with chronic transfusion protocol to keep Hgb S < 30%

For splenic sequestration?   Emergent transfusion with subsequent splenectomy

For aplastic crisis?   Supportive care; transfusion if necessary

For infection?   Appropriate antibiotics, penicillin prophylaxis, vaccines for *S. pneumoniae, H. influenzae, N. meningitidis*

What are common progressive complications?

Cardiovascular?   Cardiomegaly and cardiomyopathy secondary to serum iron overload and chronic anemia

Pulmonary?   Progressive disease with infarcts and infections

Hepatic?   Cholecystitis, hepatitis, glomerular and tubular fibrosis

Renal?   Hematuria, hyposthenuria

Ophthalmologic?   Retinopathy

Skeletal?   Codfish vertebrae, aseptic necrosis

HEMOLYTIC ANEMIAS

GLUCOSE–6–PHOSPHATE DEHYDROGENASE (G6PD) DEFICIENCY

What is G6PD?	G6PD is a dehydrogenase involved in the pentose phosphate pathway, which is important in NADPH production.
What causes its deficiency?	Mutation in the G6PD gene on the X chromosome. G6PD deficiency is an X-linked recessive disorder.
What is the physiologic effect of G6PD deficiency?	In the RBC that is deficient in G6PD, oxidative stress depletes NADPH and reduces glutathione (GSH) with subsequent oxidation of Hgb, causing cell membrane damage and hemolysis.
What are common signs and symptoms?	An asymptomatic child with G6PD deficiency usually has normal hematologic parameters, but when faced with oxidative stress, the child may have jaundice, hemoglobinuria, splenomegaly, and anemia.
What are some oxidative triggers?	Fava beans, infections, and certain drugs (e.g., sulfas, antimalarials, analgesics)
What diagnostic study is used?	Measurement of G6PD activity in RBCs of reticulocyte-poor blood
What is the treatment?	Usually supportive; with severe hemolysis, transfusion is occasionally necessary.

SPHEROCYTOSIS

What is it?	Autosomal dominant congenital hemolytic anemia with spherical RBCs
What is the pathophysiologic effect?	Loss of membrane surface area due to deficiencies in some RBC proteins (e.g., spectrin, ankyrin) leads to spherically shaped, less deformable cells, which become subject to lysis and trapping in the spleen.
List 5 signs and symptoms.	Symptoms (mild or severe) include

anemia, hemoglobinuria, jaundice, and splenomegaly. Hemolysis increases with infections.

List 3 diagnostic studies.	1. CBC: Hgb is decreased 2. Blood smear, which shows increased spheres and reticulocytes 3. Osmotic fragility test
What are 2 treatments?	1. **Supportive** usually, if the clinical course is mild. 2. **Splenectomy,** with or without cholecystectomy, if severe anemia, recurrent significant hemolysis, or cholecystitis exist. Splenectomy is usually delayed until after age 6 if possible.
List 3 common complications.	Aplastic crisis; cholecystitis; dependence on blood transfusions to maintain acceptable red blood cell levels

APLASTIC ANEMIA

What is it?	Pancytopenia secondary to decreased production of blood cells because of destruction of stem cells in bone marrow or because of abnormal bone marrow environment; may be inherited or acquired.
List the 2 classifications and their characteristics.	1. Severe: granulocyte count < 500, platelet count < 20,000, reticulocyte count < 1% after correction for Hgb; hypocellular bone marrow on biopsy 2. Mild or moderate: mild-to-moderate cytopenia; normal or increased bone marrow cellularity
What are some causes?	
Acquired? (List 5)	Drugs, radiation, viral infections, pre-leukemia, paroxysmal nocturnal hemoglobinuria
Inherited? (List 4)	Fanconi anemia (see p. 176), congenital dyskeratosis, Schwachman-Diamond syndrome, myelodysplasia

List 4 signs and symptoms.	Fatigue, pallor, and increased bleeding and infections
List 5 diagnostic studies.	1. CBC: shows pancytopenia and decreased reticulocytes 2. Bone marrow biopsy: shows hypocellularity The following studies may also be considered: 3. Viral titers 4. Screening for paroxysmal nocturnal hemoglobinuria 5. DNA breakage studies for Fanconi anemia
What are 4 methods of treatment?	1. Bone marrow transplantation—if a related matched donor is available, transplantation is the primary therapy. 2. Immunosuppressive therapy (e.g., antithymocyte globulin, cyclosporine, steroids) 3. Hematopoietic growth factors 4. Supportive care with antibiotics and transfusion therapy
What is the prognosis?	Prognosis is poor without bone marrow transplantation. **Pretransplantation transfusions should be avoided as much as possible.**

GAUCHER DISEASE

What is it?	Inherited storage disease with deficiency of the enzyme **glucocerebroside β-glucosidase**
How is it inherited?	As an autosomal recessive disorder
What is the physiologic effect?	Accumulation of glucocerebroside in reticuloendothelial (Gaucher) cells
List the 3 types and their characteristics.	1. Chronic non-neuronopathic (adult form): the clinical course is variable and may include anemia, thrombocytopenia with marrow infiltration, bleeding tendency, hepatosplenomegaly, and aseptic necrosis of bones 2. Acute neuronopathic (infantile form):

severe, with presentation in infancy; CNS infiltration with neural defects and hepatosplenomegaly; death usually occurs by 2 years of age.

3. Subacute neuronopathic (juvenile form): neurologic defects occur later in course of disease and may increase after splenectomy

In what ethnic group is the adult form commonly found?

Ashkenazi Jews

List 4 results that diagnostic studies show.

1. Bone marrow biopsy shows Gaucher cells
2. Decreased lysosomal β-glucocerebrosidase in leukocytes or cultured skin fibroblasts
3. Increased acid phosphatase
4. Increased angiotensin-converting enzyme

List 3 treatments for non-neuronopathic Gaucher disease.

1. Enzyme replacement therapy
2. Splenectomy if hypersplenism exists, but this may increase other symptoms (now only rarely performed).
3. Bone marrow transplantation

POLYCYTHEMIA

What is it?

RBC count, Hgb level, and total RBC volume all exceed the upper limits of normal. In postpubertal children, it is distinguished by Hgb > 16 g/dl and a total RBC mass > 35 ml/kg.

What is the appropriate term for high Hgb level with a concurrent decrease in plasma volume (e.g., as occurs in acute dehydration and burns)?

Hemoconcentration

What is polycythemia rubra vera?

This is a **primary myeloproliferative polycythemia**

List 3 diagnostic criteria of polycythemia rubra vera.

Increased total RBC volume, Hgb, and hematocrit; arterial oxygen saturation $\geq$ 92%; splenomegaly

List 5 laboratory findings.	Thrombocytosis, leukocytosis, increased leukocyte alkaline phosphatase, increased vitamin B_{12} or unsaturated B_{12}-binding capacity
List 2 treatments.	Phlebotomy and chemotherapy
List 2 long-term risks.	Myelofibrosis and acute leukemia
What is the prognosis?	Poor
What is secondary polycythemia?	Polycythemia due to other inciting causes

List 6 of these causes.

1. Hypoxia
2. Hemoglobinopathies
3. Neonatal conditions, such as twin-twin transfusion or maternal hemorrhage, being the infant of a diabetic mother, intrauterine growth retardation, neonatal thyroid toxicosis, adrenal hypoplasia, trisomy 21
4. Benign and malignant tumors that secrete erythropoietin
5. Excess presence of anabolic steroids caused by either adrenal disease or excessive administration of anabolic steroids
6. Familial

GRANULOCYTE DISORDERS

What is leukocyte adhesion deficiency?	It is a deficiency of a β_2 integrin. The condition is autosomal recessive and results in deficiency of leukocyte adhesion to offending agents.
List 3 clinical manifestations.	Leukocytosis, delayed separation of the umbilical cord, and bacterial infections
What is Chédiak-Higashi syndrome?	An autosomal recessive disorder affecting granule-bearing cells. Granulocytes and melanocytes are characteristically affected.
List 3 ways in which granulocytes are affected.	Defects in chemotaxis, degranulation, and bactericidal activity.

List 3 clinical manifestations.	Oculocutaneous albinism; large neutrophil granules; and recurrent bacterial infections
What is chronic granulomatous disease (CGD)?	A genetically heterogeneous condition that results in a defect in "respiratory burst" in leukocytes
What is the respiratory burst?	It is a reaction catalyzed by NADPH that forms hydrogen peroxide and hydroxyl radicals, which are thought to play a key role in killing microbes.
What is the clinical manifestation of CGD?	Recurrent bacterial and fungal infections
List 3 treatments.	There is no cure. Trimethoprim-sulfamethoxazole prophylaxis may limit infections. γ-Interferon or bone marrow transplantation may help some patients.
What is the definition of neutropenia?	Absolute neutrophil count (ANC) < 1000
What is cyclic neutropenia?	The neutrophil count cycles between a normal and low ANC.
What is autoimmune neutropenia?	A condition resulting from the presence of antineutrophil antibodies. Usually found in infants with no predisposing cause. May also be seen following transplacental transfer of maternal IgG (neonatal alloimmune neutropenia) or in neonates whose mothers have an autoimmune disease (neonatal maternal autoimmune neutropenia).
Can infection induce neutropenia?	Yes
List 4 types of infection that most commonly cause neutropenia.	Viral infections are the primary cause. Bacterial, mycobacterial, and rickettsial infections may also cause neutropenia.
What is Kostmann syndrome?	This is a rare autosomal recessive condition associated with neutropenia at birth.
What is the cause of this disease?	Unknown

What is the clinical mani-festation?	Severe, often fatal, infections
What is Schwachman-Diamond syndrome?	An autosomal recessive condition characterized by neutropenia and pancreatic insufficiency. Chemotaxis is also defective in these neutrophils.
List 5 clinical manifestations.	Pancreatic insufficiency, potential growth failure, dry skin, eczema, and ichthyosiform lesions
For which malignancy are these patients at risk?	Leukemia

List 5 treatment options for neutropenia conditions.

1. Judicious use of antibiotics to either treat or prevent serious infection.
2. Steroids may be used in autoimmune neutropenia.
3. Granulocyte colony-stimulating factor (G-CSF) may be used in some neutropenic conditions.
4. γ-Interferon may be useful in CGD.
5. Bone marrow transplantation may be used in Chédiak-Higashi syndrome, CGD, Wiskott-Aldrich syndrome, and leukocyte adhesion deficiency.

PLATELET DISORDERS

CONGENITAL PLATELET DISORDERS

What is Wiskott-Aldrich syndrome?	Thrombocytopenia, purpura, eczema, and an increased susceptibility to infection due to impaired humoral immune responses and chemotaxis of neutrophils. This syndrome is an X-linked recessive trait.
What causes the thrombocytopenia?	Uncertain—probably an intrinsic platelet abnormality or defective formation or release of platelets. However, the number of megakaryocytes is normal.
List 3 treatment options.	Splenectomy improves platelet count (post-splenectomy sepsis is a risk); administration of transfer factor; bone marrow transplantation

List 3 long-term risks of Wiskott-Aldrich syndrome.

Infections; bleeding; malignancy (about 12% of patients develop malignancies, including leukemic lymphoreticular malignancies)

What is TAR syndrome?

Thrombocytopenia associated with **A**plasia of the **R**adii. There may also be cardiac and renal anomalies. The thumbs are usually normal.

What is the clinical manifestation of thrombocytopenia?

Hemorrhage, which may be evident even in the first days of life (e.g., during circumcision)

List 3 laboratory findings.

Thrombocytopenia; normal Hgb; and possibly leukocytosis

List 2 findings of bone marrow aspirate.

Megakaryocyte count is normal; nuclear morphology may be abnormal.

What is Fanconi anemia?

A hypoplastic or aplastic anemia characterized by pancytopenia with associated skeletal, solid organ, and skin abnormalities.

What is the etiology?

Autosomal recessive inherited condition.

What are its clinical manifestations?

Usually pancytopenia beginning at 3–4 years of age, which can lead to bleeding and infection. Other manifestations include hyperpigmentation, skeletal abnormalities (including absent or hypoplastic thumbs), short stature, and other anomalies. Skeletal findings may be subtle in some patients.

List 4 major risks of Fanconi syndrome.

Hematologic malignancy, infections, bleeding, solid organ (especially liver) failure

What are the bone marrow findings?

Aplasia (similar to that seen in acquired aplastic anemia). The bone marrow may be normal if there is no pancytopenia.

What are the treatment options?

Steroids and androgens (relapse occurs in 50% of patients); G-CSF; bone marrow transplantation

What is the prognosis?

Poor. The median survival age is 16 years.

What is Kasabach-Merritt syndrome?

A condition of platelet trapping and consumptive coagulopathy associated with congenital hemangioma, usually of the liver.

What is the pathophysiology?

Trapping and destruction of platelets within the extensive vascular bed of the hemangioma

What are the peripheral blood smear findings?

Thrombocytopenia with RBC fragments

What are the bone marrow findings?

Normal megakaryocytes

What is the clinical manifestation?

Spontaneous hemorrhage

List 5 treatment options.

1. Administration of steroids
2. γ-Interferon
3. Occlusion of hepatic artery (liver hemangioma)
4. Resection or compression of hemangioma, although this might result in uncontrollable hemorrhage
5. Radiation to the hemangioma

What is hemolytic-uremic syndrome (HUS)?

A clinical syndrome of microangiopathic hemolytic anemia, thrombocytopenia, and acute renal failure (Ch 19, p. 260, for more on HUS).

What is thrombotic thrombocytopenic purpura (TTP)?

A condition characterized by thrombocytopenia and hemolytic anemia.

List 2 of the major clinical manifestations.

1. Hemorrhage
2. Neurologic sequelae—may include aphasia, blindness, and convulsions due to embolism and thrombosis of small blood vessels of the brain.

List 3 treatment options.

1. Plasmapheresis and plasma infusions (effective in 60%–70% of cases).
2. Steroids

3. Splenectomy if condition is refractory to the above therapies.

List 5 common drugs that may cause drug-induced thrombocytopenias in children.	Carbamazepine (Tegretol), phenytoin, sulfonamides, trimethoprim-sulfamethoxazole (Bactrim), chloramphenicol

IDIOPATHIC THROMBOCYTOPENIC PURPURA (ITP)

What is it?	Development of platelet antibodies with subsequent destruction of platelets
What is the peak age for ITP?	2–4 years
In whom is it most commonly seen?	Previously healthy children, often after viral illness. It can be associated with autoimmune disease and HIV.
List 4 characteristic laboratory and diagnostic findings.	1. Platelet count $< 50,000/mm^3$ 2. Sparse, large platelets on blood smear 3. Bone marrow aspirate shows an increased number of megakaryocytes, usually of immature forms 4. Anti-platelet immunoglobulins are present.
List 3 treatment options for severe ITP.	Steroids; IV immunoglobulin; possibly, splenectomy (if ITP is chronic). Platelet transfusions are usually not helpful, but may be used in conjunction with other therapy in episodes of serious bleeding or in surgery. If ITP is not severe (platelet count $> 20,000$), observation is prudent.
List 3 complications of ITP.	Severe GI hemorrhage; severe CNS hemorrhage; hematuria
What is the prognosis?	Majority of childhood ITP is benign and self-limited; 10%–15% of patients develop chronic ITP.

COAGULATION DEFECTS

HEMOPHILIA A AND B

What is hemophilia A, or classical hemophilia?	Factor VIII deficiency

What is hemophilia B, or Christmas disease?	Factor IX deficiency
What is the pathophysiology of these conditions?	Both are X-linked recessive disorders with decreased production of factor VIII or IX, respectively. There is a moderately high spontaneous mutation rate.
How is the severity of hemophilia A classified?	By the percentage of factor VIII present: Severe < 1%; moderate 1%–5%; mild > 5%
What is the physiologic result?	Inability to generate normal fibrin
What are common signs and symptoms?	1. Bleeding, including neonatal bleeding (especially with circumcision) or intracranial hemorrhage (ICH); oral, muscular, or joint bleeding 2. Easy bruising and bleeding with mild trauma
List 3 components of the diagnosis.	1. Family history 2. Prolonged partial thromboplastin time (PTT); bleeding time is usually normal, except in very severe cases 3. Decreased level of factor VIII (hemophilia A) or IX (hemophilia B)
What is the treatment?	Replacement therapy with the deficient factor: recombinant factor VIII is now available; factor IX is not recombinant; DDAVP may be useful in patients with mild hemophilia.
How much does 1 unit/kg of factor VIII raise the patient's plasma factor VIII?	1 unit/kg of factor VIII will give a 2% rise in plasma factor VIII.
1 unit/kg of factor IX?	1 unit/kg factor IX will give a 1% rise in plasma factor IX.
How much factor is appropriate for:	
Mild-to-moderate hemorrhage?	Achieve a factor level of **30%–40%.**

Major surgery or a life-threatening bleeding episode?	Achieve **100%** and maintain for **7–14 days.**
Oral bleeding?	Antifibrinolytics (e.g., aminocaproic acid) may also be used.

List 4 complications of these deficiencies.	1. Damage from repeated episodes of joint bleeding 2. Serious hemorrhage 3. Development of factor inhibitors (usually seen in factor VIII deficiency) 4. Infections (e.g., HIV, hepatitis) from factor replacement

VON WILLEBRAND DISEASE

What is it?	A disorder of von Willebrand factor (vWF) protein production; several variants are known, based on laboratory tests and platelet count. In the most severe form, there is an undetectable level of vWF and a decreased level of factor VIII. Most cases are caused by mutation of a single allele. Therefore, it can be inherited as an autosomal dominant trait. However, some patients are homozygous, so autosomal recessive inheritance is sometimes seen.
What is the physiologic result?	Inability of platelets to adhere to damaged endothelium
How common is von Willebrand disease?	It is **probably the most common inherited bleeding disorder.** The actual prevalence is difficult to determine because of its clinical variability.
List 3 signs and symptoms.	1. Easy bruising and bleeding with or without trauma 2. History of recurrent epistaxis 3. History of recurrent menorrhagia Clinical severity may vary. Some affected persons may be asymptomatic.
List 5 components of the diagnosis.	1. Bleeding time is prolonged. 2. PTT may be increased. 3. A decrease in von Willebrand antigen,

ristocetin cofactor, and factor VIII
levels
4. Platelet count may be decreased in
certain variants.
5. Normal-to-abnormal vWF multimers
Testing often has to be repeated to assure
diagnosis.

List 3 treatments.

1. DDAVP can be used to increase the
vWF in some types of the disease.
2. Cryoprecipitate or certain factor VIII
concentrates (e.g., Humate-P) can be
used in DDAVP failure, in a severe
bleeding episode, or in major surgery.
3. Patients with oral bleeding may also
benefit from antifibrinolytics (e.g., α-
aminocaproic acid).

DISSEMINATED INTRAVASCULAR COAGULATION (DIC)

What is it?

Consumptive coagulopathy that activates
the plasma coagulation system and
depletes clotting and antithrombotic
factors as well as platelets

**What is the physiologic
effect?**

Cycle of intravascular thrombosis and
fibrinolysis, particularly in small vessels

**What are some common
etiologic factors?**

Sepsis, malignancy (especially promyelo-
cytic leukemia), obstetric complications,
extensive tissue damage from trauma,
burns, hypoxia, snakebites

List 3 signs and symptoms.

Bleeding or clotting; embolic signs;
oozing from vascular access or phlebot-
omy sites

**What are the diagnostic
findings?**

Decreased platelet levels, prolonged
prothrombin time (PT) and PTT,
decreased fibrinogen, increased fibrin
split products

**What are 2 approaches to
treatment?**

1. Successful treatment is possible only
with correction of underlying etiologic
factors.
2. Symptomatic treatment includes
transfusion with platelets, fresh frozen
plasma (FFP), and cryoprecipitate.

Heparin may be used at times if thrombosis is a prevalent symptom.

What are significant complications?

Severe bleeding or thrombosis in the GI, pulmonary, and CNS systems

NEONATAL ALLOIMMUNE THROMBOCYTOPENIA

What is it?

Severe thrombocytopenia in infants secondary to having different platelet antigens from the mother, with subsequent platelet destruction by maternal antiplatelet antibodies—similar to Rh sensitization in blood groups

Is there a high risk of bleeding?

Yes. It may occur prenatally.

How is it diagnosed?

Platelet typing of mother and father

List 3 treatments.

1. Transfusion with irradiated maternal platelets
2. Steroids prenatally or postnatally
3. Possible IV immunoglobulin

What are "hypercoagulable states"?

Conditions that predispose to blood clotting.

Give 7 examples.

Examples include disseminated intravascular coagulation (DIC) (see p. 181), protein C deficiency, protein S deficiency, factor V Leiden, anti-thrombin 3 deficiency, homocystinuria (due to cystathionine synthase deficiency), and homocystinemia (due to methylene tetrahydrofolate reductase deficiency)

How are these diagnosed?

DIC should be excluded (by platelet count, D-dimer assay, peripheral smear, and a search for associated conditions). There is no simple screening test for the genetic causes of hypercoagulability. These require specific tests.

16

Pediatric Cardiology

INTRODUCTION TO PEDIATRIC CARDIOLOGY

GENERAL CONSIDERATIONS

What percent of pediatric cardiology patients have congenital heart disease (CHD)?	90%; 10% have acquired heart disease [(e.g., myocarditis (p. 201), cardiomyopathy (p. 202), hypertension)]
What is the incidence of CHD in the general population?	Almost 1% of live births are infants with CHD.
What are 2 of the most common types of heart conditions that cause clinical problems in newborns?	Cyanotic or severe obstructive lesions
What sign alerts pediatricians to potential heart defects in infants and school-age children?	Murmurs, of which a vast majority are "innocent" or functional; atrial septal defect (ASD) and ventricular septal defect (VSD) are the most common causes of organic murmurs.
In preadolescents and adolescents?	Chest pain (usually noncardiac in origin), palpitations, and hypertension
What is congestive heart failure (CHF)?	A clinical syndrome in which the heart is unable to pump adequately to support the circulation. CHF is not a common finding in children.

CYANOTIC CONGENITAL HEART DEFECTS

PERSISTENT TRUNCUS ARTERIOSUS

What is it?	A single vessel arises from the heart that

branches to form the aorta and pulmonary arteries (PAs) (1% of CHDs)

Define the four types.

1. **Type I:** a common PA arises from the truncus and divides into left and right PAs
2. **Type II:** separate right and left PAs arise from the posterior aspect of the truncus
3. **Type III:** separate right and left PAs arise from the lateral aspects of the truncus
4. **Type IV:** pulmonary blood flow originates from aortopulmonary collateral arteries (a severe form of tetralogy of Fallot (TOF)

What are 2 associated defects?

VSD; semilunar valve abnormalities

In what syndrome is truncus arteriosus seen?

DiGeorge syndrome

List 2 ways patients with truncus arteriosus present.

Most common presentation is CHF caused by either excessive pulmonary blood flow or truncal valve insufficiency. Less common presentation is cyanosis due to stenosis at the origin of the PA.

List 4 signs or symptoms.

Tachypnea, tachycardia, holosystolic murmur with loud S2; diastolic murmur may also be present

List 3 radiographic findings.

Cardiomegaly; increased pulmonary vascular markings; right aortic arch (in one-third of patients)

What 3 other diagnostic studies are used?

ECG (shows biventricular hypertrophy), echocardiography, cardiac catheterization before surgical repair

What is the treatment?

Medical: management of CHF with diuretics and afterload reduction
Surgical: Establishing continuity from the right ventricle (RV) to the PA with conduit, VSD closure

What are 2 complications of surgical repair?

Conduit failure; truncal valve insufficiency

What are the outcomes?	**Surgically untreated** patients die at < 1 year old from development of pulmonary vascular obstructive disease. **Surgical therapy** now achieves early survival rates of 80%–90%; long-term survival is also improving.

TRANSPOSITION OF THE GREAT ARTERIES

What is it?	The aorta arises from the RV and the PA arises from the left ventricle (LV). It represents 10% of CHDs (second most to VSD).
List 5 potential associated defects.	VSD; pulmonary stenosis; ASD; patent ductus arteriosus (PDA); coarctation of the aorta
In which gender is it more common?	Males by 4:1 ratio.
What is the physiologic result?	Cyanosis; oxygenated blood remains in pulmonary circulation and deoxygenated blood in the systemic circulation (**parallel** rather than normal **series** circuit). Blood mixes through a PDA, patent foramen ovale, or a VSD if present.
List 4 signs or symptoms.	Cyanosis in the newborn period; CHF (with a large VSD); there may be minimal cyanosis; murmur unless VSD is absent
What are typical radio-graphic findings?	Heart classically described as an "egg on its side" with normal heart size and narrow mediastinum. Increased pulmonary vascular markings are present.
List 3 other diagnostic studies that are used.	ECG (usually normal at birth); echocardiography; cardiac catheterization: balloon atrial septostomy (Rashkind procedure) can be done if needed for better mixing of oxygenated and deoxygenated blood (temporizing measure).
What is the treatment?	**Medical:** prostaglandin infusion to maintain patency of ductus arteriosus until septostomy or surgery

Surgical:
Pre-1980: Mustard or Senning procedure (atrial baffle), either of which may still be used in infants with severe pulmonary stenosis
Post-1980: Jatene procedure (arterial switch)

When should surgical repair be performed?

Infants with simple transposition should be repaired within 2 weeks of birth to avoid weakness of the LV muscle. Large VSD, severe pulmonary stenosis, or coronary artery anomalies may preclude an early switch.

List 5 complications of atrial baffle repair.

Atrial dysrhythmias (common); obstruction of the superior vena cava (SVC); baffle leak; tricuspid valve insufficiency; RV failure

Of arterial switch? (List 2)

Early myocardial ischemia may be caused by the manipulation necessary to re-implant the coronary arteries. Postoperative supravalvular pulmonary stenosis may be present (20% of patients).

What is the outcome of atrial baffle?

Early survival rate is about 85%. However, long-term sequelae are significant and include atrial arrhythmias, sick sinus syndrome, RV failure, and sudden death.

Of arterial switch?

Good: 90%–95% survival rate at 1 year postoperative

TRICUSPID ATRESIA

What is it?

Agenesis of the tricuspid valve (1% of all CHDs)

List 5 common associated defects.

ASD; small RV; malposition of great arteries; VSD; pulmonary stenosis

What is the physiologic result?

Cyanosis (mild to severe, depending on the size of the VSD and degree of pulmonary stenosis); all patients have right-to-left shunt at atrial level. If transposition of the great arteries is present, CHF develops early due to pulmonary overload.

List 3 signs or symptoms.

Cyanosis in the newborn period; possible excessive pulmonary blood flow and CHF (especially with associated transposition of the great arteries); murmur from VSD (holosystolic) or from pulmonary stenosis systolic ejection murmur (SEM)

List 2 radiographic findings.

Mild cardiomegaly; pulmonary segment is usually small in those infants with cyanosis

List 3 diagnostic studies.

ECG: shows tall, notched P waves consistent with right atrial enlargement, left axis deviation, and left ventricular hypertrophy (LVH); echocardiography; cardiac catheterization: enlargement of atrial communication can be accomplished if needed by balloon atrial septostomy.

What is the treatment?

Surgical treatment
1. Palliative SVC-to-PA (Glenn) shunt in late infancy
2. Blalock-Taussig shunt may be necessary in early infancy if cyanosis is severe (see Tetralogy of Fallot below).
3. A modified Fontan procedure in childhood (in which all systemic venous return is directed to the PA); this is also known as the caval–pulmonary isolation procedure.

List 4 complications of surgical repair.

Shunts may form clots or develop stenosis; pleural and pericardial effusions; supraventricular arrhythmias; left ventricular dysfunction as a late outcome

What is the outcome?

After the Fontan procedure: cyanosis is resolved; exercise capacity is less than that of the average person. The 10-year survival rate is about 65%

TETRALOGY OF FALLOT (TOF)

What are the components?

VSD; pulmonary stenosis; aortic override; right ventricular hypertrophy (RVH)

TOF represents what percent of all CHDs?

5%

What is the physiologic result?

VSD allows interventricular shunting, usually right-to-left. Degree of right-to-left shunting depends on degree of pulmonary outflow obstruction. Exercise produces or worsens shunting (cyanosis).

List 3 signs or symptoms.

Cyanosis: worsens with activity or may be spontaneous (i.e., "tet spell")

Child assumes squatting position to increase oxygenation and relieve cyanosis. It is believed that squatting increases systemic pressure and therefore relieves excessive right-to-left shunt.

Normal S_1, soft S_2, SEM

List 4 ways a cyanotic spell may be managed.

1. Calming measures, sedation, and IV fluid
2. Oxygen and either morphine or propranolol (or both)
3. Knee-chest positioning
4. If no reversal of spell occurs, then **emergency surgery**

Name an important radiographic finding.

Boot-shaped heart ("coeur en sabot")

What 2 conditions cause coeur en sabot?

RVH and absence of prominent PAs

List 3 other diagnostic studies.

ECG: shows right-axis deviation and evidence for RVH

Echocardiography: Doppler is helpful to assess flow to the PAs.

Cardiac catheterization: look for degree of stenosis of pulmonary outflow, multiple septal defects, and coronary artery abnormalities.

What is the treatment?

Primarily surgical:

Systemic-to-pulmonary shunt will temporize until child is 3–6 months old. Blalock-Taussig shunt employs end-to-side subclavian-to-PA shunt; an H graft may also be used between these two vessels (modified shunt).

Definitive repair of defect involves closing the VSD and widening pulmonary outflow tract. Sometimes this may be the primary procedure.

List 3 complications of definitive surgical repair.	Residual VSD; residual RV outflow obstruction; arrhythmias, particularly ventricular ectopy
What is the outcome?	90% of patients with definitive repair survive well into adulthood (slightly fewer than the average population). Working capacity, maximum heart rate, and cardiac output are generally less than those of the average person.

DOUBLE-OUTLET RIGHT VENTRICLE

What is it?	Both the aorta and the PA arise from the RV; this condition may be seen as part of a continuum with TOF. (Is 1% of all CHDs)
What are some associated defects?	VSD (the "outlet" for LV blood) and various malpositions of the PA and aorta
What is the physiologic result?	It ranges from VSD physiology (left-to-right shunt with increased flow to lungs) to TOF physiology (right-to-left shunt with decreased flow to lungs), depending on the size of the VSD, the position of the PA and aorta, and the amount of pulmonary stenosis.
List 2 possible signs or symptoms.	Cyanosis is present if pulmonary blood flow is decreased; CHF is present if pulmonary blood flow is increased.
What are the radiographic findings?	Similar to those in TOF. There may be fullness of the PAs with pulmonary edema if there is no pulmonary stenosis.
List 3 diagnostic studies that are used.	ECG: right axis deviation and evidence for RVH are the most common findings
	Echocardiography: distinguishes the type of VSD and its relationship to the PA and aorta
	Cardiac catheterization before surgical repair

What is the treatment?

The goal is to establish LV-to-aorta continuity and RV-to-PA continuity if possible.

Inadequate pulmonary blood flow: systemic-to-pulmonary shunt is placed in infancy, followed by VSD closure and reconstruction of right ventricular outflow tract in childhood

Excessive pulmonary blood flow: PA band (Damman-Muller procedure) in infancy, and VSD repair later in childhood

List 2 major complications of surgical repair.

Residual VSD; outflow obstruction

What is the outcome?

Good results in those with VSD physiology and simple repair

EISENMENGER SYNDROME

What is it?

The result of a CHD that allows right-to-left shunt in response to marked elevation of the pulmonary vascular resistance. This term is commonly used to describe such a shunt in VSD with pulmonary hypertension. The term is also sometimes used to describe idiopathic primary pulmonary hypertension in which the pulmonary pressure is markedly elevated in the absence of any structural cardiac lesion.

What is the physiologic result?

High pulmonary vascular resistance elevates PA pressure, and deoxygenated blood enters the systemic circulation through any existing communications.

List 3 signs or symptoms.

Cyanosis; poor exercise tolerance; risk of sudden death

List 2 radiographic findings.

Decreased pulmonary vascular markings; heart size usually normal

List 3 other diagnostic studies.

ECG: shows RVH, as well as characteristics of the particular CHD causing the syndrome

Echocardiography: ratio of right-sided pre-injection period:ejection time is increased due to elevated pulmonary vascular resistance and early closure of pulmonic valve

Cardiac catheterization: for diagnosis and to determine if the defect is operable. It will typically show a bidirectional shunt at the VSD, with equal systolic pressures in systemic and pulmonary circulations, and elevated pulmonary vascular resistance.

What is the treatment?

Medical: calcium channel blockers or prostacyclins (benefits are short term) and anticoagulation

Surgical: heart-lung transplantation offers improvement in symptoms, but long-term positive outcome is limited at present.

What is the outcome?

Prognosis is poor.

HYPOPLASTIC LEFT HEART SYNDROME

What is it?

Underdevelopment of the left heart (i.e., the mitral valve, LV, aortic valve, and ascending aorta). It represents 3%–4% of CHDs.

What is the physiologic result?

Almost uniformly fatal within first weeks of life—systemic circulation depends on right-to-left flow at ductus arteriosus.

What are 3 signs or symptoms?

Cyanosis, sometimes within hours of birth; circulatory collapse with poor perfusion; soft systolic murmur

What are the radiographic findings?

Cardiomegaly—usually mild at first and then rapidly becoming more marked, with an increase in pulmonary vascularity

What are 2 diagnostic studies?

ECG (RVH is commonly seen); echocardiogram (for diagnosis)

What is the medical treatment?

Prostaglandin infusion until surgery

What are the surgical alternatives?

1. **Norwood procedure,** which is a three-stage procedure:

Stage I: atrial septostomy, ligation of the distal main PA with connection of the proximal PA to the aorta; synthetic shunt from the aorta to the distal main PA

Stage II: connection of SVC to PAs (Glenn shunt)

Stage III: connection of the inferior vena cava to the PAs (Fontan procedure)

2. **Orthotopic heart transplant**

What are the complications of the surgical treatment?

Cyanosis, CHF, reduced exercise tolerance; complications of transplantation include infection, rejection, coronary artery disease, and malignancy

What are the outcomes?

Uniformly fatal if surgically untreated; reduced life expectancy with either surgical approach

TOTAL ANOMALOUS PULMONARY VENOUS RETURN

What is it?

The pulmonary veins do not connect to the left atrium (LA) (1% of all CHDs)

In which gender is it more common?

Males

List 3 areas into which the anomalous pulmonary veins may drain.

Supracardiac—connect to vertical vein or SVC

Cardiac—connect to coronary sinus

Subcardiac—connect to inferior vena cava below the diaphragm; obstruction of pulmonary venous return is most common in this group

What is the physiologic result?

Unobstructed flow: comparable to ASD with left-to-right shunt (enlarged right atrium [RA] and RV)

Obstructed flow: decreased filling of the LA and LV, cyanosis, and decreased cardiac output. Severe pulmonary congestion.

What are the signs or symptoms?

Unobstructed flow: tachypnea and murmur.

Obstructed flow: cyanosis and circulatory collapse.

What are characteristic radiographic findings?	Cardiomegaly with increased vascular markings; classic "snowman" shape to heart secondary to prominent vertical vein, large SVC and enlarged RA.
List 3 other diagnostic studies that are used.	ECG (RVH is commonly seen); echocardiography; cardiac catheterization (for definitive confirmation of drainage pattern)
What is the treatment?	Surgical. Connect pulmonary venous confluence to the LA and close the patent foramen ovale or ASD, to separate the pulmonary venous system from the systemic venous system
List 2 complications of repair.	Continued obstruction of pulmonary venous return to the LA; persistent pulmonary hypertension
What is the outcome?	Infants with severe pulmonary venous obstruction have the worst outcome and face a 30%–35% early and late mortality rate following surgery. If there is no obstruction, surgical results are excellent.

PULMONARY ATRESIA WITH INTACT VENTRICULAR SEPTUM

What is it?	Underdeveloped RV and a small to nearly imperforate pulmonary valve (1% of all CHDs).
What are the physiologic results?	Severe cyanosis as newborn; all affected infants have right-to-left shunt at atrial level; pulmonary blood flow is supplied by the PDA.
List 2 signs or symptoms.	Cyanosis; circulatory collapse if the PDA closes
What are the radiographic findings?	Normal-size heart with decreased pulmonary lung markings (dark lung fields) if the PDA is small or closed
List 3 other diagnostic studies.	ECG (may show LVH); echocardiography; cardiac catheterization (to plan management and document any coronary abnormalities)

What is the treatment?	**Medical:** prostaglandin infusion until surgery **Surgical:** 1. Palliative shunt 2. Right ventricular outflow patch 3. Transplant 4. RV-PA homograft 5. Fontan procedure (beyond infancy)
List 3 complications of repair.	Palliative shunts may clot or develop stenosis; the RV may fail to grow.
What are the outcomes?	Moderate mortality rate for all procedures; long-term survival rates are improving.

ACYANOTIC CONGENITAL HEART DEFECTS

ATRIAL SEPTAL DEFECT

What is it?	Hole in the septum between the right and left atria (5%–10% of all CHDs)
List the 3 types.	Secundum ASD (most common); primum ASD (associated with other endocardial cushion defects); sinus venosus ASD (rare)
Is ASD more common in males or females?	Females, by 2–3:1 ratio
What is the physiologic result?	Left-to-right shunt with overload of the RA, RV, and PA
List 2 factors that determine the volume of the shunt.	The size of the hole; the compliance of the RV
What are the signs or symptoms?	Usually asymptomatic in children; it may cause right-heart congestion in the third to fifth decades of life in untreated patients.
List 3 physical signs or symptoms.	Nonspecific SEM from increased pulmonary flow; widely (or fixed) split of S2
List 2 radiographic findings.	Cardiomegaly due to enlargement of the RA and the RV; prominent PA segment

List 3 other diagnostic studies.	ECG (may show RVH); echocardiography; cardiac catheterization (indicated if primum or sinus venosus defect is present)
What is the treatment?	Surgical closure
What is the main complication of surgical repair?	10% of patients may have atrial dysrhythmia
What is the outcome?	Very good if repaired before adolescence.

VENTRICULAR SEPTAL DEFECT

What is it?	CHD consisting of a hole in the septum between the RV and LV (20% of all CHDs—is most common)
List the 4 types.	1. Type I-supracristal (subpulmonary) 2. Type II-perimembranous 3. Type III-inlet (atrioventricular-canal type) (See Atrioventricular Canal Defect, p. 207) 4. Type IV-muscular
What is the physiologic result?	Left-to-right shunt which increases blood volume to lungs.
List the 2 factors that determine the volume of the shunt.	Size of the hole and resistance in the lung vasculature
What are the signs or symptoms of a small VSD?	No signs or symptoms, with loud holosystolic murmur
List typical signs or symptoms of moderate-to-large VSD?	Signs or symptoms of pulmonary congestion (e.g., tachypnea, poor feeding), with holosystolic murmur and diastolic rumble
What are the radiographic findings of a small VSD.	Normal
Of a moderate-to-large VSD?	Cardiomegaly with increase in vascular markings
List 3 other diagnostic studies.	ECG (may show LVH); echocardiography; cardiac catheterization to plan for surgery

What is the treatment for a small VSD?

Possibly none needed—at least 50% of VSDs close spontaneously.

For a moderate VSD?

May require diuretics until surgical repair; child will usually be allowed to grow as much as possible, with repair sometimes delayed until the early toddler years.

For a large VSD?

Requires patch closure, which is usually done when child is 3–12 months old

List 2 common complications of surgical repair.

Residual VSD; aortic insufficiency (AI)

What is the outcome?

Good survival rate, with few sequelae

PATENT DUCTUS ARTERIOSUS

What is it?

Persistent patency of the ductus arteriosus (5–10% of all CHDs)

What group of infants is at risk for PDA?

Premature infants—as many as 75% of infants of 28–30 weeks gestation have a PDA

Is it more common in males or females?

Females, by a 3:1 ratio

What is the physiologic result?

Left-to-right shunt from the aorta into the PA. With a large PDA, enlargement of the LA and the LV may occur leading to CHF. Rare association with pulmonary hypertension (Eisenmenger syndrome) (see Eisenmenger Syndrome, p. 190).

What are the signs or symptoms?

Usually asymptomatic in older children. Small infants may have signs or symptoms of pulmonary congestion. Continuous murmur may be present in the second intercostal space, with bounding pulses.

What are the radiographic findings?

Radiography may show cardiomegaly due to enlargement of the LA and LV.

List 3 other diagnostic studies that are used.

ECG (may show LVH); echocardiogram (with color-flow Doppler to demonstrate defect); catheterization (needed only if an associated defect is suspected or if pulmonary hypertension is present)

What is the treatment? Few PDAs close spontaneously after infancy. They usually require ligation and division or interventional catheterization for closure. A symptomatic PDA in a premature baby is usually successfully closed with intravenous indomethacin treatment.

What is a complication of repair? Residual shunt

What is the outcome? Excellent prognosis

PULMONARY STENOSIS

What is it? Congenital obstruction of the right ventricular outflow tract; valve or subvalve (infundibulum) obstructions are the most common. (is 5% of all CHDs)

What is the physiologic result? High right-ventricular pressure; if severe, it can produce cyanosis by right-to-left shunt at atrial level (patent foramen ovale or ASD).

What are typical signs or symptoms.
1. Mild-to-moderate stenosis: potentially no signs or symptoms
2. Severe stenosis: cyanosis, reduced exercise capacity
3. SEM: more likely with increasing severity

What are the radiographic findings? Most are normal, but some may show a prominent main PA segment.

List 3 other diagnostic studies. ECG (may be normal or may show RVH); echocardiography (Doppler assesses the severity of obstruction); cardiac catheterization (indicated if obstruction is severe; balloon valvuloplasty for therapy if severe)

What is the treatment? **Mild-to-moderate stenosis:** no treatment is indicated
Severe valve stenosis: valvuloplasty by catheterization or by open operation

Severe infundibular stenosis (characteristic of double-chambered RV): operative removal of obstructing muscle bundles

What are the complications of repair?	Complications are uncommon; possible pulmonary insufficiency.
What is the outcome?	Mild-to-moderate stenosis: normal cardiac function. Severe stenosis: good results from surgery and catheterization

COARCTATION OF THE AORTA

What is it?	A narrowed area of the aortic arch at the level of the ductus arteriosus or the ligamentum arteriosum. (8% of all CHDs)
Is it more common in males or females?	Males, by a 2–5:1 ratio
List 4 physiologic results.	Obstruction to systemic cardiac output; upper-body hypertension; LVH; collateral vessels develop to distribute blood to lower body
What are the signs and symptoms?	Mild obstruction: no signs or symptoms Moderate-to-severe obstruction: CHF
List 2 findings on examination of pulses.	Pulses diminished in the lower extremities; time delay (lag) between brachial and femoral pulse waves.
What are the radiographic findings?	1. A **reverse "3"** sign of dilated ascending aorta, coarctation segment, and descending aorta (a classic sign). 2. **Rib notching** from dilated intercostal vessels (rare in patients less than 10 years old)
List 5 other diagnostic studies.	Physical examination (feel pulses and take blood pressure readings in all extremities); ECG (may be normal; infants may have RVH; and older children may have LVH); echocardiography (may be diagnostic); catheterization (a prime standard for diagnosis); cardiac MRI

What is the medical treatment?	**Management** of CHF until surgery
List 4 options for surgical treatment.	Subclavian flap angioplasty; resection of coarctation segment with end-to-end anastomosis; resection of coarctation segment with graft placement; interventional catheterization with balloon dilatation
What are the complications of repair?	**Early:** Residual gradient (particularly if native arch is small); paradoxical hypertension in 25% of patients; post-coarctectomy syndrome: abdominal pain and bleeding **Late:** Recoarctation from scarring; residual gradient (particularly if native arch is small)
List 3 commonly associated cardiac anomalies.	Bicuspid aortic valve (50%); VSD; mitral valve disease (less often associated).
What is the outcome?	Generally good, but follow-up is necessary to monitor for recurrence of stenosis, hypertension, endocarditis, and aneurysm formation.

BACTERIAL ENDOCARDITIS

What is it?	An inflammatory process caused by a bacterial infection of a valve, the endocardium, or a blood vessel; process can be **subacute** or **fulminant,** depending on the bacterial agent.
List the 2 most common etiologic agents.	*Streptococcus viridans* and *Staphylococcus aureus,* accounting for about 80% of cases
What is the physiologic result?	Possible valvular dysfunction with subsequent CHF.
What are potential signs and symptoms?	Fever; peripheral embolization; nonspecific signs or symptoms (e.g., myalgia, arthralgia, malaise); new or changing heart murmur

List 3 other diagnostic studies.	Blood cultures (repeated blood cultures may be necessary) Measurement of acute phase reactants (elevations are suggestive, not diagnostic) Echocardiogram: diagnostic when large intracardiac vegetation is present
List 2 modes of treatment.	**Antibiotic treatment** against the identified pathogen (intravenous, generally continuing for at least 4 weeks) **Surgical valve replacement** for intractable heart failure
How can bacterial endocarditis be prevented?	**Antibiotic prophylaxis** is recommended for any surgical or dental procedures in children with any CHD or other conditions that put them at risk for endocarditis.
What are the outcomes?	Streptococcal endocarditis generally has a good outcome. Staphylococcal and fungal endocarditis have high morbidity and mortality rates.

ACUTE RHEUMATIC FEVER

What is it?	Rare inflammatory complication following infection with Group A *beta-hemolytic streptococcus* (usually pharyngitis); multiple organ systems may be affected by the inflammatory vasculitis. Acute rheumatic fever is the most common cause of acquired heart disease in children.
What is the physiologic result?	Inflammation may cause carditis (acutely) and valvular dysfunction (chronically).
What are the 2 most common results of acute rheumatic fever carditis?	Mitral and aortic valve insufficiency
List the Jones criteria.	**Major:** 1. Polyarthritis 2. Carditis 3. Chorea 4. Erythema marginatum

5. Subcutaneous nodules
Minor:
1. Arthralgia
2. Fever
3. Laboratory evidence of inflammation (such as elevated erythrocyte sedimentation rate [ESR] or C-reactive protein [CRP])
4. Prolonged P-R interval

Using Jones criteria, what is required for diagnosis?

Presence of two major Jones criteria, or one major and two minor Jones criteria with evidence of previous streptococcal infection

List some diagnostic studies.

Throat culture; antistreptolysin O titer; Anti DNase B titer; ESR; C-reactive protein; ECG; echocardiogram (to evaluate evidence of carditis, aortic valve insufficiency, mitral regurgitation)

List 3 components of initial treatment.

Treatment for streptococcal pharyngitis (primary prevention)
Treatment for inflammation with high dosage of aspirin for 4–8 weeks or steroids for 2–3 weeks
Treatment for CHF, if present

List 2 requirements of long-term treatment.

After initial treatment, patients should remain on chronic (i.e., lifelong) penicillin prophylaxis to prevent future acute rheumatic fever (secondary prevention). Patients should also receive prophylaxis for subacute bacterial endocarditis when appropriate.

What are the outcomes?

Generally very good; rarely, severe carditis may cause severe valvular dysfunction that requires valve replacement.

MYOCARDITIS

What is it?

An infection of the heart muscle

What are the most common causes?

Eighty percent of cases are **viral;** most commonly, coxsackievirus, influenza virus, and ECHO.

Bacterial agents are the second most common cause.

What is the physiologic result?

Inflammation of cardiac muscle with cellular infiltrate

List 4 signs or symptoms.

Fever, tachycardia, dysrhythmia, heart failure

List 4 diagnostic studies that are used.

ECG, echocardiography, viral or bacterial cultures, myocardial biopsy may be considered

List 2 treatments.

Supportive care and treatment of bacterial cause, if it is identified (steroid use is controversial)

What are the outcomes?

Generally good, with improvement of CHF; however, myocarditis may proceed to dilated cardiomyopathy (p. 203)

CARDIOMYOPATHY

Hypertrophic Cardiomyopathy

What is it?

Cardiac disease characterized by a markedly thickened LV

What are some etiologic factors?

Altered cardiac myosin or other ultrastructural proteins. Certain gene defects are associated with severe disease and sudden death. Some storage diseases can present with hypertrophic cardio-myopathy.

What is the physiologic result?

Impaired filling of the left ventricle as a result of a thick (stiff) left ventricle; there may also be significant left ventricular outflow obstruction.

List 4 signs or symptoms.

1. Sudden death—may be first indication of disease
2. SEM if there is significant outflow obstruction
3. Dysrhythmia
4. Decreased capacity for exercise

List 2 diagnostic studies.

ECG: may reflect LVH and T-wave abnormalities; echocardiogram

What is the medical treatment?	Some patients improve with beta-blockers or calcium channel blockers. However, agents that reduce ventricular preload or afterload or stimulate cardiac contraction may worsen the outflow obstruction. Therefore, diuretics, vaso-dilators, and digoxin are usually contra-indicated.
What is the surgical treatment?	Some centers advocate: Myotomy or myectomy for severe outflow obstruction Mitral valve replacement Placement of a pacemaker, defibrillator, or both
What is the outcome?	Variable—most cases are diagnosed when the patients are adults and remain stable; then the rate of sudden death is low. The prognosis is worse for cases diagnosed during childhood or that occur in a family with high rate of sudden death.

Dilated Cardiomyopathy

What is it?	Dilated, poorly contractile LV
What causes dilated cardiomyopathy?	There are many possible causes. Most are likely secondary to myocarditis, but metabolic disorders have been identified in some patients. Mitochondrial abnor-malities may also be a cause.
What is the physiologic result?	CHF
List 3 signs or symptoms.	Pulmonary congestion; hepatomegaly; murmur—absent, or soft S3 murmur may be present
List 2 radiographic findings.	Cardiomegaly; increased pulmonary vascular markings
List 2 other diagnostic studies.	ECG (nonspecific findings, usually LVH); echocardiogram (dilated chamber with decreased function)
List 6 medical treatments.	Digitalis, diuretics, afterload reduction, beta-blocker, aspirin, warfarin

What is the surgical treatment?	Orthotopic transplantation
What is the outcome?	Poor if condition is diagnosed when child is > 2 years old.

ARRHYTHMIAS

What is an arrhythmia?	Heart rhythm other than regular sinus rhythm
What is sinus arrhythmia?	Marked variation of the sinus rate with breathing; it is **normal and expected in children.**

Common Atrial Arrhythmias

What is sinus tachycardia?	Sinus rate greater than normal for age
What is sinus bradycardia?	Sinus rate less than normal for patient's age
In what 2 situations is a pacemaker needed?	When rate is very slow (i.e., < 30 beats/min); when cardiac output is compromised
What are premature atrial contractions?	The QRS complex occurs early, usually without compensatory pause. There may be alterations in P wave shape.
Is treatment needed?	No
What is wandering atrial pacemaker?	P wave and P-R intervals change; QRS complex is normal.
Is treatment necessary?	No; it is a normal variant.
What is atrial tachycardia (supraventricular tachycardia)?	Narrow QRS tachycardia; rate generally > 200 beats/min
What usually causes it?	It is usually idiopathic; 10%–20% of patients may have Wolff-Parkinson-White syndrome (pre-excitation may occur via accessory pathway that bypasses the AV nodes).
Is it likely to resolve without therapy?	The younger the patient, the more likely it is to resolve and not require long-term treatment.

List 4 methods of treatment.	Vagal stimulation; medical therapy with digoxin or a beta blockade; pharmacologic (adenosine) or electroshock cardioversion if condition is unstable; ablation of accessory pathways is available to older children in some treatment centers.
When does atrial fibrillation or flutter occur in children?	These are uncommon in pediatric patients; may occur postoperatively.

Ventricular Arrhythmias

Describe a common ventricular arrhythmia.	Premature ventricular contractions: isolated wide QRS beats that all have the same morphology can occur in 5% of normal children. All other ventricular arrhythmias are rare and require evaluation.
What is wide QRS tachycardia?	It is considered ventricular tachycardia until proven otherwise
What is the differential diagnosis?	Electrolyte disturbance, drug toxicity (consider digoxin), myocarditis, and myocardial ischemia

MITRAL VALVE PROLAPSE

What is it?	One of the mitral leaflets has excessive movement after closure; is commonly overdiagnosed in healthy children.
With what 2 conditions may it be associated?	Connective tissue diseases such as Marfan syndrome; secundum ASD
Is it more common in males or females?	Females
What is the physiologic result?	Normal physiology; occasionally children present with nonexertional chest pain.
What are the signs or symptoms?	Midsystolic click; late systolic murmur of mitral insufficiency may be present (louder when the child stands). Mitral valve prolapse has been associated with anxiety, palpitations, and chest pain.
What are the radiographic findings?	Normal

What 2 other diagnostic studies?	ECG (may have repolarization abnormalities or dysrhythmia); echocardiogram (for diagnosis and to assess mitral insufficiency)
List 2 treatments.	Antibiotic prophylaxis during surgical or dental procedures to prevent endocarditis if mitral regurgitation is present; treatment with beta-blockers may decrease chest pain and palpitations.
What are the outcomes?	In children, it appears to be benign in the absence of connective tissue disease. In adults, it has been associated with endocarditis, dysrhythmia, stroke, and sudden death.

AORTIC STENOSIS

What is it?	Obstruction of left ventricular output caused by a narrow aortic valve (5% of all CHDs)
List the 3 types.	Valvular, subvalvular, and supravalvular. Valvular stenosis is the most common and associated with bicuspid or unicuspid valve
Is it more common in males or females?	Males, by a 4:1 ratio
What is the physiologic result?	Obstruction causes increased LV pressure and muscle hypertrophy. The ascending aorta is dilated. Severe aortic stenosis (AS) may cause LV dilation and cardiac failure. Stenotic aortic valves are also frequently insufficient (AI).
List 4 signs or symptoms.	Mild-to-moderate AS: none Severe AS: CHF, exercise intolerance, chest pain, syncope
Physical signs or symptoms?	Harsh SEM, heard best at right upper sternal border with radiation to neck; high-pitched diastolic blowing murmur along left sternal border if AI is present
What are the radiographic findings?	May show cardiomegaly with dilated ascending aorta.

List 3 other diagnostic studies.	ECG (classically it shows LVH; severe AS has LVH criteria with negative T waves in lateral precordial leads [LVH with strain])
	Echocardiography (assesses valve anatomy, valve area, and gradient using Doppler)
	Cardiac catheterization (the standard for determining severity; data can also be used to estimate valve area).

What is the treatment?	Mild-to-moderate defect: none
	Severe defect: interventional catheterization or surgical valvuloplasty
	The goal is to reduce the AS gradient without producing AI.
	Common surgical repair options:
	1. Replacement of valve
	2. Ross procedure: Moves the pulmonary valve into aortic position and creates a RA→PA conduit.
	Mechanical valve replacement is delayed as long as possible to avoid multiple operations (as the child grows) and anticoagulation complications.

| **What are 2 complications of repair?** | Residual stenosis; valvular insufficiency |

| **What are the outcomes?** | Severe AS diagnosed in infancy has poor prognosis and requires multiple procedures throughout childhood, with fairly high morbidity rates. If bicuspid valve is present, it is generally not stenotic in childhood, but is the most common cause of AS in adults. |

ATRIOVENTRICULAR CANAL (AVC) DEFECT

| **What is it?** | A CHD derived from failure of endocardial cushion development (2% of CHDs) |

| **List the 2 types and their identifying characteristics.** | **Complete:** inlet VSD, primum ASD, and a common atrioventricular valve |
| | **Partial:** primum ASD and cleft mitral valve |

With what condition is AVC defect commonly associated?

Down syndrome (trisomy 21)

What is the physiologic result of complete AVC defect?

Left-to-right shunt at the combined atrial-ventricular septal defect, with pulmonary congestion and elevation of PA pressure

Of partial AVC defect?

Left-to-right shunt with ASD physiology

List 3 signs or symptoms of complete AVC defect.

Failure to thrive; CHF, caused by pulmonary overcirculation; murmur—often soft and nonspecific

List 2 possible signs and symptoms of partial AVC defect.

Usually asymptomatic, but may show systolic murmur of increased pulmonary flow and holosystolic murmur of mitral insufficiency

What are the radiographic findings?

Cardiomegaly with increased vascular markings

List 3 other diagnostic studies.

ECG (classically demonstrates superior QRS axis: QRS positive in lead I and negative in lead AVF)

Echocardiography (for diagnosis)

Cardiac catheterization (considered for obtaining hemodynamic data before intracardiac repair)

What is the treatment?

Manage CHF until surgery
Surgical treatment:
Complete AVC defect: patch closure of ASD and VSD, and construction of a tricuspid valve and mitral valve from common AV valve tissue
Partial AVC defect: patch closure of ASD and repair of cleft in mitral valve

What are the most common complications of repair of complete AVC defect?

Mitral insufficiency or mitral stenosis; if severe, either may require valve replacement.

Of partial AVC defect?

Residual mitral insufficiency

What are the outcomes?

Residual defects are common following surgical repair. If AVC defect is associated with trisomy 21, life expectancy is reduced to 40–50 years. Fifty percent of children with trisomy 21 have CHDs; VSD and ASD are most common, followed by AVC defect and TOF.

17

Respiratory and Thoracic Disorders

CONGENITAL DIAPHRAGMATIC HERNIA (CDH)

What is it?	A congenital defect in the diaphragm due to failure of the pleuroperitoneal canal to close at 8 weeks' gestation
What is a Bochdalek hernia and what are its main characteristics?	By far the most common CDH (85%–90%). It is a **posterolateral defect;** 15% have an intact sac.
What is a Morgagni hernia and what are its main characteristics?	An **anterior, parasternal defect.** It is usually smaller than a Bochdalek hernia, tends to have an intact sac, and does not have the pulmonary and systemic ramifications of a Bochdalek hernia.
What is the incidence of CDHs?	About 1 in 4,000 live births
What percentage of Bochdalek hernias are on the left?	85%
List 4 anatomic ramifications of Bochdalek hernia.	1. The abdominal contents herniate into the chest. 2. The lung on the involved side is small and hypoplastic, but the lung on the opposite side may also have evidence of hypoplasia. 3. The abdominal cavity may be smaller than normal. 4. There is malrotation of the bowel (see Chapter 19, Gastrointestinal Disorders, p. 238).
Of Morgagni hernia? (List 2)	The viscera may be in the hernia. Chest structures are not significantly affected.

What are the physiologic ramifications of a Bochdalek hernia? (List 2)

Bochdalek CDH was once believed to be a surgical emergency. It is now understood that **pulmonary vascular hyperreactivity** (and therefore pulmonary hypertension) and **pulmonary hypoplasia** are the major complications.

Of Morgagni hernia?

Usually none, unless the hernia is very large

List 4 signs and symptoms of a Bochdalek hernia.

Respiratory distress—usually immediately at birth; the infant's **chest appears expanded,** with **scaphoid abdomen.** Occasionally a child survives with Bochdalek CDH undetected in the perinatal stage and presents with **gastrointestinal (GI) problems** days to weeks later.

Signs of Morgagni hernia?

May be asymptomatic—or child may have mild respiratory symptoms or GI difficulties

List 2 prenatal ultrasound findings in Bochdalek hernia.

A multicystic appearance in the involved chest; there may be polyhydramnios.

What are 2 perinatal radiographic findings in a Bochdalek hernia?

1. Chest radiograph shows viscera in chest.
2. Nasogastric tube, if present, is often seen curling into the involved chest field if the stomach is herniated into the chest.

Why are radiographic findings in a Morgagni hernia more subtle?

Because the defect is anterior

List 5 elements in the initial management of a Bochdalek hernia.

Intubation, oxygenation, ventilation, sedation; paralysis is frequently used to make mechanical ventilation more efficient.

What are 2 major ventilation goals?

1. **Avoid pulmonary vascular spasm and shunting**—may require keeping postductal pH in the 7.50–7.60 range

and keeping P_{CO_2} in the 25–30 mm Hg range. Often an infant requires 100% O_2 and hyperventilation with a conventional or high-frequency oscillatory ventilator to achieve these ranges.

2. **Attempt to normalize P_{CO_2}, P_{O_2}, and pH as soon as possible**—if the infant can tolerate the attempt.

These infants are extremely tenuous, and even small changes in ventilation or oxygenation parameters may send an infant into a **lethal respiratory spiral** due to pulmonary vascular spasm.

List 4 agents used for pulmonary vasodilation.

Inhaled nitric oxide is the most commonly used agent because it may act selectively on the pulmonary vasculature. Other agents traditionally used have included **intravenous tozalozine, prostacyclin,** and **nitroprusside;** however, they have systemic effects as well. None of these agents is the panacea.

What may be necessary if conventional therapy fails?

ECMO

What is ECMO?

Extra **C**orporeal **M**embrane **O**xygenation. Essentially, it is a lung bypass machine.

What is the primary goal of ECMO?

To allow the lung to grow and the pulmonary hypertension to subside

List the 3 steps in surgical correction of CDH.

1. Subcostal (or occasionally, chest) incision
2. Reduction of the viscera into the abdomen making sure there is no volvulus
3. Closure of the diaphragm

A prosthetic patch may be needed to close the diaphragm, abdomen, or both.

When should surgical repair be performed?

Opinions are divided about the appropriate timing for surgical correction. Some measure of respiratory and hemodynamic stability is usually desired before surgery is performed. This may entail days, and in some cases, may only be obtained by placing the infant on ECMO. Repair may be undertaken prior to, during, or after ECMO (if ECMO is needed).

What is the "honeymoon period"?

After surgical correction, the baby tends to improve briefly, but then declines again.

What is treatment for a Morgagni hernia?

Treatment is **surgical closure** of the defect with routine supportive pre- and post-operative care. This surgery is usually done through a transverse substernal incision.

What is the outcome for Bochdalek hernia?

Overall survival is about 65%. Some infants may have long-term respiratory deficiency, GI reflux, or CNS sequelae from hypoxia or complications from ECMO.

What percentage of infants with CDH who are placed on ECMO survive?

Approximately 60%

What is the prognosis for Morgagni hernias?

Excellent

EMPHYSEMA

What is it?

An enlargement of the airspace distal to the terminal bronchioles due to either dilatation or destruction of the surrounding walls

List 4 potential mechanisms for emphysema.

1. **Congenital** (usually restricted to one lobe)
2. **Hyperexpansion of distal airspace** to fill space left by loss of adjacent lung volume from resection or atelectasis ("compensatory emphysema")
3. **Obstruction of gas egress** by foreign body, mass (e.g., tumor, adenopathy), mucosal edema (e.g., asthma), or vascular ring
4. **Destruction of airspace walls,** typically from presence of proteases in

excess of proteinase-inhibitor activity either because of a deficiency in inhibitor concentration or activity (as in α-1-antitrypsin deficiency) or because of an excess of protease concentration or activity (as in cystic fibrosis, bronchopulmonary dysplasia, or cigarette smoking)

List 4 signs and symptoms.
They vary with underlying etiologic factors. A child may be **asymptomatic** (e.g., compensatory emphysema following lobectomy). Alternatively, symptoms may include **cough, dyspnea, decreased breath sounds** or an **inspiratory phase lag** over the involved region.

How is it diagnosed?
By radiograph; delineation of the under-lying cause may require other measures. Obstructive emphysema can be distin-guished from the other forms by obtain-ing images (plain or fluoroscopic) during expiration, because the increase in lung volume will persist. Decubitus positioning may be used for this purpose.

What does a radiograph show?
Areas of **hyperlucency** and **decreased lung (vascular) markings.** There may be associated contiguous areas of opacity (either primary or compressive atelectasis) or mediastinal shift.

What is the treatment?
1. Congenital: remove involved lobe
2. Obstruction: remove foreign body or relieve obstruction
3. All other causes: good pulmonary toilet with management of underlying condition

LOBAR EMPHYSEMA

What is it?
Overdistention of a histologically normal lung lobe

What are the causes?
It is thought to be caused by poorly developed cartilage of the involved bronchus, creating a "ball–valve" effect. It may also be acquired.

What are 2 symptoms?	Mild-to-moderate tachypnea; failure to thrive
In what 2 ways is it diagnosed?	Chest radiograph; CT—may help diagnosis
What is the treatment?	Usually, resection of involved lobe. Acquired forms may resolve spontaneously.

LUNG CYSTS

What are they?	Simple cysts of the lung that most commonly reflect injury to the lung
List 3 common causes of injury to the lung.	Trauma; mechanical ventilation (particularly in premature infants); disease processes [e.g., infection or cystic fibrosis (CF) (p. 220)]
Treatment?	Most cysts may be observed. Occasionally, large ones should be resected.

PNEUMONIA/PNEUMONITIS

What is it?	An inflammatory (pneumonitis) or infectious (pneumonia) process involving the distal airspace. The term is also applied to processes involving the lung interstitium ("interstitial" pneumonia or pneumonitis). It should be distinguished from processes involving the trachea (tracheitis), bronchi (bronchitis), and distal airways (bronchiolitis).
What is the incidence?	Varies with age. Risk is roughly 5% per year in the preschool age group and is increased in institutional settings (e.g., dorms, the military).
What are some common signs and symptoms?	They vary with age and etiologic organism: Commonly: cough, fever, and chills, but child also may have chest pain, vomiting, diarrhea, or abdominal pain (can mimic **gallbladder disease** or **appendicitis!**) On physical exam: tachypnea, evidence of increased work of breathing (e.g., nasal flaring, retractions)

What do percussion, auscultation, and oximetry show?

Percussion may demonstrate an area of dullness, either from consolidation or associated pleural effusion. **Auscultation** may reveal areas of decreased breath sounds and inspiratory crackles or rales. However, auscultation may reveal normal breath sounds, especially in small infants. **Oximetry** usually reveals mild-to-severe oxygen desaturation, depending on severity of process.

How is it diagnosed?

Diagnosis can be made clinically, although radiograph should be used for confirmation in immunocompromised and severely ill children and children with a history of repeated episodes.

List 4 ways to determine the etiologic agent.

By **blood** or **sputum culture,** although in mild cases in an otherwise healthy child this is probably unnecessary. Identification is more urgent in the immunocompromised child, thus **bronchoscopy** or **biopsy** for diagnosis may be warranted.

What are the etiologic agents?

Viral and bacterial pathogens and other agents such as fungi. They vary with the child's age and immune status. In all groups, however, **viral pathogens are most common. Geography** or **exposure** may dictate consideration of agents such as fungi (coccidiomycosis, blastomycosis, histoplasmosis) or *M. tuberculosis.* If aspiration pneumonia is a possibility, anaerobes should be considered.

What is the most common viral pathogen?

Respiratory syncytial virus (RSV)

List the typical bacterial pathogens in the following age groups.

Newborns (List 3)

Group B streptococcus; gram-negative bacilli; *Chlamydia*

1 month–6 years (List 2)

Streptococcus pneumoniae; Haemophilus

	influenzae (H. flu is becoming less common with increasing use of vaccine)
Children older than 6 years and adolescents (List 4)	*Mycoplasma* species; *Streptococcus pyogens; Staphylococcus aureus; Streptococcus pneumoniae*
List 3 categories (with examples) of typical agents in hospitalized or immunocompromised children.	1. Gram-negative rod bacteria (e.g., *Pseudomonas, Klebsiella, E. coli, Serratia*) 2. Fungi (*Candida;* others may rarely occur) 3. Other nonbacterial agents (*Pneumocystis,* cytomegalovirus [CMV], Epstein-Barr virus)
List 2 components of treatment for most children.	Most otherwise healthy children can be treated as outpatients with: 1. Oral antibiotics (e.g., amoxicillin-clavulanate, erythromycin, cephalosporin) 2. Antipyretics Generally, cough suppressants are avoided, but they may be acceptable at bedtime to facilitate sleep.
For severely ill children?	Severely ill children (i.e., those with high fever, dehydration, intractable cough, hypoxemia) may need to be admitted to a hospital for IV antibiotics and supportive therapy (e.g., IV fluids, oxygen, chest physiotherapy). **Any immunocompromised child should be admitted.**
List 5 complications.	Pleural effusion, empyema, pulmonary abscess, respiratory failure, bronchiectasis (more common with recurrent episodes, but may occur acutely and be reversible)

ASTHMA

What is it?	A chronic lung disease defined as reversible narrowing or obstruction of large and middle airways due to hyperresponsiveness to various immunologic and nonimmunologic stimuli. Asthma is also sometimes referred to as "reactive airway disease."

What is the prevalence?

It is the most common chronic disease in childhood. Its prevalence in the United States is 5%–7%.

What is believed to be the pathophysiology of asthma?

Airway hyperresponsiveness is the central feature of asthma, resulting in bronchial smooth muscle constriction, mucus hypersecretion, and mucosal inflammation. Asthmatic lungs are believed to be more sensitive to challenges by allergens, physical stimuli (e.g., cold air, exercise) and environmental triggers (e.g., viruses).

List 5 mediators of asthma.

Mediators are released by eosinophils, mast cells, and alveolar macrophages. The mediators include histamine, eosinophil granular products, leukotrienes, prostaglandins, and thromboxanes.

What are extrinsic and intrinsic asthma?

Extrinsic asthma is caused by allergens (Ch 29, p.440)
Intrinsic asthma is nonallergic or non-IgE mediated

List 3 common allergens in extrinsic asthma.

Pollens, dust mites, animal dander

List 4 common triggers in intrinsic asthma.

Cold air, odors, smoke, viral infections

What are the signs and symptoms?

Mild?

Wheezing or coughing at night or with exercise

Moderate?

Wheezing and/or coughing at rest

Advanced? (List 8 symptoms)

Increased respiratory rate, retractions, cyanosis, decreased or absent inspiratory breath sounds, increased accessory muscle use due to the need to maintain lungs in a hyperinflated state, marked expiratory wheezing, pulsus paradoxus, agitation

List 4 typical findings on chest radiograph.

Pulmonary hyperinflation with flattening of the diaphragm; increased anteroposterior (AP) diameter; increased lung markings due to inflammation; atelectasis

List 3 stages of the expected blood pH in exacerbations of asthma.

1. Initially a **respiratory alkalosis** develops due to hyperventilation.
2. As respiratory effect worsens, CO_2 retention occurs and **respiratory acidosis** can develop.
3. Finally, increased muscular effort and poor oxygen intake lead to increased lactic acid and ketosis, resulting in **metabolic acidosis**

What is the differential diagnosis of wheezing?

Common diagnoses

Bronchial asthma, foreign body, CF, infection (especially upper respiratory infection [URI]), laryngotracheomalacia, bronchiolitis, and bronchopulmonary dysplasia

Uncommon diagnoses

Vascular rings, laryngeal webs, enlarged lymph node, and bronchostenosis

What are 4 goals of treatment of asthma?

1. To maintain normal activity levels
2. To prevent symptoms, such as cough or nighttime shortness of breath
3. To prevent recurrent exacerbations
4. To avoid adverse effects from medication

What are the 2 major classes of pharmacotherapeutic agents for treating asthma? (List 3 examples of each)

1. **Bronchodilators:** β-adrenergic agonists, theophylline, anticholinergic agents
2. **Anti-inflammatory agents:** cromolyn sodium, nedocromil sodium, corticosteroids (oral or inhaled)

List 7 signs of theophylline overdose.

Early signs are insomnia, headache, nausea, and vomiting. High theophylline levels may cause seizure, coma, and death.

List 5 factors that can affect theophylline metabolism.

Age, immunizations, smoking, other medications, infection

List 3 other treatment modalities besides medications.

Environmental control, patient education, immunotherapy

What is exercise-induced asthma?	Airway narrowing that occurs minutes (5–10) after vigorous activity (Ch 13, p. 145)
How can it be prevented?	Treatment with β_2-agonist or cromolyn before exercise (Ch 13, p. 145)

AIRWAY FOREIGN BODY

Where do aspirated foreign bodies typically lodge?	1. Usually below the carina 2. In toddlers, foreign bodies lodge with equal incidence in either mainstem. 3. In older children, they usually lodge in the right mainstem.
List 4 symptoms.	Coughing, gagging, choking, wheezing. An asymptomatic interlude may follow.
List 2 radiographic findings.	1. Either hyper- or hypo-inflation of affected lung may occur. 2. Foreign body will be visible if radiopaque, but not all are!
What is the treatment?	Removal of the object via rigid bronchoscopy.
List 5 potential sequelae if the foreign body is not removed.	Pneumonitis or pneumonia; abscess; bronchiectasis; pulmonary hemorrhage; erosion and perforation of the enclosing structure

CYSTIC FIBROSIS (CF)

What causes CF?	A defect in the cystic fibrosis transmembrane regulator protein
How is CF transmitted?	Autosomal recessive trait; about 1 in 20 Caucasians carry the gene.
How common is CF?	In the Caucasian population, about 1 in 2,000. It is also found in other populations.
What is the pathophysiology?	Abnormal, thickened secretions in a variety of organs, causing inspissation and mucous buildup
List 4 ways patients with CF may present.	1. Meconium ileus in the neonate 2. Recurrent bronchitis, pneumonia, or both

3. Malabsorption, with failure to thrive
4. Male infertility

What percentage of infants with CF have meconium ileus?

10% of CF infants have meconium ileus; 99% of infants with meconium ileus have CF.

List 2 ways CF is diagnosed.

Usually by an elevated sweat chloride concentration. DNA testing for specific mutations may also be used.

What is the most common CF gene mutation?

ΔF508, although there are over 700 other mutations. The relative frequency of specific mutations varies with ethnicity.

List 6 components of treatment.

Nutritional support, pancreatic enzyme supplementation, chest physical therapy, antibiotics, bronchodilators. Lung transplantation is now being attempted.

What is the outcome?

With appropriate therapy, many patients live into adulthood. The end-stage event is usually respiratory failure.

TRACHEOMALACIA

What is it?

Suboptimal integrity of the tracheal wall and cartilage rings that leads to partial collapse of the trachea upon inspiration

What group of children gets this condition?

Neonates; it reflects incomplete maturation of the tracheal structures

List 2 associated conditions.

It can be a primary condition or exacerbated by other conditions, such as esophageal atresia or vascular rings.

List 2 signs and symptoms.

Inspiratory stridor; in severe cases, the infant may have "**dying spells**"—periods of **prolonged apnea** resulting in **cyanosis** and requiring stimulation for resolution.

List 2 ways it is diagnosed.

Fluoroscopic examination; bronchoscopy

List 3 treatments.

1. If condition is primary, it is usually self-resolving.
2. If associated with exacerbating

process, then that process needs to be corrected (e.g., division of vascular ring).
3. Occasionally, aortopexy is done to enhance opening of the trachea.

PNEUMOTHORAX

What is it?	Separation of the visceral pleura from the parietal pleura, resulting in the presence of air in the pleural space
List the 3 most common causes in infants.	Barotrauma; respiratory distress syndrome (RDS) (previously called hyaline membrane disease) (Ch 10, p. 89); bronchopulmonary dysplasia
In older children? (List 6)	Trauma, rupture of apical bleb, CF, severe coughing, asthma; it may also be idiopathic
What are the symptoms?	Mild-to-severe respiratory distress. A small pneumothorax may be asymptomatic.
What is a tension pneumothorax?	Air collection in the pleural space under pressure, creating a shift in the mediastinum, compression of the opposite lung, and hemodynamic compromise. **THIS IS A LIFE-THREATENING CONDITION!**
How is pneumothorax diagnosed?	**Chest radiograph.** Occasionally, the supine trauma victim will have pneumothorax discovered during a CT scan, because the air is anterior in this situation.
What is the treatment?	A small, asymptomatic pneumothorax that is not the result of trauma may be allowed to resolve spontaneously. Otherwise, chest tube placement is required until the air leak seals.
List 2 ways recurrent pneumothorax is treated.	1. Instillation of a sclerosing agent, such as talc or tetracycline, via a chest tube or thoracoscopy.
	2. Resection of the apical bleb or other

site of parenchymal leak via thoracoscopy or thoracotomy.

How is tension pneumothorax treated?	**Immediate placement of a chest tube.** If a tube is not available, a large bore angiocatheter or needle should be placed in the **second intercostal space** anteriorly for decompression.

CHYLOTHORAX

What is it?	An accumulation of lymph fluid (chyle) in the thorax. It can be **congenital** or **acquired.**
List 2 common congenital causes.	Abnormalities of the thoracic duct; birth trauma
List 6 common causes of acquired chylothorax.	Trauma; operative injury (especially during cardiothoracic procedures); neoplasm; thrombosis of the subclavian vein or the superior vena cava; lymphangiomatosis; severe coughing
What are the symptoms?	Respiratory insufficiency or distress if collection is large enough
How is it diagnosed?	Chylothorax appears as a radiopaque fluid collection on chest radiograph. Diagnosis is confirmed by thoracentesis and analysis of the fluid.
List 5 typical characteristics of chyle.	Appearance is milky or straw colored; lymphocyte predominance; protein content ≥ 5 g/dl; fat content ≥ 400 mg/dl; triglyceride level ≥ 110 mg/dl
List 3 components of the initial treatment.	Thoracentesis; low-fat diet or parenteral nutrition; chest tube drainage or repeated thoracentesis as necessary
List 3 surgical options that may be used for refractory cases.	1. Right thoracotomy with ligation of thoracic duct 2. Thoracoscopy of affected side with clipping of the leak, application of fibrin glue, or both 3. Placement of pleuroperitoneal shunt

PECTUS DEFORMITY

PECTUS EXCAVATUM

What is pectus excavatum?

Also known as "funnel chest," this condition manifests as a significant depression of the sternum.

What is the cause?

Believed to be an abnormality in growth of the cartilage connecting the sternum to the ribs.

List 3 significant anatomic and physiologic effects.

1. The heart is shifted to the left
2. In severe deformities, the lungs are compressed.
3. Children may manifest symptoms of asthma or dyspnea on exertion. However, many children are asymptomatic.

List 6 common associated conditions.

Scoliosis, Marfan syndrome, club foot, syndactyly, Klippel-Feil syndrome, mitral valve prolapse (Ch 16, p. 205)

What are 2 indications for surgery?

1. Significant respiratory insufficiency
2. Significantly abnormal appearance; some children with pectus deformity may be ridiculed by their peers and be self-conscious to a degree that significantly affects their self-image and their activities.

List 2 methods of repair.

1. Traditionally, the abnormal cartilages are removed while the surrounding perichondrium is preserved. The sternum is then elevated by any of a number of different methods and secured. Often, a metal strut is placed substernally for support and is removed 3–6 months later. New cartilage grows back within the perichondrium in the appropriate position.
2. A newer procedure is now offered, in which a metal strut is placed under the sternum with thoracoscopic guidance. The strut forces the chest into a normal configuration, but must stay in place for about 2 years.

What is the outcome?	The cosmetic and the physiologic results of the traditional repair are very good. Patients return to full activity after 3–6 months. The thoracoscopic procedure shows promise, but results are still being assessed.

PECTUS CARINATUM

What is pectus carinatum?	A condition in which the sternum protrudes. It is also a result of abnormal growth of costal cartilages.
List 7 associated conditions.	Congenital heart disease, marfanoid habitus, scoliosis, kyphosis, muscular defects, skeletal defects, asthma
What is the method of repair?	Similar to the traditional repair of pectus excavatum, except with **depression** and stabilization of the sternum

ESOPHAGEAL DUPLICATION CYST

What is it?	Congenital cyst arising from an abnormality in foregut development
What is the location?	Mediastinum; it may share a common wall with the esophagus
What is the histology?	Squamous epithelial lining, but may have ciliated mucosa with some cartilage in the wall
What are two ways a patient may present?	Respiratory distress; the condition may also be found incidentally on radiograph where it appears as a solid mediastinal mass
List 2 ways it is diagnosed.	Chest radiograph; CT
What is the treatment?	**Surgical excision** via thoracotomy or thoracoscopy. If there is a common wall with the esophagus, cyst mucosa should be stripped from the common wall.

BRONCHOGENIC CYST

What is it?	Congenital cyst arising from cells that

	become isolated during bronchial development
What are the 2 locations?	1. Central: near the hilum or medias-tinum; usually solitary 2. Peripheral: may be multiple
What are 2 ways the patient may present?	1. Respiratory distress 2. The condition may be found incidentally on radiograph
What are the radiographic findings of central and peripheral cysts?	**Central:** solid-appearing mass, or cystic lesion with air-fluid level **Peripheral:** multi-loculated appearance that may be confused with congenital cystic adenomatoid malformation (see CCAM, p. 227) or even congenital diaphragmatic hernia (see CDH, p. 210)
List 2 ways it is diagnosed.	Chest radiograph; CT
What is the treatment for each type of cyst?	**Central:** surgical excision of cyst **Peripheral:** wedge resection or resection of involved lung lobe

PULMONARY SEQUESTRATION

What is it?	Mass of abnormal lung tissue receiving an abnormal (i.e., systemic) blood supply, with no communication with the tracheo-bronchial tree
List the 2 types and the 3 characteristic features of each.	1. **Intralobar** (90%): lies within the lobe of a lung; arterial supply is systemic; venous drainage may be systemic or pulmonary 2. **Extralobar** (10%): has its own pleura; arterial supply and venous drainage may be systemic or pulmonary; may have immature parenchyma or an associated congenital cystic adenomatoid malformation (p. 227)
What are the symptoms?	Child is usually asymptomatic at birth. Serial bouts of pneumonia follow after 1–2 years.
List 2 ways it is diagnosed.	Chest radiograph, CT

What is the treatment?	Surgical excision
List 3 associated anomalies.	Congenital heart defects (CHD) (Ch 16, p. 183); congenital cystic adenomatoid malformation (CCAM) (see below); arteriovenous malformation with shunting

CONGENITAL CYSTIC ADENOMATOID MALFORMATION (CCAM)

What is CCAM?	Congenital cystic changes of the lung
What are the 3 types and their characteristics?	Type I: Large, irregular cysts Type II: Smaller, more closely arranged cysts Type III: Dense, small cysts; may resemble fetal lung
What is the histology?	Cuboidal and low columnar epithelium; few mucogenic cells
By what mechanism do the cysts arise?	Excessive proliferation of bronchioles at the expense of alveoli
List 2 symptoms.	1. Respiratory distress in infants if involved area is large (usually Type II or III) 2. Older children or adults may present with infection It may be an asymptomatic finding on radiograph
List 3 ways it is diagnosed.	Chest radiograph, CT, and sometimes detected by prenatal ultrasound
What is the treatment?	Excision of affected lobe or lobes

18 Head and Neck

EPIGLOTTITIS

What is it?

Rapidly progressive bacterial infection causing acute inflammation and edema of the epiglottis and adjacent structures (aryepiglottic folds, arytenoids); also known as supraglottitis

Why is it important?

It is **life threatening!** Affected children may have sudden and complete airway obstruction.

What is the usual age at presentation?

2–6 years of age; peak incidence is at 3½ years of age. Infants, older children and adults are rarely affected.

Is there a seasonal incidence?

No

What are causative agents?

Haemophilus influenzae **type b** is the primary cause. It is rarely caused by pneumococci, staphylococci, or streptococci.

What is the classic presentation?

A previously well child with sudden onset of symptoms; 4–12-hour history of sore throat, high fever, dysphagia, irritability, or lethargy; symptoms continue to progress rapidly

What are the classic signs?

Child is febrile, toxic, and appears anxious, with inspiratory **stridor,** and in **respiratory distress.** Child often is leaning forward with an open mouth, drooling. Child usually is aphonic, but may have a muffled "hot potato" voice if speaking, and prefers to sit in the tripod position.

What is the tripod position?

A sitting position in which the arms are extended in front of the body supporting the trunk; the neck is hyperextended with the chin protruding. This position maximizes the size of the supraglottic airway.

What is the differential diagnosis?

1. Infection: bacterial tracheitis, peritonsillar abscess, retropharyngeal abscess, diphtheria
2. Foreign body aspiration
3. Angioneurotic edema
4. Anaphylaxis
5. Neoplasm
6. Trauma: burns, thermal injury, blunt trauma

What must be done first in evaluation and management?

Quickly proceed with the epiglottitis protocol that has been established at the medical facility. Protection of the airway is the primary priority.

List the key steps that are typically included in an epiglottitis protocol.

1. Keeping the patient **calm** and with the parents
2. Administering **100% O$_2$,** without further agitating the child (parents may hold the child)
3. Assembling at bedside: **CPR equipment,** including resuscitation bag and mask, intubation equipment, and instruments for emergency **cricothyroidotomy**
4. Calling senior **pediatrics, anesthesia, pediatric surgery** or **otolaryngology staff** to bedside
5. Taking patient (accompanied by parents) to the **operating room** for induction of anesthesia (if needed), placement of IVs, direct laryngoscopy, intubation, and blood and epiglottis cultures. Equipment and expertise for an emergency tracheostomy should be present.
6. Admitting to the **intensive care unit** Not every child with epiglottitis will have the classic signs and symptoms. **It is better to initiate a "false"**

epiglottitis drill than to miss this disease.

What key laboratory and diagnostic studies are ordered?	Only after the epiglottitis protocol has been performed and the patient has a secure airway: 1. **Blood culture,** which usually is positive for *H. influenzae* type b 2. **WBC count,** which may be moderately elevated with a left shift 3. **Lateral neck radiograph,** which shows a thickened epiglottis ("thumb sign") and a distended hypopharynx
What should the physician NOT do when evaluating the child's condition?	1. Do not agitate the child. 2. Do not make the child lie supine. 3. Do not try to visualize the pharynx or epiglottis with a tongue blade. 4. No laboratory procedures, needle sticks, or radiographs should be performed before establishing epiglottitis protocol. **All of these things can lead to airway obstruction, cardiopulmonary arrest, or both.**
How is the diagnosis confirmed?	Diagnosis is confirmed by seeing an edematous cherry-red epiglottis on endoscopy. Endoscopic examination should not be performed in advance of the epiglottitis protocol.
What are the main components of treatment after protection of the airway and diagnosis are established?	1. **Maintain adequate (usually artificial) airway** until inflammation and edema resolve—often 36–72 hours 2. **Parenteral antibiotics,** directed against *H. influenzae*, assuming this is the cause; classically, ampicillin and chloramphenicol have been used, but now a third-generation cephalosporin (e.g., cefotaxime or ceftriaxone) is also an option; treat for 7–10 days 3. **Rifampin prophylaxis** to treat the carrier state and prevent further spread of disease
List 3 instances in which rifampin prophylaxis is used.	When: 1. ***H. influenzae*** is the etiologic agent

	2. Patient has non-immunized or immunocompromised household contacts < 4 years of age
	3. Patient has day-care contacts < 2 years old, for > 25 hrs/wk
Who needs it?	All household and day-care contacts (if they are children) and the patient (immediately before discharge)
Is the *H. influenzae* (Hib) vaccine decreasing the incidence of childhood epiglottitis?	Yes

CROUP

What is croup?	**Viral infection** of the upper and lower respiratory tract that causes **subglottic inflammation** (laryngotracheobronchitis)
What are the 2 classic features of croup?	Stridor and barking cough
What is the usual age at presentation?	3 months to 3 years of age; peak incidence at 2 years of age
What is the epidemiology of croup?	Affects boys more often than girls. Peak occurrence is in fall and winter (epidemics); also occurs in spring.
What are the primary causative agents of croup?	**Parainfluenza virus** (especially type 1), influenza virus, respiratory syncytial virus, adenovirus, *Mycoplasma pneumoniae,* and measles virus.
List the key symptoms of croup.	Symptoms of upper respiratory infection (URI); intermittent nonproductive "barking" cough (sometimes described as "seal-like"); stridor; respiratory distress (tachypnea, nasal flaring, retractions); hypoxia; agitation Symptoms vary; children may be alert and comfortable, with only mild symptoms of upper respiratory infection (URI) and an intermittent barking cough.
What is the typical history?	It is often preceded by several days of

upper respiratory symptoms, followed by hoarseness and a deepening, nonproductive barking cough. Symptoms may fluctuate, worsening at night. Stridor and mild dyspnea may occur and usually resolve in a few hours. Most cases are mild; however, respiratory distress can become severe.

What is the differential diagnosis for croup?

See Epiglottitis, p. 228

How is the diagnosis made?

Clinically. **The physician should try not to agitate the child, particularly if the symptoms are severe.**

What diagnostic studies are used?

Perform studies only if patient is not in respiratory distress.
1. Radiograph of the anterior-posterior neck may show a "pencil tip" or "**steeple sign**" of the subglottic trachea. Do not use a radiograph to make management decisions in a patient with an unstable airway.
2. Lab studies (e.g., CBC) usually not helpful

Why do some children improve spontaneously?

Because of natural fluctuations in the disease

List 2 treatments for mild cases.

1. Humidification
2. Exposure to cold night air is thought to help, but this is largely anecdotal.

What are some treatments for severe cases of croup?

For more severe symptoms requiring hospitalization:
1. **Airway support,** including O_2, pulse oximetry, and intubation if necessary. Clinical assessment and close observation are of paramount importance.
2. **Humidification,** via cool mist wand. Avoid croup tents as they make observation of the patient difficult.
3. **Racemic** epinephrine—may cause rapid improvement in symptoms. If used, watch for **rebound phenomenon**—symptoms may abruptly return

when the effect of epinephrine wears off, usually within 2 hours.

4. **Corticosteroids (dexamethasone)**—may help in moderately severe croup; may be used in the outpatient setting if patients demonstrate maintained improvement 2–3 hours after treatment.

Do most children with croup need hospitalization?	No. Symptoms typically resolve within a few days.
What is spasmodic croup?	A benign condition with recurrent episodes of stridor and barking cough; may be associated with viral illnesses. It typically resolves spontaneously and is rarely associated with severe respiratory distress.

PIERRE ROBIN MALFORMATION

What is it?	Congenital micrognathia, with associated cleft of the soft palate and glossoptosis
What are 2 general symptoms?	1. Respiratory distress when the infant is supine. 2. Feeding difficulties (especially with palate and tongue abnormalities).
What are the treatments for the 2 components of the malformation?	1. **Micrognathia:** proper positioning (prone) and possibly a nasopharyngeal tube usually allow appropriate respiration. The mandible grows faster than the whole child and is usually no longer a problem by 3 months of age. Rarely, suturing the tip of the tongue to the lower lip is needed to support a patent airway. 2. **Palate abnormalities:** surgical intervention is necessary. A tracheostomy may be needed until repairs are completed. If feeding is difficult, a gastrostomy tube is needed.

CHOANAL ATRESIA

What is choanal atresia?	Congenital persistence of a bony membrane across the nasopharyngeal passage

How does choanal atresia typically present?	Respiratory difficulty at birth, because infants prefer nasal breathing
How is choanal atresia diagnosed?	Examiner's inability to pass a suction catheter into the pharynx via the nasal passages. The diagnosis may be confirmed by contrast nasopharyngography.
What are the 2 treatment components for choanal atresia?	1. Initial treatment: maintenance of the oral airway until the infant can breath on his/her own 2. Resection of the bony septum and placement of stents until the passage epithelializes

VOCAL CORD PARALYSIS

What is it?	Paralysis of one or both cords, which may be either **congenital** or **acquired**
What are 4 common causes of acquired vocal cord paralysis?	Birth trauma; injury to the recurrent laryngeal nerve during ligation of the patent ductus arteriosus (PDA); increased intracranial pressure; intracranial hemorrhage
Is unilateral or bilateral cord paralysis more common?	Unilateral
What are potential symptoms?	**Bilateral:** Inspiratory and expiratory **stridor** or frank respiratory distress **Unilateral:** symptoms may be minimal
What is the method of diagnosis?	**Laryngoscopy** with the infant under light anesthesia allows visualization of cord movement, or lack of movement, during spontaneous breathing.
What is the treatment?	Most cases of vocal cord paralysis resolve spontaneously after 4–6 weeks. Tracheostomy may be needed to alleviate severe symptoms.

LARYNGEAL WEB

What is laryngeal web?	Congenital abnormality of the glottic region resulting in a web-like lesion.

What is the range of symptoms?	Symptoms range from mild inspiratory–expiratory stridor to frank distress.
How are laryngeal webs treated?	1. A thin web may be lysed with cautery or a laser. 2. A thicker web may require more extensive reconstruction, and may necessitate tracheostomy.

SUBGLOTTIC STENOSIS

What is it?	Narrowing of the subglottic region, which may be either **congenital** or **acquired**
How is it acquired?	May be a sequela of a previously placed endotracheal tube (ETT)
List 2 types of symptoms.	Inspiratory or expiratory **stridor;** inflammation of any kind may cause frank **distress.**
What are the treatments for congenital and acquired subglottic stenosis?	**Congenital:** usually supportive; infant will outgrow the condition **Acquired:** if severe, may require tracheostomy, then an appropriate surgical procedure (laryngotracheoplasty or anterior cricoid split)
What is laryngeal atresia?	Complete nonformation of the laryngeal area, which is **incompatible with life** unless there is a large trachea-esophageal fistula

BRANCHIAL CLEFT REMNANTS

What are they?	Remnants of branchial arches that are embryologic sources of head and neck structures
List 4 forms they may take.	Cysts, sinuses, fistulae, and cartilaginous remnant
What are the names and locations of the commonly found remnants?	**First branchial remnant:** lies anterior to the ear and may extend to the eustachian tube **Second branchial remnant:** begins in the midneck, anterior to the sternocleido-mastoid muscle, and may extend up

through the carotid bifurcation to the pharynx

Third branchial remnant: begins superior to the medial portion of the clavicle and passes lateral to the carotid bifurcation, up toward the pharynx

What are typical features of presentation?

A draining area, dimple, or mass at one of the 3 branchial remnant sites; infection may occur as first sign.

What is the treatment for branchial cleft remnants?

Surgical excision; more than 1 incision may be needed for extensive lesions

THYROGLOSSAL DUCT REMNANT

What is it?

Remnant of embryologic path that the thyroid takes from the foramen cecum to its final position

What 2 forms may it take?

Cyst (75%); sinus (25%)

List key features of presentation.

1. The child usually has an asymptomatic mass in the anterior midline of the neck.
2. The mass may be an infected, draining site.
3. The mass moves upward with swallowing.

What is the treatment?

Surgical excision with a Sistrunk procedure: the cyst or sinus is excised widely along its tract to the base of the tongue. Excision includes the middle third of the hyoid bone.

Are thyroid function tests necessary?

Yes, if thyroid tissue is found in the excised tissue

Why?

Thyroid tissue in the excised cyst or sinus may represent the only thyroid tissue the child has, necessitating thyroid hormone replacement.

TORTICOLLIS

What is torticollis?

An intense spasm of the sternocleidomastoid muscle.

What is the cause?	Uncertain—it may be related to hematoma from birth trauma. It typically is found in infants 2–8 weeks old.
What are the symptoms?	The infant tends to keep her/his head turned to one side (i.e., facing away from the site of the spasm).
List the typical physical findings.	A mass is noted in the midportion of the sternocleidomastoid muscle; the rest of the muscle is very tight.
What is the treatment?	The goal is to stretch the sternocleidomastoid muscle and relieve the spasm. This is done in 3 ways:

1. Stimulate the infant to turn his/her head toward the side of the affected muscle. This can often be done during feeding.
2. Turn the infant's head passively toward the side of the affected muscle.
3. **Gently** massage the spasm area. (If massage is too vigorous, bradycardia may result from carotid body stimulation.)

These steps are repeated on a routine basis during daily feeding and care activities until torticollis resolves.

What is the outcome?	Torticollis usually resolves in 2–6 weeks with the therapy noted above. Only rarely is surgical intervention required.

19 Gastrointestinal Disorders

SHORT-GUT (SHORT-BOWEL) SYNDROME

What is it?

Nutrient malabsorption and excessive intestinal fluid and electrolyte losses following massive small intestine loss or resection

List the 3 most common causes of extensive small bowel loss in children.

Malrotation with midgut volvulus; small intestine atresia(s); necrotizing enterocolitis (NEC) (see p. 240)

How much small intestine does an infant have?

A full-term infant has ~ 250 cm of small intestine (an adult has 600–800 cm). The diameter increases from 1.5 cm during infancy to 3.5 cm in adulthood.

How much intestine does a child need to lose before developing short-gut syndrome?

There is no absolute amount of loss that defines short-gut syndrome. As much as 75% of the small intestine may be lost without serious long-term problems if the duodenum, terminal ileum, and ileocecal valve are spared. In contrast, the loss of 25% of the small intestine coupled with the loss of the terminal ileum and the ileocecal valve may cause significant difficulties.

What is the primary symptom?

Diarrhea

List 4 clinical results.

Growth failure, protein–calorie malnutrition, recurrent dehydration, and a variety of nutritional deficits

Does it matter which part of the bowel is lost?

Yes. Loss of much of the jejunum may cause few long-term symptoms because the ileum "adapts." The jejunum is less adaptable and unable to develop the specialized functions of any lost distal small intestine.

What conditions are caused by the loss of the terminal ileum or ileocecal valve?

Usually, **vitamin B_{12} deficiency** and **bile salt malabsorption.** Loss of the ileocecal valve may lead to bacterial contamination of the small bowel and poor regulation of flow of intestinal contents.

Describe the 2 phases of the treatment.

Therapy is often divided into 2 phases:
1. **Acute phase** (usually lasts several weeks after surgery): the child often has massive secretory diarrhea. Attention must be paid to fluid and electrolyte status. H_2 receptor antagonists may decrease intestinal secretion. Parenteral nutrition should begin as soon as possible to prevent catabolism.
2. **Chronic phase:** goal is to support normal growth and development while maximizing intestinal adaptation. Maximal adaptation may take 6–12 months after surgery. Calories are provided totally or in part from parenteral nutrition during this period.

Is enteral nutrition beneficial?

Yes. It stimulates bowel growth and adaptation. Initial feeding is usually an elemental formula provided as a constant infusion through a nasogastric (NG) tube or gastrostomy tube.

How are attempts at enteral feeding regulated?

The volume and concentration of the formula are adjusted in response to stool volume and clinical symptoms, such as feeding residuals, vomiting, and abdominal bloating.

What is the prognosis?

Outlook for long-term survival is good. Children who have more than 20 cm of small intestine and an ileocecal valve are usually ultimately capable of enteral nutrition alone.

NECROTIZING ENTEROCOLITIS (NEC)

What is it?	An acute fulminating inflammatory disease of the intestine associated with focal or diffuse ulceration and necrosis of the small bowel, colon, and, rarely, the stomach
What are common complications of NEC?	NEC is the most common cause of gastrointestinal (GI) perforation and acquired short-gut syndrome among hospitalized premature infants.
Which infants are most susceptible to NEC?	NEC is predominantly a disease of premature infants. The overall incidence is 3%–5% of all neonatal intensive care unit admissions. Full-term infants rarely acquire NEC.
What is the pathogenesis of NEC?	The pathogenesis is multifactorial. It likely represents a final common pathway of the response of immature intestine to injury rather than a distinct disease.
List 5 implicated factors in NEC.	1. Ischemia-reperfusion injury of the intestine 2. Enteral alimentation 3. Infectious and inflammatory agents 4. An immature immune system 5. Immature intestinal mucosa
What are the early GI signs and symptoms?	Early GI signs and symptoms are nonspecific and may include: vomiting, delayed gastric emptying, increased gastric residual volume, hematemesis, bright red blood from the rectum, diminished or absent bowel sounds, abdominal distension with or without tenderness, and diarrhea.
What are the non-GI symptoms?	The infant may also exhibit a number of nonspecific non-GI symptoms consistent with bacterial sepsis, including: apnea, respiratory distress, bradycardia, lethargy, temperature instability, cyanosis, mottling, systemic acidosis, and hyper- or hypoglycemia.

List 5 complications that may appear as the disease progresses.	The infant may develop septicemia, disseminated intravascular coagulation (DIC), hypotension, ascites, and intestinal perforation with peritonitis.
How is NEC diagnosed?	Primarily clinical. Confirmation can be provided by the radiographic presence of pneumatosis intestinalis (i.e., accumulation of gas within the intestinal wall), portal venous gas, or pneumoperitoneum.
What is the differential diagnosis?	Sepsis with ileus Malrotation with midgut volvulus (see p. 266) Pseudomembranous colitis (see p. 245) Hirschsprung disease (see p. 265) Gastric stress ulcer Hemorrhagic disease of the newborn Swallowed maternal blood
What are components of treatment?	1. Enteral feedings should be discontinued, and nasogastric (NG) suction and IV fluids started. 2. Broad-spectrum parenteral antibiotics. Abdominal radiographs should be performed every 6 hours to detect early perforation and to follow the radiographic course of the disease.
Do most cases resolve with medical treatment?	Yes
When can enteral feeding be reintroduced?	After 7–10 days of medical therapy in uncomplicated cases.
What are 2 absolute indications for surgery?	**Intestinal perforation or clinical deterioration unresponsive to medical therapy.**
What does surgery usually involve?	Resection of the perforated or necrotic bowel, an end stoma, and mucous fistula. The bowel may be reconnected when the infant is fully recovered. Alternatively, placement of an abdominal drain may ameliorate systemic symptoms, and allow resuscitation until a definitive procedure can be performed. Occasionally, the intestine

will heal with drainage and laparotomy will not be needed.

What are long-term complications of NEC?	1. **Short-gut syndrome:** if significant bowel resection 2. **Bowel stricture:** 18%–25% of cases; mostly left colon. Infants with chronic or recurrent GI symptoms should undergo an upper GI series, with follow-through, to look for strictures.

ULCERATIVE COLITIS

What is it?	An inflammatory bowel disease that involves rectal and colonic mucosa. The rectum is involved first, and the disease progresses proximally in a contiguous manner.
What are the characteristics of the mucosa?	Crypt abscesses form leading to mucosal ulcerations, pseudopolyps, and ultimately a denuding of the mucosa.
What are the etiologic factors?	Uncertain, but an autoimmune process with a genetic predisposition is currently the most popular theory. About 15% of patients have a family member with inflammatory bowel disease.
What are the possible associated conditions?	Ankylosing spondylitis, uveitis, growth retardation, anemia, osteoporosis, nephrolithiasis, arthralgia, skin lesions (e.g., erythema nodosum, pyoderma gangrenosum), liver lesions (e.g., sclerosing cholangitis, fatty infiltration of liver), and aphthous stomatitis.
What is the age of onset?	Usually adolescence or the third decade, occasionally earlier.
What are the signs and symptoms?	Signs and symptoms can be insidious— crampy abdominal pain can progress to diarrhea containing blood or pus. If condition is unchecked, a toxic colitis can ensue. (Occasionally, this is the initial presentation.)

List 2 components of diagnosis.

1. The diagnosis is largely one of exclusion and is confirmed by endoscopy and biopsy of colonic mucosa.
2. As many as 85% of children with ulcerative colitis have significant circulating titers of perinuclear antineutrophil cytoplasmic antibodies (p-ANCA)

What is toxic megacolon?

A fulminant presentation characterized by colonic dilatation, a low motility state, and probable bacterial overgrowth. Patients are severely ill with septic manifestations. Supportive therapy is needed with IV fluids, antibiotics, and bowel rest. Rarely, colectomy will be needed emergently.

How is ulcerative colitis medically treated?

1. Initial treatment usually includes 5-aminosalicylic acid (5-ASA) derivatives such as sulfasalazine (Azulfidine), mesalamine (Asacol, Pentasa), olsalazine (Dipentum)
2. Corticosteroids given orally or rectally
3. Other effective immunosuppressive agents are azathioprine, 6-mercaptopurine, methotrexate, and cyclosporine.
4. Anti-tumor necrosis factor antibody infusions may be helpful.

While broad-spectrum antibiotics are often used, there is little evidence to indicate they are effective. Antidiarrheal medicines should be used with care, because toxic megacolon may result. **Medical therapy is not curative.**

What is surgical treatment?

Virtually all patients need surgery. **The curative procedure is a total proctocolectomy with ileoanal pull-through** or **permanent end ileostomy.**

What are the outcomes?

Surgical removal of the colon and rectum is curative. The pull-through procedure causes an increased number of bowel movements, but with appropriate training and medical support, patients may experience as few as 4–8 bowel movements daily.

How is the large bowel at risk if not removed?	Colon cancer risk may be 3%–5% in the first decade of the disease, and as high as 20% in each subsequent decade.

CROHN DISEASE

What is it?	An inflammatory bowel condition that is transmural and marked by bowel wall thickening, ulcerations of mucosa, and "skip lesions" (i.e., lesions separated by normal portions of bowel). Characteristic granulomas are identified in only 60% of patients.
Which parts of the GI tract may be affected?	**Any part!** (Distal small bowel and colorectal regions most frequently.)
What is the epidemiology?	Incidence in boys and girls is the same. It is 5 times more common in whites than in blacks. The overall incidence has increased significantly during the past 50 years.
What age groups usually present with Crohn disease?	Adolescents and young adults
List typical signs and symptoms.	It can be insidious at onset. Typical symptoms include weight loss, abdominal pain, diarrhea, and fever. A perianal ulcer or abscess may be the initial manifestation. There may be rectal bleeding, but this is much less frequent than in ulcerative colitis.
What are the extraintestinal manifestations that may occur?	Growth failure—or growth deceleration—is common in children and often precedes the obvious GI symptoms. Other findings can include digital clubbing, delays in sexual maturation, skin lesions (most often erythema nodosum or pyoderma gangrenosum), large joint arthritis, liver lesions, uveitis, and chronic hypochromic microcytic anemia.
What are some options for medical therapy?	Medical therapy includes: 1. 5-ASA derivatives such as sulfasalazine, mesalamine, or

olsalazine administered either orally or by rectum.

2. Corticosteroids (Because of their side effects they cannot be used chronically.)

3. Other immunosuppressive agents shown to be effective include azathioprine, 6-mercaptopurine, cyclosporine, and anti-tumor necrosis factor antibodies.

4. Metronidazole may alleviate perianal or fistulous disease.

5. Ciprofloxacin

List 6 indications for surgery.

1. Failure of medical therapy to treat symptoms adequately
2. Intestinal obstruction
3. Abdominal abscess
4. Enteric fistulae or fistulae to the genitourinary tract
5. Perirectal fistula or abscess
6. Perforation of bowel (rare)

What is the surgical strategy?

Surgery is used to treat a specific problem and usually involves resection of a symptomatic section of bowel or drainage of perirectal abscesses. **Surgery is a palliative, not a curative, procedure.**

Can Crohn disease be cured?

There is currently no known cure.

ANTIBIOTIC-RELATED COLITIS (PSEUDOMEMBRANOUS COLITIS)

What is antibiotic-related colitis?

A condition in which the normal intestinal flora is altered because of the use of antibiotic medicine.

What is the primary symptom?

Generally, an increase in diarrheal stools. Stools may be bloody in severe cases.

What is the most commonly identified pathogen?

Clostridium difficile

List 3 ways in which the condition is identified.

1. Identification of a pathologic organism by stool culture

2. Identification of the toxin of a pathologic organism (primarily *C. difficile*) in the stool.
3. Sheets of WBCs are seen in the stool.

What is the treatment?

Discontinuing the antibiotic allows recovery of normal stool flora and function. If *C. difficile* is identified, metronidazole (by either mouth or IV) may be used for a cure. Other therapies include oral vancomycin, oral bacitracin, and oral bile-salt binding resins such as cholestyramine or colestipol.

CELIAC SPRUE (GLUTEN ENTEROPATHY)

What is it?

An acquired form of malabsorption. In susceptible hosts, the ingestion of gluten (e.g., wheat gluten and other similar proteins) causes immunologically mediated damage to the small intestinal mucosa.

At what age do patients typically present?

6–18 months of age.

What is the significance of the age of onset?

It correlates with the introduction of wheat, rye, or barley into the child's diet.

What are common signs and symptoms?

Diarrhea, a protuberant abdomen, wasted extremities, decreased height and weight.

What are other possible signs and symptoms?

Intermittent vomiting, irritability, abdominal pain, peripheral edema, long eyelashes, digital clubbing, and rectal prolapse.

A small number of children may present with isolated growth failure and an absence of GI symptoms.

What is the differential diagnosis?

Other causes of intestinal malabsorption: cystic fibrosis (CF), milk protein enteropathy, chronic giardiasis, Shwachman-Diamond syndrome, isolated pancreatic enzyme deficiencies, intestinal lymphangiectasia, abetalipoproteinemia, and chronic infections associated with immunodeficiency disorders.

What are 4 associated laboratory findings?	Most laboratory abnormalities in celiac sprue are caused by chronic malabsorption. Iron deficiency anemia, deficiencies of fat-soluble vitamins (prothrombin time may be prolonged because of vitamin K deficiency); abnormal 72-hour fecal fat excretion and D-xylose absorption; IgA deficiency.

List 3 ways it is diagnosed.

1. **The definitive test is a biopsy of the small intestine** revealing villous atrophy with hyperplasia of the crypts and abnormal surface epithelium.
2. Among children who are NOT IgA-deficient, the combination of anti-gliadin and tissue transglutaminase antibodies is sensitive and specific.
3. Full clinical remission after complete withdrawal of gluten from the diet.

What is the treatment?	The cornerstone of therapy is a **strict gluten-free diet,** in which wheat, rye, and barley are excluded from the diet and substituted with rice and corn. Parents must read all food labels, because wheat by-products are added to many foods. In severe cases, a **short course of corticosteroids** may help.
How long do patients have to stay on a gluten-free diet?	Celiac sprue is a lifelong disorder.
What are 2 long-term risks to affected individuals who continue to eat gluten?	**Osteoporosis** and **small bowel lymphoma**

PEPTIC ULCER DISEASE (PUD)

What is it?	The disruption of the gastric or duodenal mucosal barrier by a combination of pepsin and gastric acid
Do children get ulcers?	Yes
What is the incidence?	Overall incidence in children is unknown. It is estimated that 3–4 in 10,000 pediatric inpatients have PUD.

Do babies make enough acid to develop ulcers?

Yes—by 48 hours of life most infants have a gastric pH between 1 and 3, and by 3 years of age gastric acid secretion approximates adult values.

What are common signs and symptoms?

The most common symptom is **abdominal pain,** often most severe at night. Children older than 6–7 years of age generally complain of classic epigastric pain. Younger children usually complain of generalized or periumbilical pain, and occasionally right lower quadrant pain. Less common symptoms include **vomiting, hematemesis,** or **melena.**

Is perforated ulcer common in children?

No

What is in the differential diagnosis?

Functional abdominal pain, irritable bowel syndrome, gastroesophageal reflux, cholelithiasis, pancreatitis, urinary tract infection or obstruction, lower lobe pneumonia, Crohn disease, ovarian cysts, appendicitis, and constipation.

What is the most reliable method of diagnosis?

Flexible fiberoptic endoscopy. The sensitivity and specificity of double-contrast radiographic studies are only 60%–70%.

List 3 treatment options.

Antacids to neutralize acid; H_2 receptor antagonists or proton-pump inhibitors to inhibit acid secretion; sucralfate or bismuth compounds to provide a protective mucosal barrier. These therapies may be used individually or in combination.

How effective is medical treatment?

The most frequently prescribed therapy is a 6- to 8-week course of an H_2 receptor antagonist; effective in 85%–95% of cases.

What is the role of *Helicobacter pylori* in childhood PUD?

Unclear—about 15% of children undergoing endoscopy have evidence of *H. pylori* infection, but rates vary from 5%–75%. Children with documented *H. pylori* infection should probably be treated to eradicate the organism.

INTUSSUSCEPTION

What is it?

A segment of intestine with its associated mesentery (the intussusceptum) telescopes into an adjacent segment of intestine (the intussuscipiens) (See Figure 19–1).

What is the typical age at presentation?

More than 50% of recognized cases occur between 3–12 months of age, and more than 75% occur before 2 years of age.

Is there a gender predilection?

Boys by a 3:1 ratio.

What segments of intestine are most commonly involved?

Most cases are ileocolic, with the intussusception starting immediately proximal to the ileocecal valve. Colocolic, ileoileal, and ileoileocolic intussusceptions are much less common.

What are the causes?

More than 90% of cases are idiopathic, without an identifiable "anatomic lead

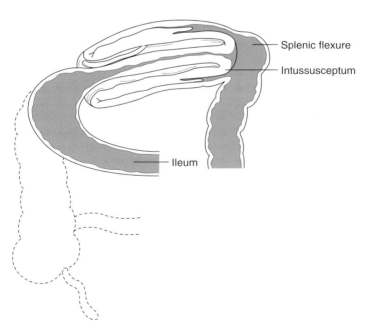

Figure 19–1. Development of intussusception.

point." Some researchers have hypothe-
sized that various viral illnesses cause
hypertrophy of Peyer's patches in the
terminal ileum, which serve as a lead
point for the intussusception.

What is the most commonly identified lead point?

Meckel diverticulum (see p. 277)

(see p. 277)

List 6 disorders that seem to predispose a child to intussusception.

CF, Henoch-Schönlein purpura, Meckel
diverticulum, juvenile inflammatory
polyps, *Ascaris lumbricoides* (round-
worm) infestation, and rotavirus infection.

What are the signs and symptoms?

Sudden onset of episodic crampy
abdominal pain, often with vomiting.
Between episodes of pain, the child may
be asymptomatic. Passage of stool and
flatus is diminished. Passage of dark blood
by rectum ("currant-jelly stools") suggests
venous congestion and mucosal slough-
ing. The intussusception may be palpable
on abdominal exam. As the symptoms
progress, the child may become lethargic
or somnolent.

How is it diagnosed?

The presentation is variable, and
clinicians must maintain a high index of
suspicion. Laboratory findings may be
nonspecific or may suggest dehydration.
Abdominal radiographs may be nonspecific or may suggest an abdominal mass,
intestinal obstruction, or rarely, free air.
The diagnosis is usually established with
an air or barium enema, which may also
be therapeutic.

What is the treatment?

Diagnosis and treatment of an intussusception is by either **an air or a barium
enema.** Pressure from the enema serves
to reduce the intussusception. Imaging of
the reduction is done with fluoroscopy
(ultrasound in some centers). The child
should receive IV hydration before the
enema. Evidence of peritonitis or a
general toxic state may be contraindications to the enema. A **surgeon should
be immediately available** when an

enema is performed in case the enema is unsuccessful or perforation occurs.

How often is an enema successful?

In about 80% of cases. The success rate is reduced if symptoms have been present > 48 hours.

What is the risk of perforation?

Approximately 1%

What is the incidence of recurrence after an enema?

Approximately 10% (usually within 48 hours of the initial episode).

What are 2 indications for surgery?

Failure of reduction by air or barium enema; signs or symptoms suggesting peritonitis or intestinal perforation.

What is involved in surgery?

The intussusception is usually approached and reduced through an open incision, although laparoscopy may be used in some cases. Occasionally, the intussuscepted section must be resected because the bowel cannot be reduced during surgery, or because the intussuscepted portion is necrotic.

ANORECTAL MALFORMATIONS

What is imperforate anus?

A spectrum of anomalies caused by an arrest of anorectal development during the cloacal stage between 4 and 12 weeks gestation

How does it manifest in boys?

There is no anal opening and, in most cases (90%), there is a fistula between the rectum and the urinary tract (urethra, the prostatic urethra, or the bladder).

How does it manifest in girls?

There is no opening in the anal region. About 80% of patients have a fistula into the perineum, vaginal fourchette, or vagina.

How are high, intermediate, and low anomalies defined?

1. High: rectal atresia is above the levator sling
2. Intermediate: atresia occurs at the level of the levator sling
3. Low: atresia is below the levator sling

On radiographs, the levator sling is determined by identifying the pubococcygeal line (upper border of the levator sling) and the line between the ischial tuberosities (lower border).

List 2 reasons the level of the anomaly is important.

1. The higher the anomaly, the less well formed are the sphincter mechanisms and the neurogenic innervation of these mechanisms.
2. High anomalies are also more likely to be associated with rectourinary fistulas in boys and high vaginal fistulas in girls.

Are boys or girls more prone to high anomalies?

Boys

What other types of anomalies are common when imperforate anus is recognized?

Duodenal atresia, esophageal atresia, vertebral anomalies, renal anomalies, Down syndrome, congenital heart disease, anomalies of the limbs. Imperforate anus represents one manifestation of the VACTERL association (see p. 272).

How is this condition managed?

In boys?

Initial end colostomy with distal stoma formation is usually needed. The extent of the anomaly is then assessed with a contrast study through the distal stoma into the atretic rectum. Voiding cystourethrogram (VCUG) is also needed to test for a possible rectourinary fistula.
Other studies look for the common associated anomalies. These include limb and vertebral radiographs, abdominal ultrasound, and echocardiography.

In girls?

If there is an external fistula to the perineum or vaginal fourchette, it can be dilated for the passage of stool. If the fistula opens into the vagina, a diverting colostomy should be considered. Assessment for other associated anomalies is needed as described above.

How is definitive treatment undertaken?

Usually the posterior sagittal anoplasty (popularized by Peña) is used to reconstruct the anus.

At what age is repair undertaken?

Most commonly, repair of imperforate anus takes place between 2–6 months of age. However, repairs are increasingly being done in the neonatal period as a 1-stage procedure without a diverting colostomy.

What are the outcomes?

Satisfactory continence is usually obtainable in infants with low-lying lesions. Continence may only be possible in about 50%–75% of patients in intermediate and high lesions.

What are cloacal malformations?

A condition in girls that represents a common opening of the vagina and rectum, or the urethra, vagina, and rectum

What is the treatment?

Assessment is performed in a manner similar to that for imperforate anus. Ultimately, all 3 pathways must be reconstructed, usually from the posterior approach.

HENOCH-SCHÖNLEIN PURPURA (HSP)

What is it?

HSP is a systemic vasculitis syndrome affecting small vessels.

At what age is HSP most common?

4–6 years of age, but can occur from 6 months to adulthood.

Are boys or girls more commonly affected?

Boys slightly more than girls.

Are there temporal or geographic predilections to HSP?

Increased incidence in the **spring** and **fall.** Most cases are sporadic, but temporal and geographic clusters occur.

What is the pathognomonic physical finding in HSP?

Virtually all patients have a characteristic skin rash: **palpable purpuric lesions** measuring 2–10 mm in diameter. Patients may also have coalescent ecchymoses and pinpoint petechiae. Typically, the purpura is concentrated on the buttocks and lower extremities, but it is not confined to those areas. New lesions appear in crops, then fade over several days. In one-third of patients, other symptoms precede the onset of the rash by several days, making it difficult to establish the diagnosis.

What is a common ortho-pedic manifestation?

Painful joint swelling (ankles, knees, and the dorsum of hands and feet) in approximately 80% of patients. The arthralgia is self-limited and usually abates with bed rest.

What are common GI manifestations?

Colicky abdominal pain, often accompanied by **vomiting,** in 50%–75% of patients. Occult or gross **GI bleeding** is present in 40% of patients. **Intussus-ception** is reported in 1%–5% of patients. Gastrointestinal involvement before the appearance of the rash may mimic appendicitis or inflammatory bowel disease.

List 3 rare but life-threatening GI complica-tions.

Bowel infarction, bowel perforation, massive GI bleeding

What is a common renal manifestation?

Nephritis in 50% of patients. Unlike joint or GI involvement, nephritis almost never precedes the onset of rash. Nephritis may be delayed for a number of weeks after the appearance of other symptoms, but usually becomes apparent within 3 months. It is manifested by microscopic or gross hematuria, pro-teinuria in two-thirds of patients, and hypertension in 25% of patients.

What are the less common complications?

Because HSP is a systemic vasculitis, any organ system may be affected. Other complications include intracranial bleed-ing, seizures, hemiparesis, coma, pancrea-titis, hydrops of the gallbladder, orchitis, pulmonary hemorrhage, ocular involvement, and carditis.

How long does HSP last?

Average duration is **2–4 weeks.**

What is the risk of recurrence?	One-third of patients will have 1 or more recurrences.
Who is most likely to have a recurrence?	Patients with nephritis
What is the usual nature of recurrence?	Usually occurs within 3 months of the original episode. Recurrences tend to mimic the original episode, but are usually milder and of shorter duration.
List 2 characteristic histologic features of HSP.	1. Biopsies of purpuric lesions show polymorphonuclear leukocyte infiltration in and around dermal vessels (leukocytoclastic vasculitis). 2. Immunofluorescent studies demonstrate granular deposits of IgA in the walls of vessels.
What characterizes the histologic changes in the kidney?	They range from minimal change to focal or diffuse mesangial proliferation. The characteristic finding on immunofluorescence is diffuse mesangial IgA deposits.
How is HSP diagnosed?	On clinical grounds—there is no diagnostic laboratory test for HSP. Laboratory studies help to exclude other conditions that resemble HSP.
What laboratory studies should be done?	CBC and platelet count; urinalysis; serum blood urea nitrogen (BUN) and creatinine; timed urine collection analysis for protein excretion and creatinine clearance in patients with nephritis
List 4 characteristic serologic findings.	**50%** of patients have **increased serum IgA.** Antinuclear antibody (ANA), rheumatoid factor (RF), and antineutrophil cytoplasmic antibodies (ANCA) are negative.
What are the etiologic factors?	Unknown—the epidemiology of HSP suggests infectious etiologic factors, and a variety of organisms have been implicated. HSP may represent an unusual immune response to a variety of infectious or environmental insults. It is

clear that IgA plays a pivotal role in the immunopathogenesis of HSP.

What is the pathophysiology of HSP?

Patients with HSP often have IgA-containing circulating immune complexes. Deposition of these immune complexes in vessel walls results in inflammatory vasculitis and accounts for the histologic and clinical features of HSP.

What is the treatment?

The mainstay of therapy is **supportive care.**

Why must hypertension be treated?

To prevent intracranial bleeding.

Which drugs should be avoided?

Salicylates and other drugs that interfere with platelet function should be avoided in patients with active GI bleeding.

Are steroids helpful?

Corticosteroids may alleviate joint and abdominal pain, but do not affect cutaneous purpura or hasten the resolution of the disease. Corticosteroids have no benefit in treating established nephritis.

What is the prognosis?

The prognosis is excellent for most patients.

Which manifestation is most prone to chronic problems?

Nephritis

What percent of patients develop end-stage renal disease (ESRD)?

$< 5\%$

What patients are at the highest risk for developing renal failure?

Patients with gross hematuria, massive proteinuria, and hypertension during the acute phase of the illness.

What is the relapse rate?

Approximately 10% of patients will have a relapse, generally within 2 weeks of completing therapy. A small number of children will experience multiple relapses. Relapses are most common in children who are immunocompromised, such as those receiving chemotherapy.

INTESTINAL TRANSPORT DEFECTS

What are they?

Isolated abnormalities of the absorption or secretion (i.e., transport) of specific ions or nutrients across the intestinal mucosa

What is the most common transport defect?

There are several defects that occur commonly. CF is most common and is related to abnormal secretion of chloride across many different tissues, including the intestinal mucosa.

What is the general presentation?

Usually **chronic diarrhea.** However, symptoms of each defect are best explained by an understanding of which ion or nutrient cannot be absorbed or transported.

What is congenital chloridorrhea?

The chloride-bicarbonate exchange mechanism in the ileum and colon is dysfunctional, causing excessive chloride secretion with resultant secretory diarrhea and hypokalemic metabolic alkalosis.

What is congenital glucose-galactose mal-absorption?

The active transport of glucose and galactose across the intestinal mucosa is defective; thus, the ingestion of any glucose or galactose causes osmotic diarrhea. Affected infants have severe diarrhea with profound growth failure.

What is X-linked hypo-phosphatemic rickets?

The renal and intestinal phosphate trans-port protein is defective, causing inade-quate intestinal phosphate absorption, excessive urinary phosphate loss, and severe rickets.

What is the treatment?

There are no specific treatments for most transport defects. Instead, the patient's symptoms and the metabolic abnormalities caused by the specific transport defect are treated.

APPENDICITIS

What is it?

Inflammation or infection, or both, of the appendix caused by occlusion of its lumen

What are some causes of occlusion of the lumen?

Stool (fecalith), inflamed or swollen lymphoid follicles, pinworm, or carcinoid tumors

What are common symptoms?

1. Abdominal pain: starts as generalized pain caused by irritation of visceral pain fibers; pain migrates to right lower quadrant as worsening appendicitis causes local irritation of peritoneum
2. Nausea and vomiting: usually follows onset of pain
3. Fever: usually, but not always present
4. Anorexia

What are common findings on physical examination?

1. Localized guarding and referred pain to the right lower quadrant; diffuse tenderness if appendix is ruptured. Tenderness may be less severe if the appendix is retrocecal or in another location if the appendix is malpositioned (e.g., malrotation).
2. Diminished bowel sounds
3. Pain upon iliopsoas extension
4. Possible mass or tenderness anteriorly on rectal exam
5. Possible palpable mass in right lower quadrant if the rupture is contained

List 6 potential diagnostic studies and what each shows.

1. WBCs: usually elevated with left shift
2. Urinalysis: a few (3–5) WBCs may be present secondary to local irritation of ureter or bladder
3. Abdominal radiograph: usually normal, but it may show fecalith, ileus or sentinel loop, loss of fat stripe in right lower quadrant, slight concavity of spine to right, air–fluid level in right lower quadrant suggestive of abscess
4. Ultrasound: may show thickened appendix or mass consistent with an abscess
5. Barium enema: nonfilling of appendix with irregularity of cecum
6. CT scan: best for delineating complex abscess. Is used in some centers routinely to diagnose appendicitis.

What is the treatment for uncomplicated appendicitis?

Surgical removal of appendix with perioperative antibiotic coverage.

For ruptured appendix?

Surgical removal of appendix and longer coverage with antibiotics (5–10 days)

For complex abscess?

May require initial drainage with later removal of appendix

PANCREATITIS

List the 4 most common causes of pancreatitis in children.

Trauma, cholelithiasis, CF, and congenital anomalies (such as choledochal cyst or pancreas divisum). Pancreatitis can also be seen in patients with inborn errors of metabolism, such as methylmalonic aciduria.

List 4 common signs and symptoms.

Midepigastric pain and **tenderness, vomiting**. A **palpable epigastric mass** may be present with extensive inflammation of the pancreas or pseudocyst formation.

What diagnostic studies are used?

Laboratory studies include serum amylase, lipase, and urine clearance of amylase. **Ultrasound** and **CT scan** are the best initial imaging studies. Magnetic resonance cholangiopancreatography (MCRP) may help define ductal anatomy. Endoscopic retrograde cholangiopancreatography (ERCP) can be performed for both diagnostic and therapeutic purposes (this is usually done when the pancreatitis has subsided and a cause is still unknown).

List 3 components of treatment.

IV fluids, cessation of oral intake, pain management; meperidine is usually the medicine of choice

Is surgical treatment needed?

Pancreatitis usually resolves with medical treatment.

List 5 indications for surgery.

1. Persistent pseudocyst may require drainage via a percutaneously placed catheter, or internal drainage via cyst-gastrostomy, cyst-duodenostomy, or cyst-jejunostomy.

2. Chronic pancreatitis with pancreatic ductal dilatation may require a pancreaticojejunostomy (Peustow procedure).
3. Extreme hemorrhagic pancreatitis may require debridement of the pancreas.
4. Trauma may disrupt the main pancreatic duct, requiring distal pancreatectomy with attempted spleen preservation.
5. Correction of congenital anomalies such as choledochal cyst or pancreas divisum that are causing pancreatitis.

HEMOLYTIC-UREMIC SYNDROME (HUS)

What is it?	A clinical syndrome of microangiopathic hemolytic anemia, thrombocytopenia, and acute renal failure. **HUS is the most common cause of acute renal failure in children** (Ch 21, p. 293).
What causes HUS?	Two-thirds of cases are preceded by an infection with vero-cytotoxin–producing *Escherichia coli* O157:H7. However, HUS may occur following infection with other bacterial pathogens, including *Shigella, Campylobacter, Salmonella,* and *Yersinia.*
What is the pathogenesis of HUS?	A variety of different bacterial toxins induce endothelial damage, which in turn initiates intravascular platelet activation, causing a diffuse small-vessel thrombosis throughout numerous organ systems.
What are the signs and symptoms?	1. 95% of HUS cases are preceded by gastroenteritis, and in nearly 75% of cases the associated **diarrhea** is bloody. 2. Diffuse **abdominal pain** and **vomiting** are common. 3. Resolution of the GI symptoms is associated with the abrupt onset of **pallor, easy bruisability, petechiae,** and **oliguria** secondary to acute renal insufficiency. (Do not confuse this with dehydration!)

4. CNS symptoms are common, including irritability and encephalopathy. **Seizures** may occur and are usually due to severe hypertension, hyponatremia, or both.

How is HUS diagnosed?

It is a syndrome diagnosed on clinical grounds.

What are common laboratory findings?

1. Thrombocytopenia
2. Anemia
3. Elevated BUN and creatinine
4. Elevated hepatocellular enzymes (50% of patients)
5. Elevated serum amylase and lipase (25% of patients)
6. RBCs and WBCs present on stool smear
7. Positive stool cultures for *E. Coli* O157:H7, *Campylobacter, Shigella,* or *Salmonella* (or *Yersinia* in some cases)

What are the radiographic and colonoscopic findings?

Barium enema generally demonstrates intestinal ischemia with "thumb printing," mucosal irregularity, and ulcerations.

Colonoscopic findings are nonspecific—primarily hyperemic mucosal edema and friability.

Barium enema and colonoscopy are not routinely performed unless the diagnosis is uncertain, as these maneuvers may exacerbate the colitis.

What is the treatment?

Supportive. Patients with severe GI symptoms receive **bowel rest** and **parenteral nutrition.** When clinically indicated, **red cell transfusions** and **diuretics** are administered and **fluid intake restricted.** Progressive renal insufficiency may require **peritoneal dialysis** or **hemodialysis**

What percent of children recover renal function?

95% within 2–3 weeks.

List 4 possible long-term complications.

Chronic renal insufficiency; intestinal fistulae or strictures; stroke with CNS deficits; chronic exocrine pancreatic insufficiency

CONSTIPATION

What is it?

A symptom, not a disease. It is the painful passage of large or hard bowel movements or the inability to expel a bowel movement.

What are normal childhood bowel habits?

    Infant?

Average stool frequency is 4 per day; 95% of children have from 1 stool every other day to 4 stools per day

    6 months to 2 years?

Average stool frequency is 2 per day. 95% of children have from 1 stool every other day to 4 stools per day.

    Older than 2 years?

Average stool frequency is 1 per day. 95% of children have from 1 stool every third day to 3 stools per day.

What is the relation between constipation and frequency of bowel movements?

The frequency of defecation is influenced by diet and social custom. "Constipation" refers to the character of the stool and the symptoms associated with defecation rather than the frequency of defecation.

How common is constipation in children?

As many as 20% of children ≤ 5 years of age will be brought to medical attention because of constipation. **Constipation is the most common reason children are referred to a pediatric gastroenterologist.**

List 3 main symptoms.

1. Pain associated with the passage of bowel movements
2. Bowel movements that are large, hard, or both
3. Infrequent bowel movements

See additional symptoms below.

List 5 additional symptoms children may experience.

Intermittent crampy abdominal pain, abdominal distension, intermittent vomiting, early satiety, decreased appetite.

What are the physical signs?

A distended abdomen with palpable stool in the colon on rectal examination. Anal fissures may be present, and the rectum is generally enlarged and filled with stool. Rectal prolapse may be present. Chronic constipation is the most common cause of rectal prolapse in children.

Why do children develop constipation?

In otherwise healthy children, more than 99% of cases have clearly no obvious cause and are called "functional constipation." In most children, constipation develops after the passage of several large or hard bowel movements with associated pain. This often occurs following weaning, a change in diet, school entry, an episode of gastroenteritis, or during toilet training.

What is the treatment?

The primary goal is to eliminate the pain associated with defecation. This generally means softening the stools.

In young children?

Fruit juices or dark corn syrup (such as Karo syrup) are effective. Alternatively, osmotic cathartics, such as magnesium hydroxide (milk of magnesia) or lactulose, are safe and effective.

In older children with chronic constipation?

Dietary measures are often inadequate, and laxatives (magnesium hydroxide, milk of magnesia), mineral oil, lactulose, senna derivatives, and dioctyl sodium sulfosuccinate (Colace) must be used.

In the most severe and chronic cases?

Several enemas to evacuate the colon may be needed before oral cathartics are effective. Rarely, manual disimpaction under anesthesia is required.

What are the risks of laxative use?

In an otherwise healthy child, the use of any over-the-counter laxative is safe. The major side effects of laxative overdosage are diarrhea, nausea and vomiting, and abdominal cramps.
Despite common belief, long-term use of laxatives does not cause dependency or "cathartic colon."

How are functional constipation and Hirschsprung disease differentiated?	In most cases they can be differentiated on the basis of the history and physical examination. Functional constipation is far more common than Hirschsprung disease. (See Hirschsprung Disease, p. 265.) A useful differentiating point is that constipated children will still pass flatus relatively easily, while children with Hirschsprung disease will not.

ENCOPRESIS

What is it?	Fecal incontinence, or soiling
How common is encopresis in children?	Among children older than 4 years of age, between 1%–3% will be incontinent of stool more than once weekly.
What is the main cause of encopresis?	Prolonged constipation with resulting overflow incontinence.
What are some of the other causes of fecal incontinence in children?	In rare circumstances, it is due to an underlying neurologic deficit (e.g., very low meningomyelocele or tethered spinal cord).
Is encopresis primarily a psychological problem?	Although many children with chronic encopresis have psychological and behavioral difficulties, many of these problems are a result, rather than the cause, of their fecal soiling.
What is a typical history?	There is usually at least a remote history of constipation. Soiling generally begins as small streaks of stool in the underwear. As the problem progresses, the volume and frequency of the soiling increase. The child denies any sense of the need to defecate prior to the accidents. If soiling occurs several times daily, it is often confused with diarrhea.
What are the features commonly found on physical examination?	A protuberant abdomen, with stool palpable throughout the colon. The rectal sphincter is often lax, and the rectum is large and filled with soft stool. An abdominal radiograph shows abundant stool throughout the colon.

List 2 components of treatment.

Treatment is essentially the same as that for severe, chronic constipation.
1. The colon must be completely evacuated with enemas, oral cathartics, or by manual disimpaction.
2. When the colon is completely empty, laxatives are started in doses sufficient to produce 1 or 2 soft stools daily.

The child should be encouraged to sit on the toilet for 5–10 minutes after breakfast and dinner. Some children may benefit from biofeedback therapy.

HIRSCHSPRUNG DISEASE

What is it?

Aganglionosis of the rectum or colon, causing a functional obstruction. The aganglionosis extends from the rectum proximally in a contiguous manner to some level, usually the upper rectum or left colon.

What is the transition zone?

The point where aganglionic bowel meets ganglionic bowel. It can be anywhere, but is usually in the rectosigmoid region. Occasionally the entire colon may be aganglionic, resulting in total colonic Hirschsprung disease.

What are common signs and symptoms?

They may be insidious. Initial manifestation may be an infant's failure to pass meconium within the first 24 hours of life (95% of patients) (see Chapter 9, Common Clinical Problems, p. 82). Subsequently, there is increasing difficulty with bowel movements leading to severe constipation, overflow diarrhea, and sometimes enterocolitis and sepsis.

List 4 associated conditions.

Down syndrome; Waardenburg syndrome; cartilage-hair hypoplasia; neonatal appendicitis

How is it diagnosed?

1. **UNPREPPED single contrast enema** is used to search for the transition zone. The ganglionic portion will be dilated. This may not be evident early in the course.

2. Definitive diagnosis is established by absence of ganglion cells and increased acetylcholinesterase staining on a **rectal biopsy** specimen. Cholinergic and adrenergic nerve endings also may be evident.

How is it treated?

1. Traditionally, when Hirschsprung is diagnosed, a leveling colostomy (i.e., a colostomy immediately proximal to the level of the transition zone) is performed.
2. Later, a colon pull-through procedure (Swenson, Soave, Duhamel) may be performed.
Currently, the pull-through is often performed as the initial operation, many times transanally with laparoscopic assistance.

What are the outcomes?

With appropriate surgical care, 85% of patients will have normal bowel function. Others may have functional motility difficulties despite presence of ganglion cells.

MALROTATION

What is it?

Failure of the gut to make its normal 270° counterclockwise rotation during in utero development

What are 3 anatomic results?

1. Unrotation of gut of varying degrees with the ligament of Treitz to the right of, or at, the midline, and a mobile cecum
2. Ladd's bands
3. Narrow mesenteric pedicle

What are Ladd's bands?

Peritoneal attachments of the now-mobile ascending colon to the right abdominal wall. They may stretch across the duodenum, causing obstruction.

What is the most dangerous aspect of malrotation?

The narrow pedicle may cause **volvulus** and subsequent loss of part or all of the bowel. **This may be lethal!**

At what age does a patient present with malrotation?	At any age! However, about 80% of patients with malrotation who have symptoms do so within the first 2 months of life.
List 4 conditions in which malrotation is commonly found.	Diaphragmatic hernia; gastroschisis; omphalocele; duodenal and intestinal atresia
List 3 potential symptoms.	1. Vomiting, usually of bilious material **(Vomiting of bilious material in an infant ≤ 4–6 months of age is malrotation with volvulus until proven otherwise!)** 2. Intermittent abdominal pain 3. Systemic collapse if volvulus has progressed to frank bowel necrosis
List 4 potential signs.	Patient may have a distended abdomen; usually no peritoneal irritation unless bowel injury is present; dehydration; weight loss
What is the definitive diagnostic study?	An **upper GI series** will identify a malposition of the ligament of Treitz and associated volvulus if present. A barium enema may show malposition of cecum, but the position may be normal even if the cecum has inappropriately oriented peritoneal attachments.
What is the treatment?	Surgical correction with the Ladd's procedure.
What is involved in the Ladd's procedure?	Ladd's bands are divided, the colon is mobilized to the left with the cecum situated near the sigmoid colon, the duodenum is mobilized and straightened, and an appendectomy is performed.
What is done if volvulus is present?	The bowel is turned counterclockwise on its mesentery until the volvulus is relieved. If there is necrotic bowel, this is resected, and anastomosis or stomas are performed as appropriate.
What is the outcome?	Usually very good. However, if volvulus is serious, an extensive loss of bowel may result in short-gut syndrome.

CONGENITAL DUODENAL OBSTRUCTION

What is it?	An obstruction of the duodenum secondary to failure of the recanalization process of the fetal duodenum. It occurs during the eighth to tenth week of development.
List the 3 most common types of congenital duodenal obstruction.	Duodenal atresia; duodenal stenosis; duodenal web
What is annular pancreas?	A failure in the proper rotation of the pancreas may cause an annular pancreas, which also causes duodenal obstruction. Some researchers theorize that annular pancreas is an anatomic phenomenon secondary to one of the primary duodenal conditions noted above.
What is the usual location of duodenal obstruction?	The first or second part of the duodenum. It may involve the entrance of the common bile duct.
What are typical signs and symptoms of duodenal obstruction?	Vomiting, which may be bilious; abdominal distension secondary to distended stomach and duodenum
What are 2 prenatal ultrasound findings?	**Polyhydramnios** and a **dilated duodenum.**
What is the characteristic radiographic finding?	"**Double-bubble**" sign of dilated stomach and duodenum
How is a definitive diagnosis made?	A contrast study shows total or partial duodenal obstruction with a rounded dilated duodenum (as opposed to the beak-like appearance found in malrotation with volvulus).
Which conditions and malformations are sometimes found with congenital duodenal obstruction?	One-third of affected infants have Down syndrome. Other anomalies include intestinal atresia, malrotation, imperforate anus, cardiac anomalies, and other anomalies of VACTERL association (see p. 272).
How is it treated preoperatively?	NG drainage with rehydration.

What are 3 surgical options?	Surgical correction may be done semi-electively unless malrotation is suspected, which makes repair more urgent.
	1. Duodenoduodenostomy (most common)
	2. Vertical duodenotomy through an involved web or stenosis with transverse duodenoplasty
	3. Duodenojejunostomy
	Malrotation or other atresia must be sought at operation.
What is the outcome?	Usually good, though return to full feeding is often slow as the duodenum recovers motility.

INTESTINAL ATRESIA

What is it?	A congenital condition in which the lumen of the bowel is interrupted
Where may an intestinal atresia occur?	Anywhere from the jejunum to the rectum; atresias may be multiple
List 5 classifications and their characteristics.	**Type I:** The mucosa is interrupted by a web, but the proximal dilated loop of bowel and decompressed distal loop are still connected at the serosal level.
	Type II: The proximal dilated bowel and distal decompressed bowel are connected by a fibrous atretic cord.
	Type IIIa: The proximal and distal portions of bowel are separated, as is the mesentery to these 2 portions of bowel.
	Type IIIb: The distal atretic bowel is spiraled around a segmental artery in an apple-peel form.
	Type IV: Multiple atresias are present. **(See Figure 19–2.)**
How do they occur?	They are believed to be the result of a vascular accident in utero.
How may a patient present?	1. Newborns generally develop a distended abdomen soon after birth, if it is not already present at birth.
	2. Bilious vomiting ensues, or if an NG

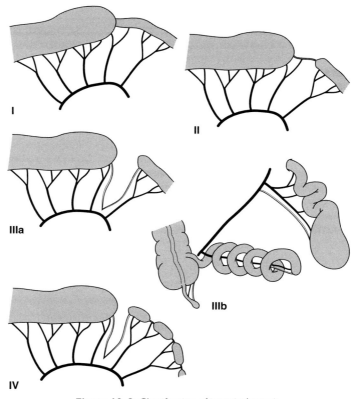

Figure 19–2. Classification of intestinal atresia.

tube has already been placed, voluminous bilious output is present.
3. Infants may pass meconium because atresias occasionally develop after meconium has passed to the distal bowel in utero.
4. Rarely, the proximal portion of bowel may perforate in utero.

What is the differential diagnosis?

Malrotation with volvulus, bowel duplication, internal hernia, adynamic ileus with sepsis, meconium ileus, Hirschsprung disease, small left colon syndrome

What is the method for diagnosis?

A contrast enema is performed in the newborn when evidence of bowel obstruction occurs. A microcolon will be visualized without connection to the proximal dilated bowel.

What is the treatment?   **Surgical correction** is necessary.

What is involved in surgical correction?   For jejunal, ileal, or proximal colonic atresia, resection of the dilated portion of the proximal bowel and the atretic portion of the distal bowel is performed, followed by anastomosis. For distal colonic atresia, an end colostomy is typically performed first, and later an anastomosis is performed.

What is the outcome?   The current survival rate is 90%–100%.

ESOPHAGEAL ATRESIA/TRACHEOESOPHAGEAL FISTULA (TEF)

What is it?   A spectrum of anomalies consisting of discontinuity of the esophagus with or without fistula(e); or a fistula between the esophagus and the trachea without esophageal discontinuity.

List the 5 types and their characteristics.   **Type A:** esophageal atresia without fistula
Type B: esophageal atresia with fistula between upper portion of esophagus and trachea
Type C: esophageal atresia with fistula between lower portion of esophagus and trachea
Type D: esophageal atresia with a fistula between the upper portion of esophagus and trachea and a fistula between the lower portion of esophagus and trachea
Type E: esophagus in continuity with isolated fistula between esophagus and trachea
(See Figure 19–3.)

Which type is most common?   Type C (85%)

What is the incidence?   1 in 3000 births, with an equal incidence between boys and girls. Prematurity is common among patients.

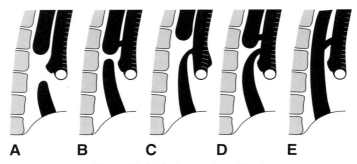

A   B   C   D   E

Figure 19–3. Tracheoesophageal fistula.

What is the VACTERL association?	A constellation of anomalies that commonly occur together, either entirely or in part, more often than would be expected by "chance." **V**ertebral **A**norectal (imperforate anus) **C**ardiac **T**racheal **E**sophageal **R**enal/genitourinary **L**imb/lumbar Infants need to be screened for all of these anomalies when any one of them is present.
List 2 other anomalies that are commonly associated with TEF.	Duodenal atresia and bowel atresias
What are the symptoms of TEF?	
Types A, B, C, D?	Excessive drooling; feeding induces choking, coughing, regurgitation, and cyanosis.
Type E?	Presentation usually delayed; feeding induces coughing and choking; repeated episodes of pneumonia
What are chest and abdomen radiographic findings for each type?	**Type A:** dilated upper esophageal pouch with gasless abdomen **Type C:** dilated upper esophageal pouch with normal bowel pattern **Types B, D, E:** may be normal

How is it diagnosed?

Types A, B, C, D: (List 3 components)	1. Inability to pass suction catheter beyond upper esophagus
	2. Presence of gas in bowel indicates fistula or fistulae between esophagus and trachea
	3. Instillation of thin barium into esophageal pouch confirms atresia of esophagus and determines presence of a proximal fistula. Bronchoscopic exam may be used to determine presence of proximal fistula.
Type E:	Barium swallow; physician may need to instill barium into esophagus with patient in Trendelenburg position to demonstrate fistula.

What is the treatment?

Type A:	1. Placement of gastrostomy tube
	2. Drainage of the upper pouch with a Replogle tube, and attempt at primary closure at around 12 weeks of age after the esophagus has had time to grow. If anastomosis is not possible, one of the options from number 3 below must be performed.
	3. Esophagostomy with later colon interposition, jejunal interposition, or gastric tube formation
Types B, C, D:	1. Thoracotomy via fourth intercostal space
	2. Extrapleural approach
	3. Division of fistula(e) with anastomosis of esophagus
Type E: (List 1)	Division of fistula via right cervical incision
List 4 possible complications.	Infection, stricture of the esophagus, leak of the esophageal anastomosis, recurrence of the fistula
What feeding precautions are necessary for children with repaired TEF?	The esophagus motility is impaired. Ultimately, feeding is normal, but chunky foods should be avoided until the child

can chew well. The esophagus caliber is
usually large enough to handle all foods
by that time.

PYLORIC STENOSIS

What is it?	Hypertrophy of the pyloric muscle, causing gastric outlet obstruction
What is the incidence?	1 in 500–1000. Male-to-female ratio is 4:1
What are the etiologic factors?	Unknown. Suggested processes include decreased number of ganglion cells, hypergastrinemia, edema secondary to feeding, and a decrease in nitric oxide synthase. It is a "multifactorial" condition.
What is the most common symptom?	Progressive, projectile, **non-bilious** vomiting that occurs after feeding. (The infant is then very hungry again.)
List 4 physical signs.	1. Abdominal protuberance possibly present secondary to gastric distension 2. Gastric waves visible through abdominal wall 3. Palpable pylorus deep in epigastrium ("olive sign") 4. Dehydration sometimes present
What metabolic abnormalities may be noted?	Dehydration; hypokalemic, hypochloremic metabolic alkalosis; and hypoglycemia. Rehydration and correction of electrolytes are necessary before surgery. Potassium and glucose need to be included judiciously in resuscitative fluid.
List 2 ways in which it is diagnosed.	Ultrasound (the best study); upper GI series: the "string sign" (i.e., a string of barium passing through pylorus) is seen. (**Caution:** pyloric spasm may mimic pyloric stenosis on upper GI series.)
How is it treated?	Ramstedt pyloromyotomy via open incision or laparoscopically.
What is the outcome?	Excellent. Babies begin feeding 4–6 hours after surgery.

INTESTINAL POLYPS

What are they?	Tumors that protrude into the lumen of the bowel
What are the most common polyps in children?	Juvenile inflammatory polyps
What are juvenile inflammatory polyps?	Mucosal lesions consisting of dilated and tortuous mucus-filled glands, with a prominent inflammatory infiltrate in the lamina propria. The glands are composed of well-differentiated, mucus-secreting cells.
What size are they?	The polyps are erythematous pedunculated masses 0.5–3.0 cm in diameter.
List 2 other characteristics.	They are often quite friable and bleed when manipulated
Where in the bowel are they most commonly found?	Although juvenile inflammatory polyps may develop anywhere in the large intestine, nearly two-thirds are located in the distal colon beyond the splenic flexure.
Are polyps solitary or multiple?	Either. More often they are multiple.
Are juvenile inflammatory polyps considered pre-cancerous?	No
What is the most common symptom?	Intermittent painless rectal bleeding in children 1–10 years of age. The blood is generally bright red and either streaked on or intermixed with the stool.
List 4 less common clinical features.	Intermittent abdominal pain; vomiting; colocolonic intussusception; prolapse of the polyp through the anal canal
How common are juvenile inflammatory polyps?	They are the most commonly identified cause of painless rectal bleeding in children 1–10 years of age.
How are they diagnosed?	Flexible colonoscopy. Polypectomy is

usually safely performed with snare electrocautery through the scope.

Must all juvenile inflammatory polyps be removed?	Most ultimately outgrow their vascular supply, and autoamputate. The diagnosis is sometimes first suspected when a child passes a polyp in the stool. Since polyps are often asymptomatic and have no malignant potential, colonoscopic intervention is not always warranted.
What other conditions may be associated with intestinal polyps in children?	Peutz-Jeghers syndrome, familial polyposis coli, Cowden syndrome, and Gardner syndrome.
Can these polyps become malignant?	Yes. In order to prevent malignancy, total colon resection with ileo-anal pull-through may be needed (especially in familial polyposis syndrome and Gardner syndrome).

BEZOAR

What is it?	A mass of ingested material, usually hair and vegetable matter, that has congealed and settled in the stomach
What is the cause?	It usually results from children (more commonly boys) eating their own hair. (Often, emotionally disturbed children will do this, although not all develop bezoars.)
List 5 symptoms.	Nausea, vomiting, early satiety, inability to eat, weight loss
What are the physical signs?	Mass in epigastrium or left upper quadrant
How is it diagnosed?	Usually with an upper GI series
List 2 treatments.	1. Removal of the bezoar is performed via open gastrotomy. 2. Meat tenderizer or removal with endoscopy may be used for small bezoars. Note: Any underlying emotional disorders should be evaluated and treated.

PICA

What is it?	Persistent eating of significant amounts of non-nutritive substances (e.g., dirt, clay, paint chips)
Does pica always indicate a serious problem?	Not always. During the first 2 years of life, mouthing and eating a wide variety of objects is normal exploratory behavior. In many older children and adults, the chewing and eating of non-nutritive substances (e.g., fingernails, pencils, ice cubes) represent a habit rather than a serious medical problem.
What are the causes?	The pathophysiology is not understood. Pica is a symptom, not a disease, and its presence may indicate an underlying disorder. Pica is most commonly observed in children with developmental disabilities, autism, or mental retardation.
What are the complications of pica?	Complications are related to the substances ingested. The most serious complications of pica are **intestinal obstruction** and **lead poisoning.** Iron deficiency anemia is seen in some patients.

MECKEL DIVERTICULUM

What is a Meckel diverticulum?	A remnant of the embryonic vitelline or omphalomesenteric duct that is a true diverticulum (contains all layers of bowel wall).
What is the incidence?	2% of the population
Where is it located?	The antimesenteric border of the ileum, usually within 2 feet of the ileocecal valve in an adult
What types of ectopic tissue may be present?	Pancreatic or gastric in 25% of cases.
What are symptoms of Meckel diverticula?	Most are asymptomatic throughout life. However, symptoms may include: 1. Profuse rectal bleeding (the most common symptom)

2. Abdominal pain caused by inflammation
3. Obstruction caused by intussusception

What causes bleeding from a Meckel diverticulum?

Erosion of mucosa opposite the diverticulum caused by production of acid from ectopic gastric mucosa

How is it diagnosed?

A symptomatic Meckel diverticulum can often be detected with a technetium-99M pertechnetate scan ("Meckel scan"), which images gastric mucosa. It may sometimes be discovered during laparotomy or laparoscopy for non-reducible intussusception or peritonitis, or incidentally at surgery.

What is the treatment?

Surgical excision of the diverticulum with primary bowel closure.

What is a Littré hernia?

An umbilical or inguinal hernia containing a Meckel diverticulum

PERIANAL AND PERIRECTAL ABSCESS

What is a perianal abscess?

An infected subcutaneous collection in the perianal region

Who is most commonly affected in the pediatric population?

Infants

What is the most common cause?

An infected diaper rash

What are typical signs and symptoms?

A firm, red, fluctuant area in the perianal region. The infant may have a fever and may be irritable.

List 2 components of treatment.

1. Lancing the area for drainage of pus.
2. Antibiotics may be necessary to resolve the surrounding cellulitis.

What is a perirectal abscess?

An infected collection that extends within the intersphincteric region

What are the signs and symptoms?

Fever and perirectal pain. External signs may be minimal initially because the infection is more recessed from the perianal region.

Who is most commonly affected in the pediatric population?

Infants—in these cases the abscess usually results from stool gathering within a violated anal crypt.

List 2 components of the treatment.

1. Lancing for adequate drainage of pus.
2. Antibiotics are necessary for perirectal abscesses.

Can perianal or perirectal abscesses recur?

Yes. If they do recur, then a fistula is present.

How are these treated?

A probe is placed through the skin opening to the open anal crypt. The overlying skin and muscle are divided and the fistula is curetted. Very deep perirectal abscesses may be better treated with a Seton wire.

List 4 conditions that can predispose older children to perianal and perirectal abscess.

Crohn disease (see p. 244), leukemia, immunodeficiency disorders, diabetes

20 Liver and Hepatobiliary Disorders

CHOLELITHIASIS (GALLSTONES)

What are the 3 types of gallstones?

Cholesterol; pigmented; mixed-type stones

Which stones are most common in children?

Cholesterol stones

What causes cholesterol stones?

An imbalance of **lecithin, bile salts,** and **cholesterol** in bile

List 3 causes of pigmented stones.

1. Breakdown products from blood in hemolytic diseases or after heart surgery
2. Abnormal absorption of bile after ileal resection
3. Cholestasis resulting from total parenteral nutrition (TPN)

What is the incidence of gallstones in children?

2 cases per 1000 children

List 5 risk factors for gallstones in neonates and infants.

Prematurity, ileal resection, cystic fibrosis (CF), TPN, prolonged fasting. Some neonates have idiopathic stones.

What are predisposing conditions in older children?

Hemolytic disorders or idiopathic cholesterol gallstones

List 3 ways in which a patient with gallstones presents clinically.

1. **Biliary colic:** intermittent right upper quadrant or epigastric pain, associated with eating, which results from obstruction of the cystic duct by a stone

2. **Cholecystitis:** inflammation of the gallbladder secondary to cystic duct obstruction from a stone
3. **Obstruction of the common bile duct:** may cause persistent right upper quadrant or epigastric pain, jaundice, acholic stools, dark urine, and cholangitis

What is the most useful imaging study?

Ultrasound is best for detecting stones within the gallbladder as well as evidence of extrahepatic ductal dilatation.

List 5 useful laboratory values and what they show.

1. **Serum bilirubin** may be elevated in hemolytic disorders, common bile duct obstruction, or cholecystitis.
2. **Alkaline phosphatase** may be elevated with common bile duct obstruction.
3. **Hepatocellular enzymes** may be elevated in cases of cholestasis.
4. **γ-Glutamyl transpeptidase** may be elevated in the presence of an obstructing common bile duct stone.
5. **Elevated serum amylase** may indicate the presence of associated pancreatitis or common bile duct obstruction, or both.

List and describe 2 kinds of treatment.

1. **Surgery**—Resection of the gall-bladder (with an intraoperative cholangiogram when indicated). If common duct stones are present, they are removed via a common bile duct exploration, through the cystic duct, or via endoscopic retrograde cholangio-pancreatography (ERCP). Surgical procedures can be performed laparoscopically or open.
2. **Expectant management**—In an infant or child who develops sludge or gallstones from TPN cholestasis, and who is otherwise asymptomatic, stones may be expected to resolve after the TPN has been discontinued. In addition, infants with idiopathic stones

can usually be observed because these stones will usually pass or resolve without symptoms.

HEPATITIS

What is hepatitis?	Inflammation of the liver (hepatocytes)
Are all types of hepatitis infectious?	No
List 5 causes of hepatitis other than viruses.	Trauma, metabolic diseases (e.g., galactosemia and α-1-antitrypsin deficiency), Reye syndrome, vascular obstruction, chemical toxicity (including certain medications)
What is chronic hepatitis?	A persistent inflammation of the liver
List 3 causes of chronic hepatitis.	Infection, immune (autoimmune) disorders, metabolic disorders
Which hepatitis viruses are associated with chronic hepatitis?	Usually the parenteral viruses: hepatitis B, C, and D
How do chronic active hepatitis and chronic persistent hepatitis differ?	Histologically, chronic active hepatitis involves the limiting plate of the portal triad, whereas chronic persistent hepatitis does not.
Which has a better prognosis?	Chronic persistent hepatitis
What is the most common cause of unconjugated hyperbilirubinemia in children?	Viral hepatitis
What viruses cause hepatitis?	Hepatitis viruses A, B, C, D, and E; herpes simplex virus; varicella-zoster virus; cytomegalovirus; Epstein-Barr virus; adenovirus; enterovirus; rubella virus; parvovirus; influenza viruses
How does a child with viral hepatitis present?	Variable. The manifestations may range from subclinical ("anicteric") to overwhelming liver necrosis and failure.

What is the typical clinical presentation of symptomatic viral hepatitis?

In the preicteric phase? (List 5 symptoms)

Fever, malaise, loss of appetite, abdominal pain, right upper quadrant tenderness

Icteric phase? (List 4)

Jaundice, light (clay-colored) stools, dark urine (secondary to bilirubinuria), increased serum levels of hepatic transaminases

HEPATITIS A

How is it spread?

Usually via the fecal-oral route

List 3 sources of infection.

Contaminated water; foods (including raw shellfish); person-to-person contact (particularly among younger children)

What is the common name for hepatitis A?

Infectious hepatitis

What is the chance of an infected child passing the disease to another household member?

About 10%–20%

What is the incubation period?

About 4 weeks, although it can range from 10–50 days

How is a child's presentation different from an adult's?

Children are more likely to have anicteric hepatitis, with subclinical disease. Most children with serologic evidence of prior hepatitis A infection have no history of clinical jaundice beyond the neonatal period.
See Figure 20–1 for the pattern of response to hepatitis A virus (HAV) infection.

What is the laboratory diagnosis?

Demonstration of **IgM anti-hepatitis A antibodies** in serum

Is demonstration of IgG anti-hepatitis A antibodies useful?

Somewhat. These titers rise later than IgM and may persist, so the positive IgG antibody does not necessarily represent acute infection.

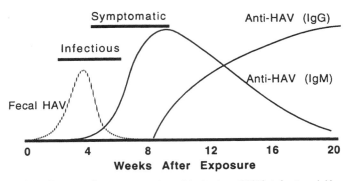

Figure 20–1. Pattern of response to hepatitis A virus (HAV) infection. *IgM* = immunoglobulin M; *IgG* = immunoglobulin G. (From Behrman RE, Kliegman RM, Jenson HB, eds: *Nelson Textbook of Pediatrics, 16th edition.* Philadelphia, W.B. Saunders Co., 2000, p 770.)

List 3 ways in which hepatitis A infection can be prevented.	1. Good hygiene practices 2. Good public health measures 3. Immune globulin injections within 2 weeks of exposure can prevent infection or reduce disease.
Is there a vaccine for hepatitis A?	Yes
Does hepatitis A lead to chronic hepatitis?	Usually not
What is the treatment of hepatitis A?	Usually supportive

HEPATITIS B

What is another name for hepatitis B?	Serum hepatitis
List 3 usual routes by which it is spread.	Usually via **parenteral** routes, including blood and blood products; sexual transmission; maternal-child transmission
What is hepatitis Be antigen?	A secreted soluble antigen that is highly associated with infectivity
What is hepatitis B surface antigen (HBsAg)?	The major envelope protein of the virus
What is hepatitis core (HBc) antigen?	The major protein in the viral capsid See Figure 20–2 for the pattern of

response to hepatitis B virus infection.

Which antigen correlates best with infectivity?

Hepatitis Be antigen

What is the risk of transplacental infection to the infant of a known hepatitis B-infected mother?

The risk depends on the mother's hepatitis Be antigen status. If positive, the risk of transplacental infection is 65%–85%. If negative, the risk is 10%–20%.

When does mother-to-infant transmission usually occur?

During delivery

What is meant by "chronic carrier state"?

Patients infected with hepatitis B who have a persistent viral infection

Who are most likely to become chronic carriers?

Infected infants

List 3 risks to chronic carriers.

Persistent infectivity; chronic liver disease; hepatocellular carcinoma

How is hepatitis B infection usually diagnosed?

Usually via serologic testing for **serum antibodies against HBsAg and HBc** and for the **presence of the HBsAg**

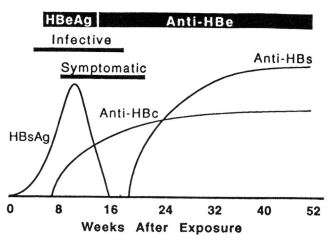

Figure 20–2. Pattern of response to hepatitis B virus infection. *HbeAg* = hepatitis Be antigen; *HBsAg* = hepatitis B surface antigen; *HBc* = hepatitis B core antigen. (From Behrman RE, Kliegman RM, Jenson HB, eds: *Nelson Textbook of Pediatrics, 16th edition.* Philadelphia, W.B. Saunders Co., 2000, p 772.)

What is the first serum marker of hepatitis B infection?	Presence of HBsAg
Which antibody usually appears first after an acute hepatitis B infection?	Anti-HBc (detectable at around 15 weeks)
List 4 ways in which hepatitis B infection can be prevented.	1. Universal precautions for health care workers 2. Decreased exposure by high-risk individuals 3. **Hepatitis B vaccine**—available and effective 4. **Hepatitis B immune globulin** for passive immunization
List 2 components of treatment for an infant born to an infected mother.	Hepatitis B immune globulin; hepatitis B vaccine within 12 hours of birth
Is hepatitis B vaccine recommended for all infants?	Yes
Is there any effective treatment for chronic hepatitis B infection?	Alpha and gamma interferons (INF-α and INF-γ) appear to have limited effectiveness. Preliminary evidence suggests that continuous treatment with the antiviral agent lamivudine is effective at suppressing viral replication. However, therapy does not usually eradicate the virus.

HEPATITIS C

List 3 ways in which it may be spread.	1. Usually via parenteral routes 2. Possibly via sexual transmission. 3. Mother-to-infant transmission—estimated to occur in fewer than 10% of cases, which is far less common than with hepatitis B
List 2 ways it is usually diagnosed.	Serology: enzyme-linked immunosorbent assay (ELISA); polymerase chain reaction (PCR)
When does the ELISA test become positive, if infection is present?	It may be up to 8–12 weeks after infection before the ELISA is positive, although it may be positive earlier.

What is the treatment?	Prolonged therapy with alpha and gamma interferons (INF-α and INF-γ) eradicates the virus in 20%–40% of cases. The addition of the antiviral agent ribavirin appears to improve cure rates in adults.
What is the risk for chronic liver disease?	Risk may be as high as 70% of infected patients

HEPATITIS D

What is another name for the hepatitis D virus?	Delta virus
By what route is it usually transmitted?	Usually via blood products
What is its relationship to hepatitis B infection?	Infection with hepatitis B virus (either previous or concurrent) is required.
In what way is it diagnosed?	Demonstration of anti-hepatitis D virus antibodies

HEPATITIS E

How is it spread?	Fecal-oral route
What is the incubation period?	2–9 weeks
How is it diagnosed?	Diagnosis is usually based on epidemiology and exclusion of other viruses.

BILIARY ATRESIA

What is it?	Abnormality of the intrahepatic or extrahepatic bile ducts, or both, in which the ducts are microscopic in size, fibrous cords, or completely absent
What is the incidence?	1 in 15,000
List 5 associated defects.	Congenital heart disease (CHD)(Ch 16, p. 183); absent inferior vena cava; preduodenal portal vein; intestinal malrotation (Ch 19, p. 266); and polysplenia
What are the etiologic factors?	Unknown at this time. Biliary atresia appears to be a condition acquired after

birth and may be due to a reovirus infection. It appears to be an inflammatory process.

What is so-called "correctable" biliary atresia?

Biliary atresia in which the intrahepatic and proximal extrahepatic ducts are patent.

What is the natural history of biliary atresia?

Biliary duct obstruction with progressive cirrhosis, portal hypertension, hepatomegaly, and jaundice. Infants with uncorrected biliary atresia are likely to die before 2 years of age.

List 6 presenting signs and symptoms.

Jaundice, hepatomegaly, acholic stools, dark urine, elevated direct bilirubin and alkaline phosphatase.

How is it diagnosed?

Ultrasound may show a contracted or absent gallbladder and no evidence of extrahepatic bile ducts. Nuclear scan shows obstruction of biliary flow. Definitive diagnosis is made at laparotomy.

What is the treatment?

Surgical correction is the first-line treatment.

Describe the 2 components involved in surgical correction.

1. **Resection** of the atretic gallbladder and biliary ducts up to the point of the liver that lies within the branches of the portal vein (the periportal plate).
2. Roux-en-Y **hepaticojejunostomy** with the jejunum anastomosed directly to the periportal plate.

What are the outcomes?

Approximately 33% of infants have a successful outcome; 66% of infants ultimately require liver transplant for survival.

When is surgical correction of biliary atresia most likely to be successful?

Before the infant is 8 weeks of age and when bile flow is established after the operation

What is the surgical procedure typically called?

The Kasai portoenterostomy

CHOLEDOCHAL CYSTS

What are they?	Abnormal dilatations of the extrahepatic biliary system, the intrahepatic biliary system, or both; thought to be congenital.
What are the etiologic factors?	Unknown. However, there is usually an abnormal entrance of the pancreatic duct into the common bile duct above the sphincter of Oddi. It is postulated that reflux of pancreatic enzymes may cause the cysts.
List the 5 types of choledochal cysts and their characteristics.	**Type I:** cystic dilatation of the common bile duct **Type II:** diverticular malformation of the common bile duct **Type III:** a choledochocele at the level of the sphincter of Oddi **Type IV:** cystic dilatation of the extrahepatic and intrahepatic common bile ducts **Type V:** single or multiple intrahepatic dilatations of the bile ducts
Who is most prone to getting choledochal cysts?	Females and people of Asian ancestry
How does an infant present with choledochal cysts?	Jaundice is usually the first presenting sign.
Older children?	A classic triad of **abdominal pain, jaundice,** and a **palpable mass** has been described. However, abdominal pain and jaundice are the 2 most common presenting signs. Older children may present with **pancreatitis.**
List 3 typical laboratory findings.	Elevated bilirubin, alkaline phosphatase, and amylase (especially with bile duct obstruction).
What is the most useful diagnostic study?	**Ultrasound.** Occasionally a biliary nuclear scan or endoscopic retrograde cholangiopancreatography (ERCP), or both, may be needed to confirm the diagnosis.

What is the treatment?

Surgical excision of the gallbladder, the dilated portion of the common bile duct and formation of a Roux-en-Y chole-dochojejunostomy. If the cyst cannot be removed in its entirety, the inner lining of the cyst should be shelled out from the outer wall. This approach works for types I, II, and IV. A type III cyst is usually simply unroofed within the duodenum. Type V cysts represent the most difficult surgical challenge. These are usually drained into a Roux-en-Y jejunal limb.

What is the risk of leaving choledochal cyst tissue behind?

Cyst epithelium can develop **adeno-squamous carcinoma.** Type V cysts are the greatest threat for this occurrence, because they cannot be entirely removed.

What are the outcomes?

The result of surgery for types I, II, III, and IV cysts is quite good. Patients with type V cysts have an increased risk of developing carcinoma and often have recurrent cholangitis.

PORTAL HYPERTENSION

List the 3 types of obstruction that may cause portal hypertension in children.

Extrahepatic obstruction (portal vein thrombosis); intrahepatic venous obstruction; suprahepatic venous obstruction (Budd-Chiari syndrome)

What is the most common type of portal hypertension in children?

Extrahepatic (portal vein thrombosis)

List 6 common causes of extrahepatic portal hypertension in children.

Neonatal omphalitis (Ch 10, p. 100), intra-abdominal infections, dehydration (Ch 3, p. 15), umbilical vein catheterization (UVC) (Ch 8, p. 65), enterocolitis, and congenital abnormalities of the portal area

What are causes of intra-hepatic portal hyperten-sion?

Usually caused by **cirrhosis,** which may be secondary to the following conditions: biliary atresia (see p. 287); congenital hepatic fibrosis (see p. 292); cystic fibrosis (CF) (Ch 17, p. 220); α-1-antitrypsin deficiency; radiation or chemotherapy changes; hepatitis (p. 282); sclerosing cholangitis; histiocytosis X; galactosemia; congenital biliary cirrhosis; hepatic hemangioma (Ch 27, p. 379); glycogen storage disease

What are the common causes of suprahepatic portal obstruction (Budd-Chiari syndrome)?

In most cases the cause cannot be identified. Occasionally, oral contraceptives and granulomatous disease (usually outside the United States) may be causes.

List the 4 most common symptoms of portal hypertension.

Esophageal variceal hemorrhage; splenomegaly with possible subsequent hypersplenism; ascites; ultimately, liver failure

TREATMENT

How is portal hypertension caused by portal vein thrombosis treated?

Esophageal variceal bleeding is usually the most troublesome complication but rarely requires emergent operative intervention. Usually, the patient is hospitalized and given **IV fluids, vitamin K, H$_2$ blockers,** and **blood transfusion,** if necessary, to provide adequate support until the bleeding stops.
In some cases, **injection of a sclerosing agent,** via direct visualization of the varices, is required.
If a portosystemic shunt is required, a **distal splenorenal** or **mesocaval shunt** are the 2 most common operations employed.

How is portal hypertension due to liver cirrhosis treated?

The ultimate course of treatment depends on the prognosis of the hepatic disease. Variceal bleeding is treated with **sclerosing agents.** Worsening hypertension may require a **distal splenorenal or a mesocaval shunt.** In some cases, **liver transplantation** is required.

How is portal hypertension due to suprahepatic obstruction treated?

Shunts from the portal system to the right atrium are occasionally successful. In most cases, **liver transplantation** is the treatment of choice.

CONGENITAL HEPATIC FIBROSIS

What is it?	A disease characterized by diffuse periportal and perilobular fibrosis. These may form duct-like structures but do not communicate themselves with the biliary system.
List 3 associated conditions.	Renal tubular ectasia; autosomal recessive polycystic renal disease; and nephronophthisis
What are 2 signs and symptoms?	This condition usually becomes evident in early childhood. **Hepatosplenomegaly** and **esophageal variceal bleeding** secondary to portal hypertension are characteristic conditions.
What is the treatment?	Usually the hepatocellular function is normal. Treatment focuses on **control of esophageal bleeding.** Bleeding episodes can be controlled by **supportive care** or **sclerotherapy** using endoscopy. In some cases, a **portosystemic shunt** may be required.
What are the outcomes?	Even if a portosystemic shunt is required, the prognosis from a hepatic standpoint is usually good. However, associated renal conditions may limit long-term survival.

21

Renal Diseases

ACUTE RENAL FAILURE

What is it?	A sudden decrease in glomerular filtration rate to a level insufficient to maintain fluid and electrolyte homeostasis
What are the most common causes of acute renal failure?	
In infants? (List 6)	Sepsis, asphyxia, hypotension, congenital heart disease (CHD), congenital urinary tract anomalies, renal arterial thrombi
In older children? (List 4)	Hemolytic-uremic syndrome (HUS); acute glomerulonephritis (usually poststreptococcal) (p. 298); trauma; sepsis
What is oliguria?	Decreased urine output
List the 3 classifications of oliguria.	1. **Prerenal:** volume depletion or poor cardiac output 2. **Renal (or intrinsic):** glomerular or tubular injury 3. **Postrenal (or obstructive):** congenital or acquired urinary tract obstruction (must be bilateral)
How can one differentiate between prerenal oliguria and intrinsic renal failure in infants?	In prerenal oliguria, the kidney responds to hypoperfusion by increasing sodium and water reabsorption. The urine is concentrated (specific gravity > 1.010) and the fractional excretion of sodium is low ($< 1\%$). When glomerular or tubular damage has occurred, these functions cannot take place. The urine will be isosthenuric (specific gravity $= 1.010$) and fractional excretion of sodium will be high ($> 2\%$).

What are the cardiac manifestations of hyperkalemia?

Peaked T waves are seen first, followed by prolonged P-R intervals, flattened P waves, widened QRS complexes and, terminally, ventricular tachycardia and fibrillation.

What is the treatment of hyperkalemia?

Membrane stabilization: calcium gluconate (100 mg/kg IV) or calcium chloride (10 mg/kg IV)

Redistribution: sodium bicarbonate ($NaHCO_3$) (1–2 mEq/kg IV) drives K^+ into cells in exchange for H^+ extruded to buffer the bicarbonate. Beta-agonists (10 mg of albuterol by nebulizer) as well as insulin (0.1 U/kg IV) plus glucose (0.5 g/kg IV) stimulate cellular uptake of K^+.

Removal: Kayexalate (Na^+–K^+ exchange resin) given by mouth or by rectum binds K^+ for later excretion; dialysis is the most effective method of removing K^+.

Why are patients with acute renal failure commonly hypertensive?

Fluid overload is the most common cause of hypertension, although acute glomerular diseases such as acute glomerulonephritis (AGN) and HUS are also associated with **high renin** output.

How is hypertension best treated in renal failure?

Appropriate **fluid management** is mandatory; diuresis if possible, and dialysis if necessary.

Vasodilators (e.g., calcium channel blockers, sodium nitroprusside, diazoxide)

Angiotensin-converting enzyme inhibitors **(must be used with care as they may actually decrease the glomerular filtration rate).**

What is the proper fluid replacement prescription for a child in acute renal failure?

Combine insensible fluid losses, urine output, extrarenal fluid losses (e.g., nasogastric drainage, stool losses), and estimated losses of Na^+ and other electrolytes.

What 2 methods of dialysis are used for children with acute renal failure?	1. **Peritoneal dialysis (PD)** is the most common, although hemodialysis may be feasible for larger children and adolescents (see p. 296). 2. **Continuous venovenous hemofiltration** utilizes a blood pump to drive fluid and electrolyte transfer across an extracorporeal membrane. It is most commonly used for children with extreme fluid overload, those with unstable cardiovascular status, or small children in whom PD is not possible.

CHRONIC RENAL FAILURE

What is creatinine clearance (Ccr)?	An estimate of glomerular filtration rate: $Ccr = UV/P \times 1.73/SA = $ ml/min/1.73 m^2, where SA = body surface area (m^2) U(mg/ml) = urinary creatinine concentration V(ml/min) = total urine volume (ml) divided by time (min) P(mg/ml) = serum creatinine A correction factor of 1.73 is used to normalize adult and child creatinine clearance values since a normal adult body surface area is 1.73 m^2.
What is a normal Ccr for an infant?	A normal newborn's Ccr is $\cong$ 20 ml/min/1.73 m^2
At what age is adult level reached?	Normal adult values (80–120 ml/min/1.73 m^2) are reached by 2 years of age.
What level of Ccr denotes end-stage renal disease (ESRD)?	Ccr < 10 ml/min/1.73 m^2
What are the most common causes of chronic renal insufficiency or renal failure in the pediatric population?	
In infants and preschool children? (List 4)	Congenital structural anomalies; obstruction; hypoplasia; dysplasia

In older children and adolescents?

Acquired glomerular diseases, including glomerulonephritis, HUS, reflux nephropathy, and systemic lupus erythematosus

Inherited disorders, including Alport syndrome and polycystic kidney disease

How well do children with chronic renal failure grow?

Poorly, both in weight gain and linear growth

List 7 potential causes of poor growth.

Steroid treatment, protein losses (in nephrotic syndrome), sodium wasting, chronic acidosis, renal osteodystrophy, recurrent illness, malnutrition

List 5 treatments of growth failure.

Aggressive nutritional support, medical management of electrolyte abnormalities, dialysis, recombinant growth hormone. **Early renal transplant may be recommended.**

What is renal osteodystrophy?

Bone demineralization caused by decreased renal function, leading to decreased production of vitamin D and elevated parathyroid hormone levels; demineralization is often severe enough to impair growth and increase the risk of fracture.

Why are patients with renal failure anemic?

Because failing kidneys stop producing erythropoietin

How is anemia treated?

Administration of subcutaneous or IV recombinant erythropoietin reduces the need for transfusions.

List 5 hallmark electrolyte abnormalities in chronic renal failure.

Hyperkalemia, uremia (increased blood urea nitrogen [BUN]), hyperphosphatemia, hypocalcemia, acidosis

List 3 treatment options for children with ESRD.

1. **PD**(the favored modality for children) utilizes the peritoneal membrane for exchange with dialysate and may be done in an automated fashion by the parents at home.
2. **Hemodialysis** is harsher, requires in-hospital treatments, and utilizes needles.

3. **Renal transplantation** (either from living relatives or cadaveric donors) provides long-term and more physiologic renal replacement; there may be problems with rejection or recurrent disease.

NEPHROTIC SYNDROME

What 4 features character-ize it?	Edema, proteinuria (> 4 mg/kg/hr), hypoalbuminemia (< 2.0–2.5 g/dl), hypercholesterolemia
List 6 causes.	Approximately 85% of children with nephrotic syndrome have "minimal-change disease." The remaining causes include: focal segmental glomerular sclerosis, membranoproliferative glomer-ulonephritis, membranous nephropathy, systemic lupus erythematosus, Henoch-Schönlein purpura (HSP) (Ch 19, p. 253)
What is minimal-change disease?	A form of nephrotic syndrome in which light microscopy and immunofluores-cence are normal, and electron micros-copy shows only fusion of the podocyte foot processes.
What is the source of the edema in nephrotic syndrome?	Not completely understood. Edema is most likely due to decreased plasma oncotic pressure secondary to protein loss into the urine. Fluid leakage into the extravascular space also causes decreased perfusion pressure, which results in increased sodium and water reabsorption by the kidney.
How is nephrotic syndrome treated?	Greater than 95% of children with minimal change disease go into remission with corticosteroid therapy within 4 weeks. Two-thirds of patients will have relapses, some frequently. A toxic reaction to steroids, steroid dependence, or both, may lead to treatment with cyto-toxic agents, such as cyclophosphamide or chlorambucil. When nephrotic syndrome is a secondary process, treatment or resolution of the primary process is usually curative.

What is the prognosis of minimal change disease?	Usually **resolves spontaneously** after puberty without renal dysfunction.
What is a complication of nephrotic syndrome?	**Infection**—pneumococcal and gram-negative infections are the most common. Increased susceptibility is due to poor nutrition, loss of immunoglobulins, and immunosuppressive therapy.

GLOMERULONEPHRITIS

What is the difference between nephrosis and nephritis?	**Nephrosis** (or nephrotic syndrome): proteinuria, hypoalbuminemia, and edema; implies no inflammation **Nephritis:** hematuria, decreased creatinine clearance, and hypertension; implies inflammation: many chronic glomerular diseases present a picture of nephritis with or without nephrosis.
List 4 features of the typical presentation of acute poststreptococcal glomerulonephritis.	Gross hematuria, hypertension, mild edema, and decreased renal function, 7–14 days following a skin or throat infection with **group A streptococcus.**
What is the lab profile of poststreptococcal glomerulonephritis?	**Decreased C3 (third component of complement) and elevated anti–streptococcal titers** (ASO, Streptozyme, or anti-DNase B)
What is the clinical course?	Varying degrees of renal insufficiency and hypertension, with resolution of clinical signs and symptoms after 1 month
How long can urinary abnormalities last?	Up to 2 years
How many children completely recover?	95%; children with severe involvement have all the risks of acute renal failure
Does penicillin help?	It may prevent further spreading of nephritogenic strains, but treatment of streptococcal infections does not significantly decrease the risk of poststreptococcal glomerulonephritis.

List 7 chronic forms of glomerulonephritis that most commonly affect children.	IgA nephropathy, lupus nephritis, membranoproliferative glomerulonephritis, membranous nephropathy, Henoch-Schönlein purpura (HSP) (Ch 19, p. 253), focal segmental glomerulosclerosis, Alport syndrome

VESICOURETERAL REFLUX (VUR)

What is it?	It is "backwash" of urine from the bladder into the ureter or kidney and is caused by incompetence of the ureterovesical junction.
How does it cause damage?	By exposing the kidney to high pressure during voiding and by increasing the risk of pyelonephritis in the presence of a lower urinary tract infection (UTI). Dilatation and scarring of the collecting system and renal parenchyma may lead to ESRD and hypertension.
What are the etiologic factors?	It may be primary and isolated (congenital incompetence) **or associated with other urinary tract abnormalities.** Secondary reflux may be caused by increased bladder pressure, inflammation, obstructing lesions (e.g., posterior urethral valves) or previous surgical procedures.
When is it usually recognized?	Usually during an evaluation for a UTI, renal insufficiency, hypertension, or voiding problems
How is it diagnosed?	Voiding cystourethrogram (VCUG), in which radiopaque dye is instilled into the bladder until full, and the dye is observed during voiding.
What is the grading system?	Grade I: reflux into a nondilated distal ureter Grade II: reflux into the upper collecting system without dilatation Grade III: reflux into a dilated collecting system without blunting of calyces Grade IV: reflux into a dilated system with blunting of calyces

	Grade V: massive reflux with gross dilatation and distortion of the ureter and collecting system
What is the natural history?	Risk of renal scarring increases with the degree of reflux. Primary Grades I and II reflux resolve spontaneously with maturation in 80% of children. Higher grades are less likely to resolve. Secondary reflux has a less favorable outcome across all grades.
What is the treatment?	Prevent infection with **antibiotic prophylaxis** (commonly, trimethoprim/sulfamethoxazole). If expectant management is undertaken, uroprophylaxis continues as long as the reflux persists. **Follow-up VCUGs** should be performed every 1–2 years to evaluate the progression or regression of the reflux. Children with severe degrees of reflux, breakthrough infections while on uroprophylaxis, or evidence of renal scarring are candidates for **surgical correction** via ureteral reimplantation.

RENAL TUBULAR ACIDOSIS (RTA)

What is it?	Systemic hyperchloremic (i.e., normal anion gap) acidosis resulting from abnormal urinary acid-base homeostasis
How does a patient usually present?	Growth failure in the first year of life
What is type 1 (distal) RTA?	The distal tubule has a deficient H^+ excretion capability, which leads to excess body H^+.
What is type 2 (proximal) RTA?	An inability of the proximal tubule to reabsorb filtered bicarbonate leads to loss of buffering capacity and acidosis.
What is type 4 RTA?	Distal tubular damage, which is commonly caused by obstructive uropathy, leads to decreased responsiveness to aldosterone. Inability to excrete H^+ and K^+ leads to hyperkalemic acidosis.

In what 3 ways can the physician differentiate among these types?	Types 1 and 2 usually cause hypokalemia, whereas type 4 tends to cause hyperkalemia. Types 1 and 2 can be differentiated in an acidotic patient by urine pH: Type 2 patients acidify urine to pH < 5.5 when serum HCO_3^- is < 16 mEq/L (patients' distal acidifying mechanisms still work). Type 1 patients cannot acidify the urine because of distal abnormalities, even in the presence of significant systemic acidosis.
How can one differentiate types 1 and 2?	By the replacement of bicarbonate: Type 1 patients typically require only 1–2 mEq/kg/day of $NaHCO_3$ to maintain acid-base balance, because of the small amount of base needed to buffer endogenously formed H^+. Type 2 patients are unable to reabsorb bicarbonate, and doses of **>10 mEq/ kg/day** may be needed for acid-base balance.

FANCONI SYNDROME

What is it?	Generalized aminoaciduria, glycosuria, and phosphaturia. It is often accompanied by bicarbonate wasting, proteinuria, and hyperkaluria, all of which are due to proximal tubule transport defects.
What are 2 common clinical manifestations?	Growth failure and vitamin D-resistant rickets.
What causes it?	It is usually idiopathic. However, it is a common feature of certain inborn errors of metabolism (e.g., cystinosis, galacto-semia, Lowe syndrome) or toxic events (e.g., heavy-metal poisoning).
List 6 laboratory findings.	Normal anion gap hyperchloremic meta-bolic acidosis, hypokalemia, hypophos-phatemia, elevated fractional excretion of phosphate (> 15%), glycosuria in the presence of euglycemia, aminoaciduria

List 3 treatments.   Evaluation of underlying abnormalities; high doses of vitamin D; phosphate and bicarbonate supplementation

DIABETES INSIPIDUS (DI)

What is central DI?   Loss of antidiuretic hormone (ADH) secretion, resulting in the inability to concentrate urine appropriately despite normal renal function

List 3 consequences.   Increased urine output, hypernatremia, and dehydration

List 9 common etiologic factors.   Idiopathic, post-traumatic, post-surgical, congenital malformation, intracranial tumors, central nervous system (CNS) infections, histiocytosis, granulomatous disease, familial factors

What are 5 signs or symptoms?   **Polyuria, polydipsia, weight loss, growth failure;** patients generally prefer water to other fluids.

What signs may indicate that DI is secondary to a tumor?   Neurologic or visual complaints

List 3 diagnostic lab results.   Morning urine specific gravity < 1.010; low urine osmolality; normal-to-high serum sodium concentration

What is the water-deprivation test?   The test is designed to assess urinary response to water deprivation. An initial water load of 500 ml/m² is given. Measurements are taken of:
1. Hourly body weight and urine output
2. Urine specific gravity and osmolality of each sample
3. Serum sodium and osmolality every 4 hours
Desmopressin (dDAVP), a long-acting analog of ADH, is given at the end of the test to document responsiveness to ADH.

List 4 indications of a positive test.   Persistence of dilute urine with osmolality less than that of plasma; a rise in serum sodium to > 145 mEq/L; a rise of serum osmolarity to > 290 mOsm/kg; weight loss of 3%–5%.

What 2 radiographic tests should be ordered?

1. **Skull radiograph** investigating for calcification, enlargement of the sella turcica, erosion of the clinoid processes, or increased width of the suture lines
2. An **MRI** to detect lesions of the pituitary gland and hypothalamic-neurohypophyseal tract.

What is the treatment?

Desmopressin (dDAVP) is given intra-nasally once or twice daily.

What is the differential diagnosis?

Nephrogenic DI; psychogenic water drinking; impaired thirst mechanism

NEPHROGENIC DIABETES INSIPIDUS

What is the difference between nephrogenic and central DI?

Patients with nephrogenic DI synthesize and secrete adequate ADH, whereas patients with central DI do not.

What is the primary defect in nephrogenic DI?

Lack of distal tubular response to ADH, with inability to concentrate the urine.

What is the etiologic factor in primary nephrogenic DI?

Primary nephrogenic DI is a rare X-linked recessive disorder with profound effects in males, although females may be mildly affected. In most families, the defect is caused by a mutation in the vasopressin receptor. Autosomal dominant and recessive DI have also been described in which aquaporin 2 (the renal water channel) is defective.

List 4 etiologic factors in secondary nephrogenic DI.

Secondary nephrogenic DI is more common and often less severe than primary DI. Causes include: obstructive uropathy, chronic renal failure, sickle cell disease, drug toxicity

How does a patient present?

In the more severe forms, signs appear within the first weeks of life, usually as the following: polyuria, polydipsia, failure to thrive, and chronic dehydration. The degree of dehydration is commonly underappreciated because the child continues to urinate. Fever, irritability, and poor feeding are also common.

What are characteristic laboratory findings?

Hypernatremia, hyperchloremia, urine osmolarity < 200 mOsm/kg in the presence of serum osmolarity > 300 mOsm/kg. ADH levels are normal, and there is no response to exogenously administered vasopressin.

List 3 treatments.

1. Maintenance of adequate fluid intake (most important).
2. Although somewhat counterintuitive, thiazide diuretics decrease urine output by causing mild sodium depletion, thereby encouraging proximal tubular sodium and water reabsorption.
3. Prostaglandin synthesis inhibitors may decrease urine output (mechanism of action is unclear).

RENAL STONES

List 3 signs or symptoms.

Hematuria (microscopic or gross); abdominal or flank pain; UTI

What is the most common chemical composition of a stone?

Calcium oxalate

List 4 other chemical compositions.

Calcium phosphate, struvite (magnesium ammonium phosphate), uric acid, cystine

List 9 predisposing conditions.

Urinary tract anomalies, recurrent UTIs, hypercalciuria, renal tubular acidosis (especially distal), immobilization, hyperoxaluria, cystinuria, hyperparathyroidism, hypocitraturia (citrate is an inhibitor of stone formation)

What are helpful imaging studies?

1. Plain abdominal radiograph shows calcium-containing stones.
2. Intravenous pyelogram or ultrasound examination (U/S) documents the location of radiopaque and radiolucent stones, as well as the degree of obstruction.
3. CT scan (special technique required)

4. U/S and VCUG help evaluate urinary
    tract abnormalities.

What are useful lab studies?

Serum: electrolytes (especially HCO_3^-),
    calcium, phosphorus, uric acid,
    creatinine, parathyroid hormone
Urine: urinalysis and culture, urine pH,
    24-hour collection for calcium,
    creatinine, phosphorus, oxalate, uric
    acid, cystine, and citrate

**What is normal calcium
excretion?**

4 mg/kg/day or urinary calcium:creatinine
ratio < 0.2

**List 4 treatments of hyper-
calciuria.**

Limit calcium intake to the recommended daily allowance; increase fluid
intake; limit sodium intake (sodium
restriction increases calcium reabsorption). If stones persist, thiazide diuretics
may help.

**Describe the therapeutic
management of renal
stones.**

Provide **hydration** and **pain management** until stone passes. **Treatment of
predisposing conditions** may prevent
future stones. If stones persist, **litho-
tripsy** can pulverize some stones without
the need for surgery. Endoscopic, percutaneous, or open **surgery** may be
needed.

HYPERTENSION

**What defines hypertension
in the pediatric population?**

Blood pressure (BP) increases with age:
Significant hypertension is defined as BP
    greater than the 95th percentile for
    age and sex.
Severe hypertension is BP greater than
    the 99th percentile.

**What is the appropriate
size for a child's BP cuff?**

The cuff bladder width should be large
enough to encircle two-thirds of the
upper arm. Bladder length should be long
enough to surround the entire arm circumference. Cuffs that are too small give
erroneously high readings, cuffs that are
too large may give erroneously low
readings.

List the 3 common causes of acute hypertension in infants.

Renal artery occlusion, medications, hypoxia

In children and adolescents? (List 3)

Acute glomerulonephritis, HUS, and medications (including illicit drugs)

List the 4 most common causes of chronic hypertension in infants.

Renal arterial thrombi (umbilical catheter complication) (Ch 8, p. 66); aortic coarctation (Ch 16, p. 198); obstructive uropathy; medications

In young children? (List 4)

Obstructive uropathy; reflux nephropathy (see Vesicoureteral Reflux, p. 299); glomerular disease {see Glomerulonephritis, p. 298); renal artery stenosis

In adolescents? (List 4)

Essential hypertension; glomerular disease (see Glomerulonephritis, p. 298); reflux nephropathy (see Vesicoureteral Reflux, p. 299); renal artery stenosis

How is the diagnosis of essential hypertension made?

By exclusion of secondary causes

What should evaluation include?

Studies of renal function, kidney anatomy, and urinary sediment

Studies for rare but correctable causes, such as pheochromocytoma (Ch 24, p. 341), Cushing disease (Ch 24, p. 340), and aortic coarctation (Ch 16, p. 198)

Nuclear scans, arteriography, or both, for diagnosis of renal artery stenosis may be needed.

What medications are used to treat chronic hypertension in children?

Essentially all forms of antihypertensives may be used if monitored appropriately.

When are diuretics used?

For patients with underlying renal disease and fluid overload, diuretics are often used in conjunction with other medications.

22

Genitourinary Disorders

HYPOSPADIAS

What is it?	Malformation of the penis with abnormal ventral placement of the urethral meatus along the penile shaft, scrotum, or perineum
What is the incidence?	About 1 per 300 male births; it is the most common penile malformation
What are some associated malformations?	Chordee (curvature) of the penis, hernias, and cryptorchidism are common. Chromosome abnormalities are uncommon in patients with uncomplicated hypospadias, but more common with complex malformations.
What is the treatment?	Surgical repair, sometimes in stages for severe hypospadias
List 3 common complications.	Chordee, fistula, stricture

CRYPTORCHIDISM

What is it?	Lack of normal descent of the testicle. Unilateral in 75% of cases, bilateral in 25%.
What is the incidence?	About 1 in 100 male infants
At what age is a boy's testicle considered truly undescended?	After 1 year of age
Why?	Testicles undescended at birth usually descend into the scrotum within the first year

What are 2 consequences of an undescended testicle?	1. After the second year, testicular degeneration occurs, resulting in low spermatogonia counts and degeneration of germinal epithelium. Seminiferous tubules become fibrous. This overall degeneration can cause the formation of sperm antibodies, which can adversely affect fertility even if there is a normal descended testicle on the opposite side. 2. There is an **increased incidence of cancer,** particularly **seminoma,** in an undescended testicle.
What is the treatment?	Hormone therapy may be used to induce descent of the testicle, but is usually unsuccessful. The major treatment is **orchiopexy,** through an inguinal incision or with laparoscopic assistance. Occasionally, the spermatic vessels may need to be divided high in the retroperitoneum as a first procedure (laparoscopic or open inguinal approach) to allow the testicle to be brought down into the scrotum. Collateral vessels then form along the vas deferens, and the testicle is brought into the scrotum as a second procedure.
When should orchiopexy be performed?	No later than 2 years of age. Current recommendations suggest that orchiopexy should be performed between 6 and 12 months of age.

EPIDIDYMITIS

What is it?	Inflammation of the epididymis
What are the 2 most common causes?	Reflux of infected urine; sexually transmitted diseases (STDs) caused by gonococci and *Chlamydia*
How does the patient present?	With unilateral pain in the scrotum
What are the physical findings?	A large, tender, and firm epididymis with a normal testicle

What is the treatment?	Antibiotics appropriate for the identified pathogen
What should be suspected if epididymitis occurs in a nonsexually active child or a prepubertal child?	A urinary tract abnormality. They should be evaluated with a renal ultrasound and a voiding cystourethrogram (VCUG).

TESTICULAR TORSION

What is it?	The testicle twists upon its blood supply and the vas deferens. The testicle may become ischemic and necrotic.
What are the 2 types of testicular torsion?	1. **Extravaginal;** torsion is outside of the tunic vaginalis (predominantly in neonates) 2. **Intravaginal;** torsion is within the tunic vaginalis (aka "Bell-clapper" anomaly–predominantly in older boys)
How do patients with torsion present?	Usually with significant scrotal pain and swelling unilaterally. The testicle may also be high in the scrotum due to the twisted cord.
What is the differential diagnosis?	Epididymitis, orchitis, acute hydrocele, torsion of the appendix epididymis or appendix testes
What is the evaluation for testicular torsion?	If testicular torsion is highly suspected, the patient should be brought directly to the operating room. If duration of symptoms is approaching or exceeding 6 hours, it is likely that the testicle is necrotic. If the time from onset of the symptoms is shorter and there is a suspicion that an alternative diagnosis is possible, **Doppler ultrasound or testicular radioisotope imaging may confirm viability of the testicle and rule out torsion.**
What is the treatment?	Surgical exploration of the scrotum is performed through a midline incision in the scrotum. If viable, the affected testicle is unrotated and is fixed in 4 points in the scrotum. If the testicle is

necrotic, it is removed. In either case, the opposite testicle is fixed in the opposite side of the scrotum at 4 points as well.

TESTICULAR TUMORS

What are the 4 common types of testicular tumors that affect boys (with examples where appropriate)?

1. **Germ cell tumors,** including yolk sac tumor (endodermal sinus tumor), teratoma, seminoma (rare in children)
2. **Gonadal stromal tumor (non-germ cell tumor)** including Leydig cell tumor, Sertoli cell tumor, gonadoblastoma
3. **Leukemic and lymphomatous infiltrates**
4. **Rhabdomyosarcoma**

Which of these types is the most common?

Germ cell tumor

Which is the most common testicular cell tumor in prepubertal males?

The yolk-sac (endodermal sinus) tumor

What is the typical sign of a testicular tumor?

Presence of a painless testicular mass. Sometimes a hydrocele may be caused by the tumor and may delay diagnosis.

What are common chemical markers of germ cell tumors?

The most common is α-fetoprotein (AFP). However, β-HCG may also be secreted.

What is the surgical workup and treatment?

Biopsy should be performed through an inguinal incision if possible. Traditionally, positive biopsies obtained through a scrotal incision have required scrotal resection. However, greater attention is now paid to scrotal preservation in these instances. Orchiectomy is performed through an inguinal incision. If the tumor is isolated to the testicle, surgical resection (orchiectomy) is all that is required. Retroperitoneal lymph node dissection is required if there is evidence of clinically suspicious nodes on CT scan. Extensive tumor will require chemotherapy.

In which patients do gonadoblastomas arise?

Male pseudohermaphrodites and patients with mixed gonadal dysgenesis. These patients are usually not phenotypic males.

What is the treatment?	Usually only orchiectomy, because these tumors are encapsulated and slow-growing
In which patients do seminomas most commonly arise?	Males with cryptorchid testes
What are the 2 components of treatment of seminoma?	Surgical resection with radiation therapy. These tumors are particularly sensitive to radiation therapy.
How are leukemic and lymphomatous infiltrates treated?	After a transscrotal biopsy, these lesions are treated systemically according to the type of disease found.
Which tumors cause precocious puberty?	These are usually the gonadal stromal and sex cord tumors, such as the Sertoli cell and Leydig cell neoplasms. Leydig cells, in particular, secrete excessive testosterone. (Ch 24, p. 329, precocious puberty)
What is the treatment?	Surgical resection (orchiectomy)
How is testicular rhabdomyosarcoma evaluated and treated?	Similar to yolk-sac tumor. Bone scan and bone marrow aspirates are needed as well. Radiation therapy may be adjunctive, but is rarely needed.
What are the outcomes for rhabdomyosarcoma?	Favorable, about 95% 5-year survival rate
What is the treatment for teratoma?	Simple orchiectomy

OVARIAN TUMORS

What are the 4 major categories of ovarian tumors in children?	1. **Germ cell tumors,** including teratoma, dysgerminoma, endodermal sinus tumor, embryonal carcinoma, and choriocarcinoma 2. **Gonadoblastoma** 3. **Sex cord stromal tumors,** including granulosa-theca tumor and Sertoli-Leydig tumor 4. **Epithelial ovarian tumors,** including mucinous, serous, clear cell, endometrioid, mixed, and undifferentiated

Which is the most common ovarian tumor in children?	Teratoma
Are most teratomas benign or malignant?	Benign
How does a child with teratoma present?	With an abdominal mass, pain, or both
What may be a pertinent radiographic finding?	The presence of calcification—in 50% of cases
What is the treatment?	If the tumor is within the capsule of the ovary, unilateral salpingo-oophorectomy is all that is needed. However, if the tumor is grade II or greater, there is an increased chance of malignancy, and chemotherapy will be required.
What are dysgerminomas?	Malignant tumors derived from primordial (i.e., sexually undifferentiated) germ cells.
In what age groups are they most common?	Prepubertal and adolescent girls.
Are these tumors biologically active?	Minimally
List 3 treatments.	**Surgical resection**. Most patients with low stage are treated without adjuvant therapy. However, these tumors are very radiosensitive. Adjuvant therapy with **radiation** and **possibly chemotherapy** is warranted in extensive or recurrent disease.
What is an endodermal sinus tumor?	An aggressive malignant germ cell tumor that originates from undifferentiated and multipotential embryonal cells. It grows rapidly and metastasizes early.
In what age groups do they most commonly present?	Teenage girls and young adult women
Is there a tumor marker?	Yes, AFP.
What is the treatment, based on stages?	Stage I and IA: Unilateral salpingo-oophorectomy

Stage II and above: Total abdominal hysterectomy and bilateral salpingo-oophorectomy.
All stages require adjuvant chemotherapy after surgical therapy.

What is the outcome?

4-year survival rate of approximately 50%–70%.

What is an embryonal carcinoma?

A rare malignant germ cell tumor that is quite biologically active. It resembles embryonal carcinoma of the adult testis.

What are the tumor markers?

AFP and β-HCG

List 3 characteristics of the typical presentation.

Abnormal vaginal bleeding, hirsutism, and precocious puberty due to elevated β-HCG.

What are 2 components of treatment?

Surgical resection, chemotherapy

What is a choriocarcinoma?

An aggressive germ cell tumor differentiated toward trophoblastic structures. It generally is hormonally active.

What is the tumor marker?

β-HCG

With what symptoms does the patient present?

Precocious puberty or menstrual irregularity

What are 2 components of treatment?

Surgical resection, chemotherapy

What is a gonadoblastoma?

A tumor that arises in dysgenetic gonads. Most patients have a 46 XY or 45 X/46 XY karyotype.

What is the treatment?

Surgical resection of the gonadoblastoma as well as the opposite ovary, because it is also at risk for malignant degeneration

What is a granulosa-theca cell tumor?

A tumor that has its origin in sex cord or stromal tissue.

With what symptoms does the patient present?

An abdominal mass and precocious puberty

What is the tumor marker?	Inhibin
What is the treatment?	Surgical resection
What is a Sertoli-Leydig cell tumor?	Another ovarian tumor of sex cord or stromal origin. These tumors were formerly called arrhenoblastomas.
What is the characteristic presentation?	An abdominal or pelvic mass with masculinization (because these tumors typically secrete testosterone).
What is the treatment?	Surgical resection
What are epithelial ovarian tumors?	Tumors of typical ovarian tissue; infrequent in children.
What are the 2 tumor markers?	CA-125 antigen; carcinoembryonic antigen (CEA)
What is the most typical presentation in children?	Presence of an abdominal mass
How is surgical staging undertaken?	1. Peritoneal washings for cytology 2. Examination of all peritoneal surfaces and liver 3. Biopsies of the diaphragm and peritoneum 4. Omentectomy 5. Sampling of para-aortic and pelvic lymph nodes
What is the treatment?	Total abdominal hysterectomy, bilateral salpingo-oophorectomy, and omentectomy with the staging procedures as outlined above. Adjuvant chemotherapy is needed in all stages above stage I as well as in some stage I cases.
What are 3 indicators of poor prognosis?	Advanced stage; aneuploidy; C-fms oncogene

VAGINAL ANOMALIES

What is vaginal atresia?	A condition in which the müllerian ducts fail to reach the urogenital sinus, which results in failure of vaginal canalization. Atresia may be proximal (i.e., virtually no

vaginal formation) or distal (proximal
canalization with distal obstruction).

In vaginal atresia, what is the status of the other reproductive organs?

The ovaries and fallopian tubes are normal. The uterus is usually normal.

What is proximal vaginal atresia due to?

Dysplasia of the müllerian ducts.

What is the status of the reproductive organs?

The fallopian tubes and ovaries are normal. The uterus and cervix are hypoplastic or absent.

What is hydrocolpos?

Filling of the vagina with mucus

What is hydrometrocolpos?

Filling of the vagina and uterus with mucus

What is hematocolpos?

Filling of the vagina with menstrual blood discharge

What is hematometrocolpos?

Filling of the vagina and uterus with menstrual blood discharge

With what symptom does a patient with distal vaginal atresia commonly present?

Colicky abdominal pain once menarche begins, due to collection of menstrual blood (i.e., hematocolpos or hematometrocolpos)

How is distal vaginal atresia treated?

Perineal vaginoplasty

How does proximal vaginal atresia present?

It is more likely to present as lack of menstrual periods, because of the hypoplasia or agenesis of the uterus.

Can abdominal pain occur with proximal vaginal atresia?

Yes, in cases in which the uterus is well formed enough to produce menstrual blood

How is this treated?

Drainage of the uterus and formation of a vagina using any vaginal tissue that may be present, using a pull-through of a portion of bowel, or a combination of these measures.

VAGINAL TUMORS

What are the 2 most typical vaginal tumors of childhood?	Rhabdomyosarcoma, endodermal sinus tumor
How do patients with these tumors present?	Vaginal mass or swelling with possible vaginal bleeding.
List 3 components that the workup for an endodermal sinus tumor should include.	Serum tests for AFP and β-HCG; CT scan of the vagina, pelvis, and abdomen; chest radiograph
What is the treatment?	Usually biopsy of the tumor is performed with subsequent chemotherapy and completion resection. Resection may include removal of the uterus if the tumor extends that far.
List 5 components included in the workup of rhabdomyosarcoma.	Chest radiograph, CT scan of the pelvis and abdomen, bone marrow aspiration, bone scan, cystoscopy
How is this tumor treated?	Usually biopsy is followed by chemotherapy to reduce the tumor and then completion resection. Hysterectomy or pelvic exenteration is rarely required.
What is the 5-year survival for rhabdomyosarcoma of the vagina?	Approximately 85%

IMPERFORATE HYMEN

What is imperforate hymen?	Persistence of an epithelial membrane at the opening of the vagina. It is the most common cause of vaginal obstruction.
How does a patient with imperforate hymen usually present?	It is often not apparent until adolescence. The girl experiences episodes of lower abdominal pain but no menstruation. After a time, a lower abdominal mass may be present, representing hydrometrocolpos, hematometrocolpos, or hematocolpos.
How is this treated?	The hymen is incised with a cruciate incision. The raw edges of the hymen ring are then sutured with absorbable sutures to promote epithelialization of the edges of the new open hymen ring.

23

Hernias and Abdominal Wall Defects

HERNIAS

What is a hernia?

Protrusion of a body component or organ outside its normal respective compartment. They can involve the inguinal canal, abdominal wall, diaphragm, fascia, and mesentery among other areas.

What is the most common type of hernia?

Inguinal hernia

INGUINAL HERNIAS

What is an inguinal hernia?

A protrusion through the inguinal canal in the groin region. There may also be weakness of the muscle comprising the inguinal canal and floor.

What is an indirect inguinal hernia?

A herniation of the peritoneal sac through the inguinal ring itself. An indirect hernia does not imply any weakness of the muscle in the inguinal region.

What is the most common sign of an indirect inguinal hernia?

A bulging in the groin region or protrusion into the scrotum. This may be unilateral or bilateral.

Which side is more commonly involved?

The right side

What are the common symptoms.

Most indirect inguinal hernias manifest as a **painless bulge**. If a hernia is symptomatic, **pain** is the most common symptom. If intestines are incarcerated within a hernia sac, **nausea** and **vomiting** may be symptoms.

What is the treatment of an indirect inguinal hernia?	Surgical ligation of the hernia sac at the level of the internal inguinal ring.
List 3 reasons an inguinal hernia needs to be repaired.	1. It does not resolve on its own. 2. It can become larger over time. 3. Most important, intestines can be entrapped within the hernia thus causing a **surgical emergency**.
What is a hydrocele?	A collection of fluid along the testicular cord or within the scrotal sac. Most hydroceles are isolated within the tunica vaginalis and resolve prior to 1 year of age.
What is a cord hydrocele?	A hydrocele that is isolated within a remnant of the processus vaginalis along the spermatic cord structures. These **tend not to resolve** and usually need to be removed.
What is a communicating hydrocele?	A hydrocele in which the fluid is moving back and forth within the sac through the patent processus vaginalis.
What is a direct inguinal hernia?	In children, this manifests as weakness in the inguinal muscle floor medial to the inferior epigastric vessels.
What are the signs and symptoms of a direct inguinal hernia?	Similar to indirect inguinal hernias; can be difficult to distinguish from indirect inguinal hernias on physical examination.
What are risk factors for direct inguinal hernias?	Conditions that result in chronic abdominal pressure, such as chronic coughing, constipation, heavy lifting, or ascites.
Are direct inguinal hernias common in infants and children?	No. However, when encountered in these age groups, they are usually in premature infants.
How are direct inguinal hernias treated?	The hernias are repaired surgically. If a sac is present, it is ligated. In addition, the musculature of the inguinal ring and floor can be repaired through a variety of techniques. Mesh is rarely used in children.

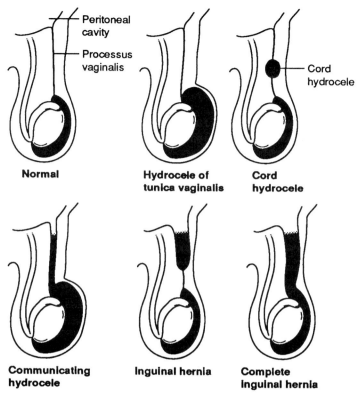

From left, configurations of hydrocele and hernia in relationship to patency of the processus vaginalis.

What is an epigastric hernia?	A weakness in the midline fascia which exists between the area of the umbilicus and the xiphoid process. It generally is between 0.5 and 1.0 cm in diameter.
How does a patient with an epigastric hernia present?	A small bulge will be noted in the involved area. There may be associated pain due to entrapment of preperitoneal fat (this condition is sometimes termed **"epipolocele"**). It is rare that intestines will be involved in such a small hernia.
How are these hernias treated?	By surgical closure of the fascia
What is a Richter's hernia?	A hernia involving an intestinal loop such

that only a portion of the intestinal lumen is entrapped by the hernia.

What is a sliding hernia?

A hernia in which a portion of the hernia sac is composed of an adjacent organ such as a loop of bowel or a portion of bladder.

What is a Littré hernia?

A hernia in which a Meckel diverticulum is protruding into the hernia sac (Ch 19, p. 277).

UMBILICAL HERNIA

What is it?

Congenital fascial defect that persists in the umbilical region—cause unknown

What is the incidence?

1 in 6 children

In what 2 groups of children is it most common?

African-American children—occurs 9 times more often than in other populations, and premature infants

What is the natural history of an umbilical hernia?

They usually close spontaneously by 3–5 years of age. However, fascial defects > 1.5 cm are not likely to close.

What is the treatment?

Surgical fascial closure

List 5 indications for surgery.

1. Lack of closure by 5 years of age
2. Fascial defect of 1.5 cm or greater
3. Large umbilical proboscis resulting in skin excoriation or other difficulty
4. Discomfort from the hernia
5. Incarceration (rare)

CONGENITAL DIAPHRAGMATIC HERNIAS

(See Ch 17, p. 210.)

ABDOMINAL WALL DEFECTS

OMPHALOCELE

What is an omphalocele?

A centrally located abdominal wall defect that results from the failure of closure of the abdominal wall during development. Omphaloceles can be small or large. The larger the omphalocele the less well formed is the abdominal wall and abdominal cavity. Omphalocele defects are covered by an intact sac (Wharton jelly) in most cases. The umbilicus extends from the apex of the Wharton jelly.

What is the incidence?

About 1 in 4000 live births

List 5 associated conditions.

Congenital heart defects, lung hypoplasia, chromosomal abnormalities, renal abnormalities, malformation syndromes (e.g., Beckwith-Wiedemann syndrome)

List 2 ways omphaloceles are diagnosed.

Prenatal ultrasound (this allows time for prenatal counseling of parents and investigation for other potential anomalies during the prenatal stage); clinical exam at birth

List 4 components of the initial management of an infant with an omphalocele.

Management is mainly supportive.
1. IV access is established and IV fluids are administered.
2. Antibiotics are administered by IV.
3. A nasogastric tube (NGT) is placed for gastric decompression.
4. The omphalocele is dressed with a moist gauze.
Cardiac and renal ultrasounds can be obtained.

How is an omphalocele repaired?

If the omphalocele is small?

If no contraindications, soon after birth.

If the omphalocele is large?

1. The Wharton jelly can be removed and a temporary silo of prosthetic material such as Silastic can be placed. The silo is then reduced over a 10- to 14-day period and the abdominal wall is closed, primarily with fascia or with a small prosthetic patch of a material such as Gore-Tex
2. Alternatively, a large omphalocele can be left intact and be treated with any of a variety of topical agents such as

silver sulfadiazine or antibiotic ointment. The Wharton jelly then epithelializes. The abdominal wall defect can then be closed months or even years later when a primary closure can be assured and the patient's medical status is stable (if there are medical contraindications at infancy).

Is the presence of an omphalocele a surgical emergency?	No, if the **Wharton jelly of the omphalocele is intact**. The Wharton jelly protects the abdominal contents. All other necessary evaluation and management issues should be addressed first. If the **Wharton jelly has been disrupted** in utero or during birth, **surgical treatment is emergently needed**.
What is the outcome of treatment of omphalocele?	Generally quite successful. Outcome depends more on associated conditions.

GASTROSCHISIS

What is a gastroschisis?	Gastroschisis is an opening in the abdominal wall that is present to the right of the umbilicus. The intestine is exposed. The opening is usually small and the abdominal wall and cavity are usually quite well formed.
What are the etiologic factors?	Unknown. A common theory is that the defect occurs in the position where a second umbilical vein degenerates during fetal development.
What is the incidence?	About 1 in 6000–10,000 live births.
List 2 ways gastroschisis is diagnosed.	Gastroschisis is often diagnosed on **prenatal ultrasound** or is immediately apparent at birth.
List 2 associated conditions.	**Atresia of the intestine** or **in utero intestinal perforation**.
List 5 components of the initial management of gastroschisis.	1. IV fluid administration 2. Administration of IV antibiotics 3. Nasogastric suction

4. Placement of a plastic bag around the infant's body up to chest level. This maintains a moist atmosphere for the exposed bowel.
5. The infant should be lying on the right side so that the mesentery of the bowel is not compromised by hanging over the umbilical region of the abdominal wall.

How is gastroschisis repaired?

Reduction of the exposed intestines should be achieved after the **supportive measures** noted above are instituted. This is generally done in the operating room with the infant under general anesthesia and the abdominal wall relaxed. If the intestines can be reduced without significantly compromising the infant's respiratory status and without compromise of renal perfusion, the abdominal wall can then be closed primarily.

If reduction cannot be achieved due to bowel swelling, then a **prosthetic silo** (e.g., Silastic) can be placed. Reduction of the intestines can be accomplished gradually over a 7- to 10-day period as bowel swelling resolves. The abdominal wall can then be closed surgically.

What is the outcome for infants with gastroschisis?

Survival is about 98%. Any adverse sequelae are due to the presence of intestinal atresia or perforation and the surgical treatment required for those conditions.

24

Endocrine Disorders

DIABETES

DIABETES INSIPIDUS (SEE CH 21)

DIABETES MELLITUS

What is it?

Absent or diminished insulin secretion or action resulting in hyperglycemia and abnormal energy metabolism

What are the two types?

Type 1: insulin-dependent diabetes mellitus (IDDM); there is a loss of pancreatic cell function, resulting in a loss of insulin secretion; **it is the most common type seen in childhood.**

Type 2: non-insulin-dependent diabetes mellitus (NIDDM); there is continuous insulin production but at a decreased rate or there is insulin resistance; more common in adults.

What are the etiologic factors?

Unknown; probably associated with a combination of genetic and environmental factors. Autoimmune processes are important in most cases.

How does a patient with Type 1 diabetes mellitus (DM) present?

Most commonly—with **polyuria, polydipsia, and weight loss;** symptoms often occur insidiously over weeks to months. Patients present less often with diabetic ketoacidosis (DKA).

How is Type 1 DM diagnosed?

Random blood sugar > 200 mg/dl or fasting blood sugar > 126; elevated glycosylated Hgb level; islet cell antibodies as well as other autoantibodies may be present.

Why is glycosylated Hgb important?

It provides an estimate of the average blood glucose level for the preceding 2–3 months.

What are the goals of Type 1 DM management?

Normal growth and development and prevention of early and late complications; specific goals for blood sugar ranges and glycosylated Hgb vary by age.

List the 4 main components of management of Type 1 DM.

1. **Insulin:** given as a combination of short-acting (regular or lispro) and long-acting (NPH, lente, or ultralente) 2–4 times daily before meals. Recombinant human insulin is less immunogenic and thus generally preferred over beef or pork insulin. Continuous insulin infusion (via insulin pump) is recommended in special cases.
2. **Diet:** limited intake of simple sugars; attention to fat intake; appropriate distribution of and total number of calories; consistency in meal and snack times.
3. **Exercise:** aerobic exercise lowers blood sugar without additional insulin and aids overall fitness; patients should exercise after a meal or snack to avoid hypoglycemia.
4. **Glucose monitoring:** 4 times daily before meals or snacks.

List 2 acute complications of Type 1 DM and their causes.

1. **Hypoglycemia** can occur with overinsulinization or vigorous exercise, or if the patient skips meals.
2. **DKA** may be caused by poor patient compliance with insulin therapy or by a severe illness.

List 8 signs and symptoms of hypoglycemia.

Hunger, diaphoresis, and tremulousness due to sympathetic discharge.
Deprivation of glucose to the central nervous system (CNS) can lead to lethargy, bizarre behavior, slurred speech, loss of consciousness, and seizures.

What is the treatment of hypoglycemia?

If the patient is awake and alert: oral glucose-containing fluids and foods or glucose tabs or gel.
If the patient is unconscious: intramuscular glucagon or intravenous glucose in water.

List 5 late complications of Type 1 DM.	Retinopathy, nephropathy, neuropathy, large-vessel atherosclerosis, ulcers on lower legs and feet
Can these be prevented?	Good glucose control can decrease the frequency of these complications by up to 75% and potentially prevent them.
What is diabetic ketoacidosis (DKA)?	A **potentially life-threatening** condition occurring in Type 1 DM that is characterized by **severe hyperglycemia,** with resulting **electrolyte disturbances** and **metabolic acidosis**
What are typical signs or symptoms of DKA?	Polyuria, polydipsia, fatigue, dehydration with tachycardia and hypotension, abdominal pain, nausea and vomiting; Kussmaul respirations, obtundation, and coma may occur
What are causes of DKA?	DKA may be the initial sign of Type 1 DM. In patients with known diabetes, DKA may be triggered by illnesses or noncompliance with insulin therapy.
List 6 metabolic derangements in DKA.	Severe hyperglycemia $\downarrow$ serum CO_2 (with respiratory compensation) $\uparrow$ Blood urea nitrogen (BUN) and hematocrit (dehydration with hemoconcentration) Normal or low Na^+ (pseudohyponatremia is artifact, due to lipemic serum or hyperglycemia) Normal or increased **serum K^+** due to cellular shifts from acidosis; however, **total body K^+ depletion is present and is potentially life-threatening.** Presence of ketones in serum and urine
List 4 components of DKA treatment.	1. **IV fluids and correction of electrolytes** (especially K^+) 2. **IV insulin:** infusion at 0.1 U/kg/hr. **Do not give IV insulin bolus.** 3. **Dextrose** (5%–10%) is added to IV fluids when the glucose level reaches 250–300 mg/dl 4. **$NaHCO_3$** is reserved for severe

acidosis (serum CO_2 < **5 or pH < 7.0**)

What are the cautions in DKA treatment?

SLOW correction of hyperglycemia and dehydration is essential. Too much fluid too quickly or rapid shifts in osmolarity may cause cerebral edema and herniation. The insulin dosage should be tapered to avoid hypoglycemia during the latter phase of DKA treatment.

What is the treatment of Type 2 DM?

Diet and exercise are first-line treatments. If these are unsuccessful, treatment includes oral hypoglycemic agents and then insulin.

PARATHYROID HORMONE (PTH) DISORDERS

HYPERPARATHYROIDISM

What is it?

Elevated levels of PTH, causing hypercalcemia and hypophosphatemia

What does PTH do?

PTH mobilizes calcium from bone and causes decreased renal tubular reabsorption of phosphorus

List 9 signs and symptoms.

Symptoms related to hypercalcemia include: nausea, vomiting, constipation, lethargy, weakness, confusion
Symptoms secondary to kidney stones: hypertension, renal colic
Fractures also may occur

List 3 diagnostic lab findings.

Elevated serum calcium (total and ionized); low phosphorus; elevated PTH (relative to elevated serum calcium)

What might radiographs show?

Subperiosteal bone resorption

List 2 etiologic factors.

Genetic (familial) hyperfunction of all the parathyroid glands (**hyperplasia**) or a solitary **adenoma** in nonfamilial cases

What are the treatments?

Hyperplasia: subtotal parathyroidectomy (usually $3\frac{1}{2}$ glands); or total parathyroidectomy with reimplanta-

tion of pieces of half gland in sternocleidomastoid or brachialis muscle
Adenoma: removal of adenomatous
gland

List 2 types of associated syndromes.	Multiple endocrine neoplasia: **Type I:** tumors of the parathyroids, anterior pituitary, and pancreatic islet cells **Type IIa:** hyperparathyroidism, pheo-chromocytoma (p. 341), and medullary thyroid carcinoma
List 3 causes of secondary hyperparathyroidism.	Chronic renal disease, hepatic disease, and vitamin D deficiency

HYPOPARATHYROIDISM

What is it?	Low levels of PTH
List 2 metabolic results.	Hypocalcemia and hyperphosphatemia
What are typical signs and symptoms?	Symptoms related to hypocalcemia, including: tetany, seizures, abdominal pain, numbness of the face or extremities, carpopedal spasm. Chvostek and Trousseau signs may be elicited.
What is Chvostek sign?	Twitching of the muscles innervated by the facial nerve; it is elicited by tapping 1–2 cm anterior to the earlobe just below the zygomatic process
What is Trousseau sign?	Carpal spasm that occurs after inflating a blood pressure cuff on the upper arm to above systolic pressure for up to 3 minutes
What is the treatment for hypoparathyroidism?	Vitamin D (or 1,25 dihydroxycholecalci-ferol) and calcium supplementation
What are the etiologic factors in children?	Sporadic, autoimmune, or DiGeorge syndrome
What is DiGeorge syndrome?	Dysgenesis of the third, fourth, and fifth pharyngeal pouches, resulting in hypo-plasia of the thymus and parathyroid glands and anomalies of the great vessels;

	frequently associated with a submicroscopic deletion of chromosome 22
What is transient neonatal hypoparathyroidism?	Decreased parathyroid responsiveness due to prematurity, hypomagnesemia (in infants of diabetic mothers, malabsorption), or maternal hyperparathyroidism
What is the differential diagnosis of transient neonatal hypoparathyroidism?	High dietary phosphate load (cows' milk or swallowed maternal blood); intestinal calcium malabsorption; hypomagnesemia; hypoparathyroidism

PRECOCIOUS PUBERTY

What is it?	Onset of puberty before 8 years of age (females) or 9 (males). (The age for females will probably be changed to 7 years in whites and 6 years in African Americans.)
What is usually the first sign of puberty in males?	Enlargement of the testes
What is the first sign of puberty in females?	Breast enlargement
Is precocious puberty more common in boys or girls?	Girls
What is the most common cause of precocious puberty in girls?	Idiopathic precocious puberty
What is meant by central precocious puberty?	Precocious puberty secondary to increased release of gonadotropin releasing hormone
List 4 causes of central precocious puberty.	1. Idiopathic true precocious puberty 2. CNS trauma, tumor, hamartoma, or malformation 3. Postinfectious or postinflammatory conditions 4. Chronic exposure to sex steroids
What is pseudoprecocious (incomplete, or peripheral) puberty?	Puberty caused by release of hormones by mechanisms other than the usual hypothalamic-pituitary-gonadal axis

List 3 causes of pseudo-precocious puberty.

Exogenous hormones; hormone-producing tumors (e.g., adrenal, ovarian, testicular); congenital adrenal hyperplasia

What is premature adrenarche?

Premature appearance of secondary sexual hair

List 2 ways in which premature adrenarche differs from precocious puberty.

1. Premature adrenarche has no other features of puberty, such as physical changes in genitalia or breasts or linear growth.
2. The bone age is not very advanced.

How is premature adrenarche evaluated?

Most patients require no laboratory testing. Careful clinical follow-up is key to excluding precocious puberty. Sometimes tests of bone age and adrenal androgen levels help.

What is premature thelarche?

Premature breast development

In what way does premature thelarche differ from precocious puberty?

In premature thelarche, there are no other signs of pubertal development.

How should premature thelarche be evaluated?

By careful and frequent clinical follow-up; most patients require no additional testing unless there are other changes suggestive of puberty

List the 2 components of an initial evaluation of precocious puberty.

Detailed history (including evaluation of growth data); physical examination

What is included in the laboratory evaluation?

Laboratory studies may include serum levels of follicle-stimulating hormone (FSH), luteinizing hormone (LH), estradiol, testosterone, adrenal androgens (DHEAS and 17-OHP).

What radiographic studies are indicated?

Plain radiographs to assess bone age may be helpful. Depending on clinical and screening lab test findings, MRI of the head and ultrasound or CT examination of the pelvis (ovaries) or abdomen (adrenal glands, other masses) may be indicated.

GYNECOMASTIA

What is it?	Breast tissue enlargement in the male
What are the four types of isolated gynecomastia?	1. Benign adolescent hypertrophy: is characterized by a small (approximately 3 cm) subareolar mass that ultimately resolves spontaneously 2. Physiologically induced gynecomastia: may be due to sporadic elevation in estrogen or other causes (e.g., hormone ingestion) 3. Gynecomastia stimulated by obesity 4. "Apparent gynecomastia" is due to pectoral muscle hypertrophy. Gynecomastia may be associated with other symptoms in various endocrine and genetic conditions.
What are treatments of the various isolated types?	Excision of breast tissue through a submammary incision may be used for physiologically induced gynecomastia and, in some cases, benign adolescent hypertrophy when it is too bothersome for the adolescent. Obesity-induced gynecomastia should be evaluated after the patient has adhered to a diet and exercise regimen to lose weight. If gynecomastia persists, resection of breast tissue may be necessary. No treatment is needed for pectoral muscle hypertrophy.

DELAYED PUBERTY

What is it?	Delay in the onset of development of secondary sexual characteristics
After what age is puberty considered delayed?	If there has been no development of secondary sexual characteristics by **13 (females) or 14 (males) years of age**
What is hypergonadotropic hypogonadism?	Delayed puberty associated with increased levels of FSH and LH
What is its pathophysiology?	The pituitary is functioning, but there is lack of peripheral (end-organ) response
What is hypogonadotropic hypogonadism?	Delayed puberty associated with inadequate levels of FSH and LH

What is its pathophysiology?

It implies a central problem in gonadotropin production or release; it may include a structural abnormality, tumor, hypopituitarism, or nutritional problem.

What is the most common cause of delayed puberty in boys?

Constitutional delay of puberty (a variation of normal)

List 6 other causes in males.

Gonadal failure or dysgenesis, Klinefelter syndrome, hypopituitarism, CNS tumors, certain malformation syndromes, nutritional disturbances

List 5 causes of pubertal delay in girls.

Turner syndrome, gonadal dysgenesis from other causes, gonadotropin deficiency, CNS abnormality, inadequate nutrition (including that resulting from anorexia nervosa)

List 4 ways delayed puberty is evaluated.

A careful history and physical examination, hand and wrist radiograph to determine bone age (if patient is of short stature), thyroid tests, serum gonadotropins

In the evaluation of delayed puberty in boys, what 3 findings indicate the need for chromosome studies?

1. Evidence of poor testicular development
2. Dysmorphic features
3. Unexplained mental retardation or developmental delay

In girls? (List 4)

Short stature, features of Turner syndrome, dysmorphic features, and unexplained mental retardation or developmental delay

What is the treatment of delayed puberty in boys?

Treatment of the underlying cause. If this is not possible, the physician may consider a brief course of **long-acting testosterone esters** by injection. A longer course may be indicated if puberty does not develop within 12 months.

What is the treatment of delayed puberty in girls?

Treatment of the underlying cause. If this is not possible, the physician may consider a **low-dose conjugated estrogen,** increasing the dosage gradually over about 1 year to mimic natural pubertal levels. Menarche can be achieved later by adding a progestational agent.

GROWTH HORMONE (GH) DEFICIENCY

What is GH?

It is an anterior pituitary hormone that causes growth of all tissues, especially bone and cartilage. It promotes mineralization of bones and has a role in carbohydrate and lipid metabolism.

What are common causes of GH deficiency?

1. Idiopathic or congenital
2. Histiocytosis, sarcoidosis, craniopharyngioma
3. Secondary to CNS trauma or infection
4. An effect of surgery, chemotherapy, or irradiation for CNS tumors

Are newborns with GH deficiency usually of normal size?

Yes, because GH is not necessary for fetal growth

What are some potential presenting signs and symptoms of GH deficiency in childhood?

Short stature with growth velocity < 5 cm/yr; mild truncal obesity; frontal bossing; flat nasal bridge; high-pitched voice; delayed dental development; sometimes hypoglycemia; microphallus in males; a decrease in growth velocity after 6–12 months of age.

List 3 diagnostic findings.

1. Delayed skeletal development (shown by bone-age radiograph)
2. Low serum insulin-like growth factor (IGF-1 and IGF-BP3)
3. Abnormal response to GH stimulation tests (random GH levels are not helpful because of pulsatile secretion)

List 2 potential associated conditions.

Panhypopituitarism; septo-optic dysplasia

What is the differential diagnosis?

Genetic short stature; constitutional delay of growth and adolescence; Turner syndrome; chronic diseases; psychosocial dwarfism; nutritional dwarfism; chronic glucocorticoid therapy; skeletal dysplasias

What is the treatment for GH deficiency?	Recombinant GH via daily subcutaneous injection

PANHYPOPITUITARISM

Which hormones are affected in panhypopituitarism?	Anterior pituitary hormones, including adrenocorticotropic hormone (ACTH), GH, thyroid-stimulating hormone (TSH), LH, FSH, and prolactin
What are the causes?	Idiopathic; effects from treatment of CNS tumors; trauma; congenital midline defects; familial causes Hypothalamic disease can produce symptoms identical to primary pituitary disorders.
What is septo-optic dysplasia?	Panhypopituitarism associated with optic nerve hypoplasia and absence of the septum pellucidum; posterior pituitary hormones may also be deficient
List 6 complications of panhypopituitarism.	Hypoglycemia; prolonged jaundice; apnea; hypotonia; microphallus in males; glucocorticoid insufficiency
How is panhypopituitarism diagnosed?	Low GH concentration (< 10 ng/dl) in response to GH stimulation tests, low TSH and thyroxine (T_4), and a low morning cortisol level with abnormal response to ACTH stimulation In newborns, low TSH, LH, and FSH levels (LH and FSH normally are low in children after the newborn period until puberty— therefore, not helpful prior to adolescence)
What is the treatment?	Replacement hormones: hydrocortisone, GH, L-thyroxine Estrogen or testosterone at puberty: easier than achieving pulsatile patterns of LH and FSH that are needed for gonadal steroid synthesis

THYROID DISORDERS

HYPERTHYROIDISM

List 6 common causes of hyperthyroidism.	Graves disease; autonomous thyroid nodules; subacute thyroiditis; McCune-

Albright syndrome; chronic lymphocytic thyroiditis; in infants, neonatal thyrotoxicosis due to maternal Graves disease

What is Graves disease?

Hyperthyroidism secondary to diffuse thyroid hyperplasia ("diffuse toxic goiter")

What causes Graves disease?

Autoimmune etiologic factor: circulating thyroid-stimulating immunoglobulins bind to TSH receptors

What are the findings on thyroid function tests?

Elevated T_4 levels; TSH is very low or undetectable due to feedback suppression by high T_4

Which sex is affected more often?

Females, approximately 4:1

At what age are children affected?

Two-thirds of childhood cases occur in patients 10–15 years of age.

What are the signs and symptoms of Graves disease?

Increased appetite; heat intolerance; diaphoresis; weight loss; frequent loose stools; difficulty sleeping; weakness and inability to participate in sports; emotional lability; deterioration of school performance; nervousness; proptosis, exophthalmos; tachycardia; warm, moist, smooth skin; tremor; thyroid gland that is diffusely enlarged, smooth, nontender, and homogenous

How is Graves disease diagnosed?

Elevated T_4, T_3, and T_3 resin uptake; low or suppressed TSH

What is Graves ophthal-mopathy?

Lymphocytic infiltration of the conjunc-tiva, extraocular muscles, and retrobulbar tissues; this infiltration may cause redness and edema of the conjunctiva, decreased mobility of the eye, and proptosis; severity of these conditions is not necessarily associated with the disease course

What is thyroid storm?

A rare, **life-threatening complication** of Graves disease; uncontrolled exag-gerated hyperthyroidism leads to marked hyperthermia, tachycardia, vomiting, diarrhea, and CNS symptoms (apathy, confusion, coma); cardiac failure may occur

List 4 factors that can cause thyroid storm.

Infection, surgery, trauma, or non-compliance with antithyroid medications

What is the natural history of Graves disease?

Waxing and waning hyperthyroidism; eventual hypothyroidism resulting from autoimmune destruction of thyroid tissue

What is the treatment of Graves disease?

Antithyroid medications to block thyroid hormone production:
Propylthiouracil, which also blocks peripheral conversion of T_4 to T_3
Methimazole
Propranolol for relief of adrenergic symptoms

List 2 treatments that should be considered for failure of medical therapy, patient noncompliance, or recurrent hyperthyroidism.

Radioactive iodine (I^{131}) or subtotal thyroidectomy

What is the differential diagnosis of Graves disease?

Hyperthyroidism due to: subacute or Hashimoto thyroiditis (early phases); autonomous thyroid nodule(s); factitious hyperthyroidism (excessive ingestion of thyroid hormone preparations); excessive TSH production (pituitary adenoma or pituitary resistance to thyroid hormone)

What is neonatal Graves disease?

Neonatal hyperthyroidism due to trans-placental passage of thyroid-stimulating immunoglobulins

List 7 presenting signs or symptoms of neonatal Graves disease.

Jitteriness, hyperactivity, stare, increased appetite, poor weight gain, tachycardia, and thyroid enlargement in an infant born to a woman with Graves disease

List 3 treatments of neo-natal Graves disease.

Propylthiouracil; iodide solution (Lugol solution); propranolol

What is the natural course of neonatal Graves disease?

It resolves over the first few months of life as maternal immunoglobulins are cleared from the infant's circulation.

HYPOTHYROIDISM

List 2 categories of hypothyroidism in children.	**Congenital hypothyroidism** due to thyroid gland agenesis, dysgenesis, or enzymatic defects **Juvenile hypothyroidism,** which is acquired and usually occurs after the first year of life
Which is more serious?	Congenital hypothyroidism
Why?	Thyroid hormone is required for normal brain growth and development during at least the first 2 years of life.
What may occur if diagnosis is delayed?	Delay in diagnosis past 6 weeks of age can lead to **mental retardation.**
How do infants with congenital hypothyroidism present?	At birth, infants most often appear normal but may have prolonged jaundice. If infants are untreated, symptoms develop over 1–2 months and include: poor feeding; lethargy; hypotonia; constipation; coarse facial features; large protruding tongue; large open fontanel; coarse cry; umbilical hernia; cool, dry, mottled skin; developmental delay.
What constitutes newborn screening for congenital hypothyroidism?	A battery of screening tests are performed (which differ slightly by state). Blood specimens are obtained by heel-stick. Samples are taken before a newborn is discharged but repeated later if discharge occurs before 48 hours of age because there are hormonal fluctuations around the time of birth. Thyroid hormone [i.e., thyroxine (T_4)] is screened for in every state. If low, a serum thyroid panel is obtained to document hypothyroidism (i.e., low T_4, low T_3 resin uptake, elevated TSH).
What is the incidence of congenital hypothyroidism?	1:4000 births
What is the treatment for congenital hypothyroidism in a newborn?	L-thyroxine as soon as possible!

What is the differential diagnosis?	Transient hypothyroidism due to maternal blocking antibodies (low T_4, elevated TSH); thyroxine-binding globulin deficiency (i.e., low total T_4, normal free T_4, normal TSH); sick euthyroid syndrome, characterized by sick preterm infants (low T_4, normal TSH)
What is the treatment strategy?	Due to the risk of the infant developing CNS abnormalities, L-thyroxine administration should continue until 2–3 years of age, then it should be stopped and T_4 and TSH should be checked in **4 weeks**. If results are abnormal, the patient should be treated for life. If test results are normal, therapy can be discontinued, but follow-up tests in 2–3 months should be performed.
What are signs and symptoms of juvenile hypothyroidism?	Slow growth; cold intolerance; decreased energy level; decreased appetite; constipation; coarse puffy face; flattened nasal bridge; stocky habitus; dull, dry, thin hair; rough, dry, sallow skin; delayed relaxation phase of deep tendon reflexes; school performance is usually not impaired.
List 4 etiologic factors.	Most commonly, autoimmune destruction secondary to chronic lymphocytic thyroiditis (**Hashimoto's thyroiditis**). Other conditions include: surgical or radioactive iodine ablation for Rx of hyperthyroidism; goitrogens (iodides in cough syrups, antithyroid drugs); ectopic thyroid dysgenesis
List 3 diagnostic findings.	Low T_4, low T_3 resin uptake, elevated TSH; thyroid antimicrosomal and anti-thyroglobulin antibodies often positive in Hashimoto thyroiditis; delayed bone age, which can indicate duration of hypothyroidism
What is the treatment for juvenile hypothyroidism?	Oral L-thyroxine

SIADH

What is it?	**S**yndrome of **I**nappropriate **A**ntidiuretic **H**ormone: excess antidiuretic hormone results in expansion of vascular volume and hyponatremia.
What are common causes?	Pulmonary and CNS diseases (e.g., pneumonitis, pulmonary TB, bacterial meningitis, intracranial tumors or trauma) and some chemotherapeutic agents. In preterm infants, SIADH occurs in association with positive-pressure ventilation and bronchopulmonary dysplasia.
What are the signs and symptoms?	**Water retention** and **weight gain;** symptoms may progress to **lethargy, confusion,** and **seizures** secondary to **hyponatremia**
List 2 components of treatment.	Fluid restriction; symptomatic hyponatremia may require careful infusion of hypertonic (3 normal) saline

ADRENOCORTICAL INSUFFICIENCY

What is it?	Adrenal insufficiency resulting in decreased cortisol and aldosterone production
What is Addison disease?	Primary adrenocortical insufficiency usually due to an autoimmune process
List 8 other common causes of adrenocortical insufficiency.	Congenital adrenal hypoplasia, bilateral adrenal hemorrhage (Waterhouse-Friderichsen syndrome), trauma, thrombosis, infection (TB), tumors, drugs, adrenoleukodystrophy
List 11 signs and symptoms.	Weakness, fatigue, anorexia, abdominal pain, nausea, vomiting, weight loss, salt-craving, hypoglycemia, postural hypotension, and increased pigmentation (especially at pressure points, lips, nipples, buccal mucosa, and scarred areas of skin)

What are diagnostic findings?	Elevated ACTH and a low morning serum cortisol level that fails to rise with ACTH stimulation There may be fasting hypoglycemia, hyponatremia, hyperkalemia, and elevated plasma renin activity
What is the treatment?	Glucocorticoid and mineralocorticoid replacement
When must glucocorticoid dosage be increased above normal replacement levels?	It must be increased 2–3 fold during illnesses and up to 5 fold for trauma and surgery.
What is an adrenal crisis?	A **life-threatening episode** that may be triggered by an illness or injury; it is characterized by fever, weakness, abdominal pain, vomiting, hypotension, dehydration, and shock.
List 3 ways it is treated.	Rehydration; correction of hyponatremia, hyperkalemia, and metabolic acidosis; intravenous glucocorticoids in stress doses

CUSHING DISEASE AND SYNDROME

What is Cushing disease?	Bilateral adrenal hyperplasia secondary to increased ACTH production caused by pituitary adenoma, resulting in increased cortisol production
What is Cushing syndrome?	Increased cortisol production due to adrenal tumors (including carcinomas), ectopic ACTH production by nonpituitary tumors, or exogenous glucocorticoids
What characterizes these conditions? (List 7 signs or symptoms)	Signs and symptoms are due to excess cortisol production or exogenous glucocorticoids and include rounded face ("moon facies"), obesity, striae (stretch marks), a hump on the upper back ("buffalo hump"), impaired growth, hypertension, abnormal glucose metabolism
What are 2 laboratory findings in these conditions?	Elevated serum cortisol levels with loss of diurnal rhythm; elevated 24-hour urinary-free cortisol

What is the treatment?	**Cushing disease:** transphenoidal surgery; other options are radiation and medical or surgical adrenalectomy.
	Cushing syndrome: therapy depends on the etiologic factors.

PHEOCHROMOCYTOMA

What is it?	A rare tumor of chromaffin cells, which are derived from neural crest tissue
Location of the tumor?	Most commonly in the adrenal medulla; most of the remainder occur along the abdominal sympathetic chain, including the organ of Zuckerkandl and renal hilus. Extra-adrenal tumors may be referred to as paragangliomas.
List 9 signs and symptoms.	Hypertension (sustained or paroxysmal), headache, vomiting, pallor, sweating, visual disturbances, weight loss, and sometimes tachycardia and tremor; hypertensive encephalopathy can be life-threatening
What are 2 laboratory findings?	Abnormally high serum levels of catecholamines (e.g., epinephrine and norepinephrine); high urine levels of their metabolites (e.g., metanephrine, nor-metanephrine, and vanillylmandelic acid)
What is the treatment?	Surgical excision of the tumor (**pre-operative control of hypertension with alpha-blockers is mandatory**)
What are associated conditions?	Multiple endocrine neoplasia: **Type IIA:** Pheochromocytoma, medullary thyroid carcinoma, hyperparathyroidism **Type IIB:** Pheochromocytoma, medullary thyroid carcinoma, multiple mucosal neuromas

AMBIGUOUS GENITALIA

What does ambiguous genitalia refer to?	A constellation of conditions, with a variety of causes, in which the genitalia are not phenotypically normal for either sex

What are the 4 major classifications?	1. Female pseudohermaphroditism 2. True hermaphroditism 3. Male pseudohermaphroditism 4. Mixed gonadal dysgenesis
What are the typical karyotypes and gonads for each classification?	1. Female pseudohermaphroditism; 46 XX, normal ovaries 2. True hermaphroditism: 46 XX, testes, ovaries, or ova-testis 3. Male pseudohermaphroditism; 46 XY, testes 4. Mixed gonadal dysgenesis; 45 X or 46 XY, dysgenetic and streak ovaries
What is the cause of female pseudohermaphroditism?	Congenital adrenal hyperplasia due to deficiencies of 21-hydroxylase (the most common deficiency), 11-hydroxylase, or 3-beta-hydroxysteroid dehydrogenase. The deficiency causes an excess formation of intermediate steroids, which cause masculinization of external genitalia.
List 2 other conditions that are associated with female pseudohermaphroditism.	The enzyme deficiencies cause deficiency of mineralocorticoids and glucocorticoids, which can result in **salt wasting** and **hypertension**.
What is male pseudohermaphroditism?	The genotypic male develops as a phenotypic female because of inadequate testosterone production, inadequate conversion of testosterone to dihydrotestosterone caused by 5-alpha reductase deficiency, or deficiencies in androgen receptors
List 3 ways this condition may be discovered.	1. A female may present with virilization of external genitalia. 2. Testes may be discovered during repair of inguinal hernia in a female. 3. A female may present with lack of menses at puberty.
For what are these patients at risk?	The testes are at risk for seminoma or gonadoblastoma if left in place. Therefore, both testicles should be removed after appropriate discussion with the family and the patient.

What is mixed gonadal dysgenesis?

It is a condition associated with a mixed karyotype pattern of 45 X or 46 XY.

For what are these patients at risk?

Gonadoblastoma, seminoma, or dysgerminoma.

What is the recommended treatment?

Removal of gonads; hormone replacement at puberty

List 7 components that should be included in the general diagnostic approach for any patient with an intersex abnormality.

1. A history for any maternal drug ingestion that may suggest the presence of progestational agents.
2. A history of any genital abnormalities in relatives or unexplained infant deaths (which may have been due to electrolyte abnormalities caused by salt wasting).
3. Physical examination to assess gonadal symmetry, phallus size and shape, and evaluation of vaginal size.
4. Karyotype
5. Serum electrolytes
6. Retrograde genitogram
7. Determinations of hormonal levels

In general, what do the genitalia in patients with ambiguous genitalia look like?

Usually the genitalia show a phallus that is suggestive of a hypertrophic clitoris with a small vagina. When the phallus is large enough to be a penis, it often has a chordee and hypospadias.

As what gender should a child with an intersex anomaly be reared?

Traditional opinion has been that if there is a question about the ability to provide an adequate phallus the patient should be reared as a female. However, some people believe that genetic status should determine gender assignment. If the anomaly is present at birth, it is imperative to assign a gender as soon as practical, so that the appropriate operative procedure and social development can occur.

What are appropriate phallus sizes for a male infant?

As measured along the dorsum from the base to the tip of the stretched glans:
At term: 3.5 ± 1 cm (mean ± 2.5 SDS)
At 34 weeks gestation: 3.0 ± 1 cm (mean ± 2.5 SDS)

At 30 weeks gestation: 2.7 ± 1.2 cm
(mean ± 2.5 SDS)

What is the surgical approach to perineal reconstruction?

For infants who will be raised as females?

Cystoscopy is used to assess the urethral and vaginal openings because, in many of these patients, these two orifices join to form a common opening at the perineum. If the vaginal opening is distal to the urethral opening, reconstruction is performed at about 6 months of age. For more proximal openings, reconstruction is performed in a staged fashion with clitoral recession and labial-scrotal reduction at approximately 6 months of age and vaginal repair at 2–3 years of age.

For infants who will be raised as males?

Reconstruction is performed in a staged manner. The first stage involves a release of the chordee; subsequent operations repair the hypospadias.

25

Neurologic Diseases

SEIZURE

(Also see Ch 6, p. 36,
re seizures and Ch 9, 78,
re neonatal seizures.)

What is a seizure?

A paroxysmal event arising from synchronized electrical discharges of CNS neurons within cerebral gray matter that interferes with normal brain function

What features characterize a tonic-clonic seizure?

Rhythmic, generalized, jerking movements and loss of consciousness. Incontinence is common. Postictal lethargy is characteristic.

What is an absence seizure?

A brief episode (5–10 seconds) of staring and loss of consciousness, often easily induced by hyperventilation. There may be eye fluttering. These spells occur many times each day. There is no postictal state, and the patient is unaware of the seizure.

What are the characteristics of a partial complex seizure?

A sensory (smell, taste) hallucination and often an affective experience (e.g., fear, depersonalization) and is followed by loss of consciousness while the patient engages in repetitive, meaningless motor activity (automatism). A postictal state follows.

Are seizures dangerous?

Not necessarily. Prolonged seizures may cause damage through hypoxia, hypoglycemia, and other mechanisms but the main danger is the underlying cause of the seizure or the accidents that may occur during the seizure.

What causes seizures?

Seizures are symptoms. The physician must check for a CNS infection or metabolic problem, especially hypoglycemia. Seizures may also be triggered by fever. However, in children the underlying cause is frequently never found; this constitutes an idiopathic seizure disorder, commonly called epilepsy. (See Table 6–2.)

Are brain tumors a cause of seizures?

Rarely

Is an EEG helpful?

It will help characterize a seizure, but does not diagnose nor rule out seizure disorder. These objectives must be carried out clinically.

Should treatment be started after the first seizure?

It depends on the setting, but many clinicians do not treat a "single" seizure.

How are seizures treated acutely?

Severe seizures may require a benzodiazepine but, if possible, the physician should treat the underlying cause (Ch 6, p. 38).

When should a child diagnosed with seizure disorder be treated with chronic anticonvulsants?

It is a matter of clinical judgment, but therapy is often started after a second seizure occurs, especially if it occurs soon after the first.

List 4 drugs commonly used to treat seizure disorder.

Phenytoin, carbamazepine, valproic acid, and phenobarbital

What is the prognosis for seizure disorder?

Most seizure problems in children resolve spontaneously. If a child is seizure-free for 2 years on therapy, then gradual withdrawal of therapy can be considered.

ARNOLD-CHIARI MALFORMATION

What is it?

Elongation and downward displacement of the medulla and cerebellum into the spinal canal

What are its consequences?

Obstruction of the fourth ventricle, resulting in obstructive hydrocephalus and possibly brain stem compression

What are associated conditions?

Neural tube defects, especially myelomeningocele (see p. 351)

List 2 ways it is treated.	Shunting, to relieve hydrocephalus; posterior fossa decompression if necessary

CEREBRAL PALSY (CP)

What is it?	A nonprogressive movement and posture disorder due to brain injury or malformation that occurs early in development. It is not an etiologic diagnosis but a clinical syndrome (a manifestation of static encephalopathy) that refers only to **motor** disability.
What are some etiologic factors?	
Prenatal? (List 4)	Genetic factors, toxins, placental factors, and infection
Perinatal? (List 2)	Prematurity and its sequelae, asphyxia
Postnatal? (List 3)	Infection, trauma, and asphyxia
What is the incidence?	Approximately 2 per 1000 children
What are some signs and symptoms?	Delay in motor development with abnormalities in muscle tone, movement patterns, and reflexes
How is the diagnosis made?	**Clinical history** and **physical examination. Laboratory and imaging tests** are often needed to confirm suspected brain injury (e.g., porencephalic cyst), to rule out a progressive or degenerative neurologic process (e.g., astrocytoma, metachromatic leukodystrophy), or to define etiology (e.g., chromosome analysis).
What are the 3 classifications of CP and their characteristics?	1. **Spastic:** subclassified topographically by the distribution of spasticity—diplegic, hemiplegic, triplegic, or quadriplegic 2. **Extrapyramidal:** subclassified by the quality of muscle tone or movement disorder—hypotonic, choreoathetoid, dystonic, or ataxic 3. **Mixed:** which includes both spastic and extrapyramidal components

What are some associated disabilities?	Mental retardation, seizures, hearing or visual impairments, learning disabilities, attention deficits, dysphagia, malnutrition, poor growth, constipation, gastroesophageal reflux, and joint contractures and scoliosis
Does CP range in severity?	Yes, from minimal, with little or no functional disability, to severe, with total dependence for mobility, self-care, and feeding.
What is the treatment?	Treatment is supportive and geared toward maximizing functional abilities, managing concurrent medical problems, and preventing secondary disabilities. Many disciplines are involved (pediatrics, neurology, orthopedics, speech pathology, physical and occupational therapy, special education, psychology, audiology, and orthotics).

INTRACRANIAL HEMORRHAGE (ICH)

(Also see Periventricular-Intraventricular Hemorrhage, Ch 10, p. 88.)

List 5 causes of ICH in the newborn.	Trauma, asphyxia, primary hemorrhagic condition, congenital vascular anomaly, and prematurity
What commonly causes subdural hemorrhages in the infant?	A large-for-gestational-age (LGA) term infant with cephalopelvic disproportion relative to the mother.
What are common predisposing factors for intraventricular hemorrhage in infants?	Mostly prematurity. Other risk factors include: respiratory distress syndrome (RDS) (Ch 10, p. 89), hypoxia or hypotension, reperfusion of ischemic tissue, pneumothorax (Ch 17, p. 222), ECMO, hypertension
When do most cases of intraventricular hemorrhage occur?	Between birth and day 3 of life.
What are the common clinical manifestations?	A bulging fontanel, decreased muscle tone, lethargy, apnea, somnolence, seizures, hypotension, and bradycardia. In

some cases, there may be no clinical
manifestations.

How is the diagnosis made?   Head ultrasonography. CT or MRI may
be used to further delineate the
hemorrhage.

What are the 4 grades of intraventricular hemorrhage and their characteristics?   Please see page 348.

What is the prognosis for intraventricular hemorrhage?   Risk for neurologic sequelae and fatal
outcome increases significantly with
increased grade.

What are 3 long-term sequelae for survivors?   Hydrocephalus requiring ventriculo-
peritoneal shunt; long-term seizure
disorder; significant development delay

GUILLAIN-BARRÉ SYNDROME

What is it?   An acute demyelination of peripheral
nerves. It is an autoimmune syndrome
and often follows a trivial viral infection.

What are 4 signs and symptoms?
1. Extremity weakness usually begins
   distally and extends proximally, progressing over several days.
2. Painful sensory complaints
3. Areflexia
4. Autonomic involvement (e.g.,
   hypotension, arrhythmias) may occur
   and is dangerous.

Which diagnostic studies may be helpful?   CSF (elevated protein); electromyogram
(EMG); nerve conduction velocity
studies; pulmonary function tests (predict
respiratory failure)

What is the differential diagnosis?   Diphtheria-associated polyneuropathy;
tick paralysis. The physician must avoid
misdiagnosing early Guillain-Barré as
conversion reaction.

What are 4 treatments?   General supportive care; plasma
exchange (if symptoms are severe or
rapidly progressing); intravenous immu-

noglobulin (IVIG); mechanical ventilation if required

What is the prognosis? Usually complete recovery.

MYASTHENIA GRAVIS

What is it?
An autoimmune disorder with neuromuscular junction dysfunction that leads to weakness

What are 3 symptoms?
Rapidly fatigable weakness (characteristic), double vision, upper airway weakness.

How is it diagnosed?
Largely on a clinical basis, by eliciting a history of fluctuating weakness and by physical findings of rapidly fatigable weakness.

What does EMG show?
Rapid loss of activity following repetitive stimulation of the same muscles

What is edrophonium chloride (Tensilon)?
A very short-acting acetylcholinesterase inhibitor administered intravenously

How is Tensilon used in assessing myasthenia gravis?
In myasthenia, Tensilon usually produces a rapid, dramatic increase in strength. A positive test is consistent with (but does not diagnose) myasthenia gravis.

What are 3 treatments?
Acetylcholinesterase inhibitors (e.g., pyridostigmine); immunosuppressive drugs (e.g., steroids); thymectomy

NEURAL TUBE DEFECTS

What are they?
Defects secondary to abnormal closure of the neural tube

List 4 examples of neural tube defects.
Anencephaly, encephalocele, meningocele, myelomeningocele

What causes neural tube defects?
Not known. Most are isolated (sporadic). There is an increased recurrence risk in families, suggesting multifactorial inheritance.

What is the incidence of neural tube defects?

Varies with geography, ethnicity, and other factors; possibly 1–4 of every 1000 births.

What is anencephaly?

Failure of the cranial portion of the neural tube to close, with associated cranial and brain malformations

What is the prognosis for anencephaly?

Most infants are stillborn or die shortly (within days) after birth.

What is encephalocele?

A defect in the cranium (usually posterior) with herniation of membranes (and sometimes brain tissue) through the opening

What is the prognosis?

Varies, depending on the amount of brain tissue involved in the process and any underlying brain abnormalities.

How is it evaluated?

Imaging studies (e.g., ultrasound, MRI, CT scan) to assess the brain and plan for surgery, if indicated.

What is a meningocele?

A defect involving vertebral arch malformation with protrusion of the meninges

Is the spinal cord usually normal?

Yes

How is a meningocele evaluated?

CT scan and MRI to rule out neural tissue involvement. A head CT should also be performed to rule out hydrocephalus.

What is myelomeningocele?

A defect usually involving malformation of the vertebral arches with involvement of the spinal cord

What are the complications of myelomeningocele?

They depend on the location of the defect and the degree of spinal cord and nerve involvement. They include Arnold-Chiari malformation and hydrocephalus, neurogenic bladder, loss of motor function below the "neurologic level" of the lesion, lack of sphincter control, and clubfoot or contractures.

What is spina bifida occulta?	A general term referring to an interrupted vertebral column in the posterior midline (usually lower lumbar and sacral level) and intact skin. Tethering of the spinal cord may be a component of these lesions.
List 5 conditions that may be associated with spina bifida occulta.	Syringomyelia, diastematomyelia, tethered cord, dermoid cyst, dermal sinus tract
How can neural tube defects be prevented?	Women who take folic acid before pregnancy and during early pregnancy have a lower incidence of infants with neural tube defects.

MACROCEPHALY AND HYDROCEPHALUS

What is macrocephaly?	Large head size (i.e., greater than 95th percentile), regardless of the cause
What is hydrocephalus?	Increased CSF within the cranium
What are 2 types of hydrocephalus?	Communicating and noncommunicating
What is the difference?	**Communicating** hydrocephalus is caused by decreased absorption or overproduction of CSF. **Noncommunicating** hydrocephalus is caused by obstruction of CSF flow.
What is X-linked hydrocephalus?	A genetic form of hydrocephalus, usually affecting males, in which there is stenosis of the aqueduct of Sylvius. The gene is located on the X-chromosome.
What is the most common congenital cause of hydrocephalus?	Neural tube defects

COMMON MUSCULAR DYSTROPHIES

What is Duchenne muscular dystrophy?	An X-linked recessive disorder characterized by progressive muscle weakness, pseudohypertrophy of the calf muscles, and elevation of muscle enzymes, particularly creatine phosphokinase (CPK)

What is the molecular defect?	An abnormality (usually a partial deletion) of the dystrophin gene on the short arm of the X chromosome
When does it present?	Between 2 and 6 years of age
What is Becker muscular dystrophy?	Another disorder involving the dystrophin gene. It has a milder onset and rate of progression.
What are 3 other types of muscular dystrophy?	Myotonic, limb-girdle, and fascioscapulo-humeral

MISCELLANEOUS NEUROLOGIC CONDITIONS

What is spinal muscular atrophy (SMA)?	Disease of anterior horn cells, frequently progressive. Most are inherited as autosomal recessive traits.
What is Werdnig-Hoffmann disease?	Also known as spinal muscular atrophy type I, it is an early-onset progressive disorder. The age of onset is usually before 6 months of age, with survival beyond 3 years uncommon. A late infantile and more slowly progressing disease is called SMA type II.
What is Kugelberg-Welander disease?	A juvenile-onset form of spinal muscular dystrophy. Age of onset is usually in the child's first decade, but it may be later; also known as SMA type III.
What is Reye syndrome?	A mitochondrial metabolic encephalopathy, frequently associated with liver dysfunction and fatty changes in the liver. Many inborn errors of metabolism may present with features similar to Reye syndrome.
What is the cause?	Unknown; it is often seen following viral infections (e.g., varicella, influenza). A relationship to aspirin use has been suggested. All suspected patients should be exhaustively evaluated for underlying metabolic disease.
What are components of diagnosis?	1. Elevated hepatocellular enzymes in serum

2. Hyperammonemia
3. Exclusion of other diagnoses (such as medium-chain acyl-CoA dehydrogenase deficiency or other fatty acid oxidation defects)

26

Neoplastic Diseases

NEUROBLASTOMA

What is it?
An embryonal tumor of neural crest cell origin

What is the incidence?
8.5 cases per 1 million children (about 500 new cases in the US). It is the **second most common solid tumor of infancy and childhood** (brain tumors are the most common).

Where does neuroblastoma arise?
In the sympathetic nervous system: adrenal medulla (50%), para-aortic sympathetic ganglia (24%), mediastinum (20%), neck (3%), pelvis (3%)

List 5 groups of children who may be at increased risk for neuroblastoma.
Those with **other neural-crest conditions** (neurocristopathies), Beckwith-Wiedemann syndrome, adrenal hyperplasia, fetal alcohol syndrome, or those whose mothers took dilantin during pregnancy

List 4 associated neural-crest conditions.
Hirschsprung disease, Klippel-Feil syndrome, Waardenburg syndrome, and Ondine curse

What is the most common presenting symptom?
Abdominal mass, found in > 50% of children with neuroblastoma.

List 8 other presenting symptoms.
Respiratory distress, Horner syndrome, proptosis, bilateral orbital ecchymosis ("panda eyes"), paraplegia, cauda equina, bladder or vascular compression, or myoclonus with opsoclonus and nystagmus (dancing-eye syndrome).

What typical diagnostic studies are used?
CT or MRI to evaluate the primary tumor and detect metastases.

Metastatic workup also includes bone scan, long-bone radiographs, and bone marrow aspiration. Metaiodobenzylguanidine (MIBG) scanning may be helpful in identifying primary tumor and metastases if the origin is unknown; however, a biopsy of the primary tumor is usually needed for definitive diagnosis.

Tumor markers are also obtained for prognostic purposes.

What are useful tumor markers?

Urine vanillylmandelic acid, homo-vanillic acid, and **metanephrine levels.**

Other tumor markers include:

Serum neuron-specific enolase (NSE), ferritin, and **lactate dehydrogenase (LDH).**

Markers from the tumor itself include:

N-*myc* oncogene, TRKA proto-oncogene, DNA ploidy, integrity of chromosome 1p, CD44

What are the stages and their characteristics?

The International Neuroblastoma Staging System:

Stage I: localized tumor with complete gross excision

Stage IIa: unilateral tumor with incomplete gross excision, microscopic residual, and negative lymph nodes

Stage IIb: unilateral tumor with or without complete gross excision, with positive local lymph nodes

Stage III: tumor infiltrating across the midline, or unilateral tumor with contralateral lymph node involvement, or midline tumor with bilateral extension by infiltration or by lymph node involvement.

Stage IV: dissemination of tumor to distant lymph nodes, bone, bone marrow, liver, or other organs

Stage IV-S: localized primary tumor as defined for Stage I, IIa, or IIb with dissemination limited to liver, skin, or bone marrow (limited to infants < 1 year of age)

[There are a variety of staging systems similar to the International Neuroblastoma Staging System. Of these historically, the more widely used systems include the Pediatric Oncology Group (POG) and the Evans System.]

What is unique about Stage IV-S?

Most newborns and 30% of infants younger than 1 year present with this stage, which has an unusually good survival rate despite dissemination. Usually no treatment is needed other than excision of the primary tumor. Chemotherapy or radiation therapy may be required if an enlarged liver compromises the infant's respiratory or nutritional status.

List 8 favorable prognostic factors.

1. Low stage (I or II)
2. Patient age less than 1 year
3. Less than 3 n-*myc* copies
4. Normal serum NSE, ferritin, and LDH levels
5. DNA aneuploidy or hyperploidy
6. High TRKA proto-oncogene expression
7. Intact heterogenous chromosome 1p
8. High expression of CD 44

What is the treatment for Stages I and II?

Primary surgical excision and follow-up chemotherapy

For Stages III and IV?

Preoperative chemotherapy may be needed to shrink the tumor before resection. Radiation may be part of the postoperative regimen. Bone marrow transplantation (BMT) with prior total body irradiation may be used in Stage IV tumors.

What is overall survival rate?

Overall survival rate for infants younger than 1 year of age is 72%, and for older than 1 year is 32%. However, survival is about 90% for children with Stages I and II in both age groups, with significantly worse prognosis for Stages III and IV. Stage for stage, children younger than 1 year of age have a better prognosis.

WILMS TUMOR

What is it?	An embryonal tumor of renal origin
What is the incidence?	500 new cases in the US each year. Wilms tumor represents slightly more than 10% of all childhood cancer cases.
What is the age at diagnosis?	Usually 1–4 years of age

List 9 conditions with an increased risk of Wilms tumor.

1. Sporadic aniridia
2. Hemihypertrophy
3. Beckwith-Wiedemann syndrome
4. Neurofibromatosis
5. Genitourinary (GU) tract anomalies
6. Drash syndrome
7. Klippel-Trenaunay syndrome
8. Perlmann syndrome
9. Abnormal expressions of 11p15, 12p15, 16q, 1p, p53 genetic sites

List 3 signs and symptoms.

Large, palpable, painless abdominal mass, gross hematuria may be noted in 10%–15% of cases, elevated blood pressure (BP) may be noted in 20% of cases.

List 4 components of diagnosis.

1. The tumor is usually identified via CT scan
2. Ultrasound to assess extension of tumor into the vena cava.
3. Chest radiograph or CT scan rules out pulmonary metastases.
4. Diagnosis and staging are determined during surgical excision.

What are the stages and their characteristics?

Stage I: unilateral tumor without capsular involvement; it is completely resected

Stage II: unilateral tumor with renal capsule or perivascular involvement; it is completely resected. Localized spill confers a Stage II on an otherwise Stage I tumor.

Stage III: unilateral tumor with incomplete resection, regional lymph node involvement, preoperative tumor rupture, or significant intraoperative tumor spill (i.e., beyond localized area)

Stage IV: metastasis to lung, bone, brain, liver, or distant lymph nodes
Stage V: bilateral renal tumors

What is the treatment?

Surgical excision is followed by chemotherapy, depending on the stage. Radiation is needed for advanced-stage tumors. Preoperative chemotherapy or radiation, or both, is sometimes used for very large tumors or tumors with extensive caval or atrial involvement.

List the 2 main pathology categories, with examples of types included in each.

1. Favorable histology (89% of cases) includes blastema, epithelial, mixed, cystic, and glomerular types.
2. Unfavorable histology includes anaplastic types.
(Clear cell sarcoma and rhabdoid histology were earlier considered unfavorable histology but are now considered individual tumor types separate from Wilms tumor.)

What is the prognosis?

Overall survival rate for patients is 80% (90% for favorable histology). Survival rate approaches 95%–100% for Stage I and II tumors.

What is mesoblastic nephroma?

A renal tumor that usually presents in infants younger than 3–4 months of age. Presentation may be similar to that of Wilms tumor. 95% are benign and surgical resection is the only treatment necessary.

What is nephroblastomatosis (nodular renal blastema)?

A capsular nest of primitive metanephric epithelial rests around the rim of the kidney. These may progress to Wilms tumor. Patients are treated with chemotherapy when these rests are found.

HODGKIN DISEASE

What is it?

A malignant lymph node disorder of unknown etiology

What is the incidence?

5% of childhood malignancies; 6 cases per 1 million children

At what ages is it most common?

The first peak is 15–40 years of age, and the later peak is 45–55 years of age; 15% of patients are younger than 16 years of age.

What is the most frequent presenting finding?

Painless cervical lymphadenopathy

List 3 other groups of presenting signs and symptoms.

1. Enlarged axillary or inguinal lymph nodes
2. Mediastinal involvement may cause respiratory distress, but this is more common in non-Hodgkin lymphoma.
3. Fever, night sweats, and weight loss (i.e., the "B" symptoms).

How is the diagnosis made?

By histologic examination. Reed-Sternberg cells must be found.

List the 4 histologic types.

Lymphocyte predominance, nodular sclerosing, mixed cellularity, lymphocyte depletion

Which is the most common histologic type in children?

Nodular sclerosing ($> 65\%$)

Which histologic type has the best prognosis?

Lymphocyte predominance

Which histologic type has the worst prognosis?

Lymphocyte depletion

What are the stages and their characteristics?

The Ann Arbor Classification:

Stage I: involvement of a single lymph node region or a single extralymphatic organ

Stage II: involvement of 2 or more lymph node regions on the same side of the diaphragm, or localized involvement of an extralymphatic organ or site and its regional lymph nodes with involvement of 1 or more lymph node regions on the same side of the diaphragm

Stage III: involvement of lymph node regions on both sides of the diaphragm; other lymphatic organs may be involved

Stage IV: diffuse or disseminated disease (Stages are further classified as "A" or "B" depending on whether or not "B" symptoms are present.)

What are the components of staging?

Staging involves clinical assessment, chest radiograph, abdominal CT, chest CT, bone marrow biopsy and, in some cases, lymphangiography and staging laparotomy.

When is staging laparotomy considered?

Staging laparotomy was formerly imperative in all cases since it will "upstage" a patient from Stage I or II in approximately 25% of cases and "downstage" a patient from Stage III in approximately 25% of cases. However, with improved imaging and greater emphasis on systemic chemotherapy and less emphasis on radiation therapy, outcome is not greatly affected. If only radiation therapy is being considered, staging laparotomy should be considered.

List 4 steps involved in a staging laparotomy.

1. Splenectomy
2. Core liver biopsies of each lobe
3. Lymph node biopsies from the celiac region, splenic hilum, porta hepatis, para-aortic region, and bilateral iliac regions
4. Oophoropexy in girls (i.e., move the ovaries to the midline so that if radiation is needed, they are not in the field of radiation to the iliac regions)

List 8 complications of staging laparotomy.

The most common complication is intestinal obstruction. Others include post-splenectomy sepsis, atelectasis, wound infection, pleural effusion, abscess, pancreatitis, and thrombotic episodes.

How is Hodgkin disease treated?

Treatment depends on disease stage. Chemotherapy is the primary treatment. Radiation is avoided, if possible, for children still undergoing growth, and for females because of an increased risk of breast cancer. In some older children with Stage I or II disease, radiation therapy alone may be sufficient.

What are the complications of therapy?

Most complications are due to the specific agents used in treatment and include:

Myelosuppression and cardiac toxicity (Adriamycin)

Pulmonary fibrosis (bleomycin)

Gonadal dysfunction or sterility (alkylating agents)

Neurologic impairment (vincristine, vinblastine)

Complications from radiation therapy include:

Growth impairment, solid tumors, gonadal dysfunction, and toxicity to lungs, heart, intestine, and other organs.

List 9 possible second neoplasms.

Acute nonlymphoblastic leukemia
Non-Hodgkin lymphoma
Thyroid carcinoma
Parathyroid adenoma
Soft tissue sarcoma
Osteogenic sarcoma
Breast carcinoma
Basal cell carcinoma
Melanoma

What is the prognosis for Hodgkin disease?

Overall survival of children with Hodgkin disease reaches 98%. The youngest children have the best prognosis. Even children and adolescents with Stages III and IV disease can expect a 60%–85% 5-year survival rate.

NON-HODGKIN LYMPHOMA

What is it?

It is a heterogenous group of lymphoid tumors.

What is the incidence?

7%–10% of all pediatric malignancies; it is the third most common pediatric malignancy (after leukemia and brain tumors)

List the 3 most common types in childhood.

1. Lymphoblastic lymphoma
2. Small non-cleaved cell (Burkitt and non-Burkitt lymphoma)
3. Large-cell lymphoma (histiocytic)

What are 2 possible causes of non-Hodgkin lymphoma?	**Viral infections** and **immunodeficiency** have been implicated. Burkitt lymphoma of the endemic type, normally found in Africa, is usually associated with Epstein-Barr virus. In the United States, where sporadic Burkitt lymphoma occurs, the Epstein-Barr virus is involved in only 10%–20% of cases.
List 7 of the associated immunodeficiency conditions.	1. HIV 2. Wiskott-Aldrich syndrome 3. Bloom syndrome 4. Ataxia-telangiectasia 5. Severe combined immunodeficiency disease 6. X-linked lymphoproliferative syndrome 7. Patients immunosuppressed for organ transplantation
What are presenting signs and symptoms:	
In lymphoblastic lymphoma?	Usually presents as an anterior mediastinal mass with respiratory symptoms or superior vena caval syndrome
In non-Burkitt lymphoma or Burkitt lymphoma of the sporadic type?	Usually presents with abdominal symptoms, which represents tumor involvement of the bowel, manifesting as intussusception or obstruction; the endemic type of Burkitt lymphoma presents with involvement of the eye or the jaw
In large-cell lymphomas?	They are usually extranodal and patients present with widely disseminated disease.
How is the diagnosis made?	By biopsy and evaluation of an involved lymph node, bone marrow, or pleural fluid or ascites
List 5 ways in which non-Hodgkin lymphomas are classified.	Morphology, immunophenotype, histochemical staining, cytogenetic markers, and molecular analysis
List 7 tests that are needed for a complete workup.	1. Complete blood count (CBC) with differential

2. Liver and renal function tests
3. Serum uric acid, calcium, phosphorus, LDH, and electrolytes
4. Chest radiograph
5. Chest or abdominal CT (or both)
6. Bone scan
7. Spinal tap

How is non-Hodgkin lymphoma treated?	It depends on the type of lymphoma. 1. Generally chemotherapy is used. 2. Radiation therapy may be needed to reduce large mediastinal tumors when respiratory distress is present. 3. Bone marrow transplant may ultimately be needed.
What is tumor lysis syndrome?	This can result from an overload of lysed tumor material into the bloodstream when the tumor is destroyed during treatment. Hyperuricemia may result, which can compromise renal function. This syndrome is particularly characteristic during treatment of lymphoma.
How is tumor lysis treated?	During treatment, hydration is very important. If tumor lysis occurs, allopurinol is given and $NaHCO_3$ is added to the IV fluid to alkalinize the urine and increase the solubility of uric acid to facilitate renal clearance. If hyperphosphatemia occurs, alkalinization must be halted because calcium phosphate may precipitate. Diuretics must be used with caution; they may lower the urine pH, enhancing hyperuricemia.

LEUKEMIA

What is the incidence of leukemia in childhood?	1 case in 2800 children before 15 years of age
List 12 clinical features that may exist on presentation.	Fatigue, fever, pallor, petechiae, purpura, lymphadenopathy, hepatosplenomegaly, bone pain, joint pain, weight loss, anorexia, headache
List 3 laboratory findings on presentation.	Thrombocytopenia, anemia, low (or high) total WBC count

What are 4 predisposing conditions?	Down syndrome, Fanconi anemia, Bloom syndrome, Wiskott-Aldrich syndrome
List 5 ways leukemias are classified.	According to: cell morphology, chromosome abnormalities, staining properties, surface antigens, clinical behavior (rapidity of onset)
What is the most common leukemia in childhood?	Acute lymphoblastic leukemia (ALL)

ACUTE LYMPHOBLASTIC LEUKEMIA (ALL)

How common is ALL?	ALL accounts for 85% of childhood leukemias.
At what age is the peak incidence of ALL?	4 years of age
List 3 good prognostic features.	Child is 3–7 years of age; WBC count $< 10,000/\mu L$; high DNA index
List 3 poor prognostic features.	Child < 1 year or > 10 years of age; WBC count $> 50,000/\mu L$; certain chromosomal abnormalities
List 3 ways leukemia is diagnosed.	By examination of bone marrow aspirate; cell surface marker studies; karyotype
List the 4 types of ALL.	Early pre-B cell, Pre-B-Cell, B-cell, T-cell. Several classification systems exist and some will identify rare sub-types (e.g., "Infant early pre-B cell" and "Transitional pre-B cell")
What is induction?	Initial treatment phase
List 4 usual medications for induction in ALL.	Usual medications include a corticosteroid, vincristine, and L-asparaginase with or without anthracycline
How successful is induction in ALL?	98% of patients achieve remission.
What is consolidation (intensification)?	Treatment regimens in some protocols that lead to further reduction in malignant cells

What constitutes remission?	Absence of leukemia cells in bone marrow, with normalization of peripheral blood counts and marrow precursors
What is maintenance therapy?	Longer-term treatment designed to further reduce the chance of recurrence of the leukemia
List 4 commonly used maintenance drugs.	Methotrexate, 6-mercaptopurine, prednisone, vincristine
What is central nervous system (CNS) prophylaxis?	Treatment to prevent leukemia relapse in the CNS
Why is this necessary?	The CNS is a sanctuary for leukemia cells, and systemic medications may not adequately penetrate the CNS.
List 3 methods of CNS prophylaxis.	Intrathecal medications (e.g., methotrexate, hydrocortisone, ARA-C), radiation, higher dosage of systemic methotrexate
What is the overall cure rate for ALL?	About 80%

ACUTE MYELOCYTIC LEUKEMIA (AML)

What is the incidence of AML?	1 in 15,000 children each year; it accounts for 15%–20% of childhood acute leukemias
List 9 presenting signs and symptoms.	Fever, anemia, pallor, pain (particularly bone pain), bleeding, bruising, hepatosplenomegaly, disseminated intravascular coagulation (DIC), skin nodules
List 4 poor prognostic features at presentation.	Organomegaly, high WBC count, DIC; certain chromosome abnormalities indicate a poor prognosis
How many subtypes of AML are there?	At least 8 (based on French-American-British [FAB] classification system)
List 4 conditions that predispose a child to AML.	Fanconi anemia, Down syndrome, Bloom syndrome, Kostman syndrome

What is the significance of chromosome abnormalities in AML?	Chromosome abnormalities are common in AML, and some may be associated with an improved prognosis. Chromosome 7 abnormalities are associated with a relatively poor prognosis.
What is the treatment for AML?	Treatment is usually more intensive than that for ALL. Induction medications may include ARA-C, daunorubicin, and other more experimental drugs. Bone marrow transplantation should be considered if there is a suitable donor.
What is the outcome of AML?	Most patients achieve an initial remission, but long-term survival is worse than that for ALL. Survival approaches 70% if there is a suitable bone marrow donor. Survival is about 50% if only chemotherapy is used.

RETINOBLASTOMA

What is it?	The most common childhood eye tumor. It arises from primitive cells of the retina prior to differentiation.
What is the incidence?	About 1 in 20,000 children
List 2 symptoms with which patients may present.	Strabismus; abnormal red reflex (the reflex actually appears white [leukocoria] because of reflection of light off the tumor surface)
Is retinoblastoma hereditary?	About 40% of cases are familial; the remainder are sporadic.
What causes retinoblastoma?	Loss of function of both allelic copies of the retinoblastoma gene (RB1), a tumor-suppressor gene on chromosome 13.
What are the 2 goals of treatment?	Eradication of the tumor and retention of vision.
List 3 treatments of unilateral retinoblastoma.	1. Enucleation if no potential for vision exists. 2. If tumor is small, laser or cryotherapy is preferred. 3. If tumor is large, chemotherapy is

employed with possible radiation or brachytherapy as required.

How is bilateral retino-blastoma treated?

Chemotherapy and subsequent local control with laser, cryotherapy, or hyper-thermia

What is the prognosis?

A 90% survival rate may be expected when enucleation of a unilateral tumor can be performed. Good survival is also expected with vision-sparing strategies.
Bilateral disease has a poorer outcome. Potential side effects of therapy include adverse radiation effects (cataracts, impaired orbital growth, lacrimal dysfunction, retinal vascular injuries) and secondary malignancies induced by chemotherapy.

For what other type of tumors are patients with retinoblastoma at risk?

Osteosarcomas, particularly in patients with hereditary retinoblastoma

RHABDOMYOSARCOMA

What is it?

It is a soft tissue tumor of skeletal muscle origin

What is the incidence?

250 new cases per year in the US. It is the most common soft tissue sarcoma in infants and children. 70% are younger than 10 years at diagnosis. There is a slight male predominance.

List 5 conditions that predispose a child to rhabdomyosarcoma.

Li-Fraumeni syndrome (familial cancer syndrome with p53 gene mutation), Werner syndrome, basal cell nevus syndrome, tuberous sclerosis, neuro-fibromatosis

Is there family clustering of cases?

There may be familial occurrences. Also, female relatives of children with rhabdo-myosarcoma may have an increased risk of breast cancer.

What are the most common ages at presentation?

Two peak age spans: 2–5 years and 12–18 years.

List 3 important prognostic criteria.	Site, histology, stage
List 12 of the primary sites of rhabdomyosarcoma in children.	Orbit, paratesticular, vagina, uterus, extremity, bladder, prostate, perianal, retroperitoneal, chest wall, head, and neck
Which 2 sites are the most common?	Head and neck
List 4 sites for which prognosis is relatively favorable.	Orbit, vagina, vulva, and paratesticular sites
What are the 6 histology types and their relative prognoses?	**Favorable:** botryoid, spindle cell **Intermediate:** embryonal, pleomorphic **Poor:** alveolar, undifferentiated
What is the most common histologic type?	Embryonal (~60% of rhabdomyosarcoma cases)
List the "Groups" (i.e., stages) of rhabdomyosarcoma, with their characteristics.	**Group I:** completely resected localized disease **Group II:** grossly resected tumor with residual microscopic disease or positive lymph nodes (removed) **Group III:** gross residual disease **Group IV:** metastatic disease
What are the signs and symptoms?	They vary according to the site of tumor.
List 2 ways in which it is usually diagnosed.	By biopsy or at excision of the tumor after primary workup
How is further tumor evaluation carried out?	This also depends on the site of the tumor. 1. Usually MRI or CT imaging is required. 2. Chest radiographs and bone scan are used to rule out spread.
What are treatment options and when are they used?	Surgical excision is desired, but this may not be possible if the tumor involves vital structures. In these cases, chemotherapy

and radiation may be required before tumor resection. Overall, the trend has been away from radical surgery. When the tumor can be primarily resected, chemotherapy and often radiation therapy are needed as adjuvant treatment. A significant exception is when the primary tumor arises in the orbit. In these cases, chemotherapy and radiation, without surgery, will result in a 90% survival rate.

What is the prognosis?

Overall survival rate during the third Intergroup Rhabdomyosarcoma Sarcoma (IRS) trial was 70% for 5 years.

OSTEOGENIC SARCOMA

What is it?

A bone tumor characterized by spindle cells.

List 6 cytologic forms in which it may occur.

It may occur in various cytologic forms, including osteoblastic, chondroblastic, fibroblastic, telangiectatic, giant-cell type, and malignant fibrous histiocytoma-like.

How common is osteogenic sarcoma?

Fewer than 500 new cases yearly, but it is the most common malignant bone tumor in children.

List 8 risk factors for osteogenic sarcoma.

Loss of retinoblastoma (RB1) gene; Li-Fraumeni syndrome; Rothmund-Thomson syndrome; radiation for other malignancies; enchondromatosis; Paget disease; fibrous dysplasia; hereditary exostoses

List 3 sites that are most commonly affected.

Distal femur, proximal tibia, proximal humerus

Is there a gender difference in incidence?

Males outnumber females by as much as 2:1.

Which 2 portions of the bone are most commonly affected?

Medullary cavity, metaphysis

How do patients with these tumors typically present?

Persistent pain after minor trauma is the typical history. A mass may be palpable.

What is the characteristic radiographic finding?	Periosteal elevation with a "**sunburst**" pattern of soft tissue calcifications.
What is the most common mode of spread for these tumors?	To the lung via hematogenous route.
What is the tumor marker for osteogenic sarcoma?	Alkaline phosphatase
What are the components of the most common treatment strategy?	Although surgical resection was often the initial treatment, preoperative chemotherapy and resection using limb salvage techniques are now the most common treatment strategy.
What is the outcome?	Overall survival rate is 60%–75%.

EWING SARCOMA

What is it?	A sarcoma that normally develops in the bone marrow and consists of small blue round cells.
List 4 bones that are most commonly affected.	The femur, humerus, ribs, and flat bones (e.g., the scapula); however, any bone may be affected
What part of the bone is most commonly affected?	The midshaft
In what age group and gender does Ewing sarcoma most commonly appear?	Male adolescents
What are typical presenting symptoms?	Bone pain followed by swelling is usually the initial symptom. Bone necrosis can ensue, causing fever, and thus Ewing sarcoma is often misdiagnosed as osteomyelitis.
What are typical radiographic findings?	Disruption of the bony cortex with layers of new periosteal bone formation resulting in an "onionskin" appearance.
What is the typical treatment strategy?	Usually a combination of chemotherapy and radiation is undertaken before

surgical resection of the involved bony region.

What is the outcome?

Usually limb salvage can be achieved. The overall survival rate is approximately 75% for localized tumors. Prognosis is worse for pelvic tumors and metastatic disease.

To what site does the tumor most commonly metastasize?

The lungs

MEDULLOBLASTOMA

What is it?

It is a tumor of the **posterior fossa**. It is characterized by "small round blue cells" of the primitive neuroectodermal tumor (PNET) type.

Where does it originate?

From the **roof of the fourth ventricle**

What are typical symptoms?

Signs and symptoms of **increased intracranial pressure (ICP)** including: headache, vomiting, diplopia, and papilledema; **in infants, a bulging fontanel** may be present.

What is the most useful diagnostic study?

MRI

What is the age of onset?

Generally, younger than 7 years of age

What is the typical treatment strategy?

Surgical removal with associated radiation therapy; if there is residual tumor after surgical removal, chemotherapy may also be needed

What is the outcome?

In favorable risk groups, 70%–90% 5-year survival.

ASTROCYTOMA

What is it?

It is a tumor of glial origin that tends to be cystic in nature.

List 2 regions in which it occurs.

In the cerebellar and intracerebral regions

What are the symptoms and signs?

They depend on the location of the tumor.

Cerebellar tumors? (List 5 symptoms)	Headache, vomiting, diplopia, papilledema, or hydrocephalus.
Tumors of the cerebral tissue? (List 3)	Epilepsy, upper motor neuron signs, or even arrested growth of the opposite extremity.
What is the most useful diagnostic study?	MRI
What is the treatment?	Surgical removal of the tumor. Follow-up radiation therapy may be required for high-grade astrocytoma or tumors that show residual progression postoperatively.
What is the outcome?	Cerebellar tumors have a much better outcome than cerebral tumors. Five-year survival for cerebellar tumors is 90%; for cerebral tumors 30%–80%. The worse the grade, the poorer the prognosis.

HEPATOBLASTOMA

What is it?	A malignant liver tumor of embryonal origin.
List the 5 types.	1. Fetal or well-differentiated 2. Embryonal (immature and poorly differentiated) 3. Mixed epithelial and mesenchymal 4. Macrotrabecular 5. Anaplastic
At what age is hepatoblastoma most commonly seen?	Usually before 4 years of age. Median age is 18 months.
List 10 potential risk factors.	Hemihypertrophy, Beckwith-Wiedemann syndrome, familial polyposis, Gardner syndrome, Fanconi anemia, fetal alcohol syndrome, cirrhosis, tyrosinemia, TPN-cholestasis, Type I glycogen storage disease
What are typical signs and symptoms?	A large right upper-quadrant mass. Nausea and vomiting may also be present.

What are pertinent laboratory values?	Serum bilirubin, alphafetoprotein (αFP) and human chorionic gonadotropin (HCG) are commonly elevated.
What are the components of the diagnostic workup?	Serum tumor markers, a plain chest and abdominal radiograph, ultrasound examination to rule out involvement of surrounding structures or the vena cava, a CT scan of the abdomen, bone marrow aspirate, and bone scan. MRI may further delineate anatomy and tumor involvement of vascular and biliary structures.
How is hepatoblastoma treated?	Tumor resection is the primary treatment. Chemotherapy may be initial treatment for exceptionally large tumors to reduce the tumor to a resectable size. **Complete surgical resection of the primary tumor, either before or after adjuvant therapy, is required for survival.** If a tumor is confined to the liver, but not to a resectable area, liver transplantation is considered.
What percentage of children with hepatoblastoma have surgically resectable tumors?	Fewer than 50%
List the stages of hepatocellular tumors and their characteristics. (Note – this system is the same for hepatoma)	**Stage I:** total resection of the specimen with clean margins **Stage II:** total gross resection with microscopic residual disease **Stage III:** unresectable tumor or gross residual disease **Stage IV:** metastatic disease
What is the outcome?	Children with Stage 1 disease who undergo a complete resection and chemotherapy may have an 85%–90% survival rate. Survival rate may be slightly higher if histology is purely fetal. Overall survival rate for all cases of hepatoblastoma is 50%.

HEPATOMA

What is it?	Hepatocellular carcinoma is an epithelial malignancy similar to that seen in adults.

It accounts for about 25% of pediatric liver tumors but is rare in infants and young children.

List 16 risk factors for hepatoma.

Chronic hepatitis from hepatitis B and C viruses; cirrhosis; hemihypertrophy; Beckwith-Wiedemann syndrome; Fanconi anemia; fetal alcohol syndrome; type I glycogen storage disease; tyrosinemia; aflatoxin ingestion; hemochromatosis; hepatic venous obstruction; androgen and estrogen exposure; Alagille syndrome; α1–antitrypsin deficiency; neonatal hepatitis and biliary atresia

In which lobe of the liver is hepatoma commonly found?

The right lobe

How and to what sites does the tumor commonly spread?

It first spreads intrahepatically via lymphatic and vascular channels. It may then extend along the hepatic veins and vena cava. Hematogenous spread is to the lung, brain, and bone marrow.

What are typical manifestations of hepatoma?

Right upper quadrant mass, nausea, vomiting, abdominal pain, weight loss, anemia

List 7 important laboratory tests.

1. CBC
2. Serum glutamic-oxaloacetic transaminase (aspartate aminotransferase)(SGOT)
3. Serum glutamic-pyruvic transaminase (alanine aminotransferase)(SGPT)
4. Alkaline phosphatase
5. Bilirubin, which is almost always normal except in advanced cases
6. Serum αFP, which is elevated in 50% of childhood cases
7. Serum ferritin, which is elevated in virtually all cases

What are key diagnostic tests?

1. Ultrasound determines that the mass is solid.
2. CT delineates extent of the tumor and vascular involvement.
3. Bone marrow aspirate

4. Bone scan
5. A hepatic angiogram or MRI may help determine liver and tumor anatomy and vascular variations.

What is the preferred treatment?

Complete resection is required for cure. If the tumor is too large for resection initially, chemotherapy may be used to try to shrink the tumor. Postoperative chemotherapy is always needed.

List 3 major metabolic concerns following hepatic resection.

Hypoalbuminemia, hypoglycemia, hypothrombinemia

What is the overall survival rate for children with hepatoma?

Less than 15%

SACROCOCCYGEAL TERATOMA (SCT)

What is it?

A teratoma is a tumor consisting of tissue from some or all of 3 primitive germ-cell layers (i.e., endoderm, mesoderm, ectoderm). Tissue may reveal itself in varying degrees of maturity. The sacrococcygeal area is the most common site for teratomas.

List 2 occasions when a sacrococcygeal teratoma (SCT) is usually noted.

Prenatal ultrasound exam or at birth

List 6 other sites teratomas may be found.

Ovary, testicle, head, neck, mediastinum, retroperitoneum

List 3 signs and symptoms.

1. In sacrococcygeal area, tumor protrudes from presacral space and pushes the rectum forward. The tumor may weigh as much as the infant!
2. Tumors in other sites may manifest as physical deformities.
3. Tumors may manifest as a result of compression of surrounding structures, such as the lung or trachea.

What are characteristic radiologic findings?	Calcifications in 50% of cases
What is the malignant potential?	Low in infants, but the potential increases with age
What are 2 serum tumor markers for SCT?	HCG (choriocarcinoma) and αFP (yolk sac carcinoma) These markers are monitored in follow-up to detect recurrence.
What is the treatment?	Surgical removal
What is the vascular source of an SCT?	Presacral vessels; these must be removed with the coccyx to minimize the potential for recurrence and malignancy.
What is the outcome?	If the tumor is benign, outcome is excellent (but it is necessary to monitor for recurrence of malignant tissue). If malignancy is present, outcome is poor. If the primary tumor has malignant components, recurrence is common, even if original tumor is thought to be completely excised.

MELANOMA

What is the incidence of melanoma in children?	It accounts for 1%–3% of all pediatric malignancies and 1%–4% of all melanomas.
List 10 risk factors for melanoma.	1. Fair skin 2. Familial atypical mole melanoma (FAMM) syndrome 3. Xeroderma pigmentosum 4. Increased numbers of melanocytic nevi 5. Acquired nevi, especially in areas of chronic irritation or trauma 6. Giant congenital nevus 7. Atypical nevi 8. Excessive (especially intense and intermittent) sun exposure 9. Family history 10. Immunosuppression **NOTE: In 30%–50% of cases, melanoma will occur at a site without a previous nevus.**

List Clark's levels of tumor invasion, with their characteristics.

Level I: tumor cells above basement membrane (i.e., in situ)
Level II: invasion of papillary dermis
Level III: tumor cells at junction of papillary and reticular dermis
Level IV: invasion of reticular dermis
Level V: invasion of subcutaneous fat

List Breslow's classifications of tumor thickness.

In situ
< 0.76 mm
0.76–1.5 mm
1.5–4 mm
> 4 mm

What determines prognosis?

Thickness of tumor and evidence of metastases.

What is the overall mortality rate?

40%

List 3 treatments.

1. Local excision with an appropriate margin may be all that is needed.
2. For extensive tumors, adjuvant chemotherapy is needed.
3. The role of lymph node dissection is controversial, although resection of the appropriate nodal group may benefit survival in early-stage lesions.

List 2 preventive measures.

Avoidance of intense sun and use of protective clothing and sunscreen; regular surveillance of questionable nevi by a dermatologist

27

Skin, Soft Tissue, Nail, and Hair Disorders

SKIN

LYMPHANGIOMA

What is it?
A benign tumor of the lymphatic system that consists of large or small saccules of lymph fluid

What is "cystic hygroma?"
This term is usually used to describe a large, primarily cystic lymphangioma of the neck.

When do patients usually present with lymphangiomas?
At or soon after birth

Where are lymphangiomas located?
Anywhere in the body, but most commonly the neck, axilla, mediastinum, groin, and lower abdomen

What are the symptoms?
Usually presents as a painless mass, but lymphangiomas of the neck, tongue, or glottic regions may cause respiratory distress. Occasionally, a lymphangioma may present as an acutely enlarging mass due to infection or inflammation.

Do lymphangiomas regress?
No

List 2 treatments.
Surgical excision (re-excision may be necessary in 10%–15% of cases); sclerosing agents (mixed results)

HEMANGIOMA

What is it?
Abnormal proliferation of vascular endothelial cells, resulting in tumors of

varying sizes and types composed of abnormal blood vessels

How do people with hemangiomas present?

Although most are visible on the skin, hemangiomas may involve any organ. Presentation may relate to the effect on the involved organ. In addition, large hemangiomas (particularly of the liver) may cause heart failure due to arteriovenous shunting, or purpura due to consumption of platelets (Kasabach-Merritt syndrome)

List 3 ways they are diagnosed.

Cutaneous lesions are easily diagnosed by **physical examination**.
Ultrasound or **CT** may be required for intracorporeal lesions.

May hemangiomas be multiple?

Yes! Discovery of one hemangioma should prompt a search for others. The examiner should ask about any evidence of airway obstruction.

What is the typical course of a hemangioma?

Growth of the hemangioma over the first 1–1½ years, followed by involution; 80% are gone by 5 years of age.

List 2 treatments.

If functional difficulties should arise, oral or injected steroids may be used initially; alpha interferon (INF-α) has also been effective.

List 7 indications for medical therapy.

1. Obstruction of vision
2. Thrombocytopenia
3. Obstruction of luminal organs
4. Uncontrollable hemorrhage or ulceration
5. Repeated infection
6. Cardiac compromise because of arteriovenous shunting
7. Increasing size causing symptoms (e.g., enlarging liver hemangioma impeding diaphragmatic excursion).

List 2 indications for surgical resection.

Any indication listed above that does not respond to medical therapy; symptoms too severe to wait for medical results

ATOPIC DERMATITIS (ECZEMA)

What is it?	A common inflammatory skin disorder of infancy and childhood in which the acute phase is characterized by an **itch-scratch** cycle; usually noninfectious
How does the patient usually present?	With an erythematous, papulovesicular eruption that can progress to a scaly, lichenified dermatitis over time. It is worse in the winter and is usually seen on the face, neck, and antecubital and popliteal fossae.
What is the prevalence?	1% of the general population and 3%–5% of children younger than 5 years of age; 90% of patients present before 5 years of age.
What is the pathogenesis?	Unknown; patients with moderate-to-severe atopic dermatitis frequently have elevated IgE as a result of altered regulation of its synthesis.
What are the phases of atopic dermatitis?	The distribution of the rash varies among 3 distinct phases: infancy phase, childhood phase, and adult phase.
What is the distribution of the rash?	
In infancy?	Cheeks, scalp, trunk, and extensor surface of the extremities.
In the childhood phase?	Flexor surfaces, especially the antecubital and popliteal fossae, wrists, and ankles.
In the adult phase?	Face, back, feet, and neck.
Individuals with atopic dermatitis are often prone to what 5 types of skin infections?	*Staphylococcus aureus*, β-hemolytic streptococci, herpes simplex, *Molluscum contagiosum*, fungal infections
With what is atopic dermatitis associated?	Families with a high incidence of allergies, asthma, or both.

What is the differential diagnosis?	Seborrheic dermatitis, psoriasis, scabies, contact dermatitis, drug reactions, zinc deficiency, severe combined immunodeficiency
What is the prognosis?	80%–90% of patients outgrow it by puberty.
What is the treatment?	Therapy is directed at controlling dryness (bath oils, mild soap, moisturizers, emollients), inflammation (topical corticosteroids), and itching (antihistamines). Environmental control is important. Antibiotics or antifungals are used for infections as needed.
What types of steroid treatment should be avoided in infants?	Strong fluorinated steroids on the face

IMPETIGO

What is it?	A cutaneous infection of either staphylococcal or streptococcal origin
What are the 2 types?	Bullous and nonbullous
Which type is more common?	Nonbullous—accounting for approximately 70% of cases of impetigo
What are the characteristics of nonbullous impetigo?	A small vesicle or pustule forms on a predisposing lesion and may spread to a honey-colored, clustered lesion of approximately 2 cm. Is usually more common during warm weather.
List 5 predisposing lesions.	Chickenpox, insect bites, abrasions, lacerations, burns
What is the treatment?	Lesions usually resolve on their own within 2 weeks. Antibiotic therapy is usually not needed.
Who typically gets bullous impetigo?	Infants and young children
What is the most common bacterial cause?	Staphylococcus (80% of cases)

What are the characteristics of bullous impetigo?	Transparent, flaccid bullae develop on the affected skin.
What is the treatment?	Either topical or oral antibiotics
List 5 potential complications of impetigo.	Cellulitis, osteomyelitis, septic arthritis, pneumonia, septicemia
What is a rare renal complication?	Poststreptococcal glomerulonephritis (Ch 21, p. 298)

CELLULITIS

What is it?	Acute inflammation of the dermis and subcutaneous fat, usually caused by bacterial invasion of the skin
What are some etiologic agents?	*Streptococcus pyogenes* (group A) and *Staphylococcus aureus* are most common. *Streptococcus pneumoniae, Haemophilus influenzae,* Group B *streptococcus,* and *Escherichia coli* also cause cellulitis.
Which are most common in newborns? (List 2)	Group B *streptococcus, E. coli*
In infants and young children? (1)	*H. influenzae*
List 3 features of the clinical picture.	1. Skin that is red, tender, edematous, warm, and may be indurated; borders of the lesions are indistinct and not elevated. 2. Enlarged, tender regional lymph nodes, lymphangitis 3. Fever, chills, malaise, poor appetite
List 3 mechanisms of spread.	1. **Local spread:** break in skin (e.g., wound, bite, excoriation, impetigo, folliculitis, carbuncle, varicella) 2. **Hematogenous spread** 3. **Direct extension** from deeper infection
List 4 groups of patients in which blood cultures are useful for determining the offending organism.	Those with systemic illness or facial cellulitis, newborns, immunocompromised patients. In most others, blood cultures are usually unrevealing.

Is tissue aspiration useful?	A positive culture may be obtained in up to 50% of patients (higher in immunocompromised patients). (Note: This is painful. The physician should consider carefully.)
What is the treatment?	**Antibiotic therapy** is aimed at the most likely causative organisms. Adjunctive therapies include warm compresses, bed rest, elevation, and pain control.
Which patients require IV antibiotics?	Newborns; immunocompromised patients; patients with high fever, systemic toxicity, vomiting, or periorbital or orbital cellulitis; or patients who show no improvement after 2 days of oral therapy. Outpatient therapy with intramuscular (IM) ceftriaxone is an alternative for patients with capacity for reliable follow-up.
What is erysipelas?	A skin infection usually caused by group A β-hemolytic *streptococcus*
In what 2 segments of the pediatric population does it most often occur?	Neonates and infants
What are the clinical features of erysipelas?	Malaise, myalgia, and systemic illness followed by development of a characteristic skin lesion.
List 4 characteristics of the skin lesion.	1. Rapid expansion 2. Sharply demarcated erythematous and elevated advancing edge. 3. Irregular, fluid-filled blisters. 4. Often involves the umbilical stump in neonates.
What is periorbital cellulitis?	Inflammation of soft tissues of the eye superficial to the orbital septum
List 6 causes.	Trauma, insect bites, severe conjunctivitis with spread of infection to the surrounding area, bacteremia, sinusitis, and hematogenous spread.

List 4 causative organisms.	*S. aureus:* usually when trauma, insect bite, or other skin infection (e.g., impetigo) is present *H. influenzae:* with bacteremia *S. pneumoniae:* with bacteremia Group A β-hemolytic *streptococcus*
What is the clinical presentation?	Eyelid, conjunctiva, and the surrounding area are swollen, red, warm, and indurated. A purple hue to the skin may be associated with *H. influenzae.* Fever and systemic toxicity may be present.
What is involved in the evaluation of periorbital cellulitis?	CBC, blood culture, and culture of the wound or lesion (if appropriate). The physician must rule out true "orbital" cellulitis clinically or by formal ophthalmology evaluation, a CT scan, or both, looking for orbital involvement (e.g., extraocular muscle (EOM) entrapment, proptosis, swelling of the optic nerve). Lumbar puncture should be performed if meningitis is suspected.
What is the treatment?	**Intravenous antibiotics**
What are 3 possible complications of true orbital cellulitis?	Compression or stretching of the optic nerve and loss of vision; cavernous sinus thrombosis; meningitis (Ch 28, p. 396)
What is buccal cellulitis?	Infection of the skin and subcutaneous tissues of the cheek
In what age group is this most common?	In children 6 months to 3 years of age.
What are 2 common causative organisms?	Hematogenous spread of *H. influenzae* or *S. pneumoniae.*
What other condition is commonly associated with buccal cellulitis?	Up to a 90% incidence of accompanying **meningitis**
What is the treatment?	Usually IV antibiotics.

HYPER- AND HYPOPIGMENTATION

What are hyper- and hypopigmentation?	An excess or deficiency in skin pigmentation, respectively.

What are the causes of pigmentation changes?	Pigmentation changes may be local or generalized and are due to a wide variety of defects, including: Absence of melanocytes; defective melanocytes; overproduction of melanin; pigmentation changes induced by hormones; focal developmental defects; postinflammatory sequelae
What are freckles?	Light or dark brown macules with poorly defined edges, usually less than 3 mm in diameter, that occur in sun-exposed areas of the body.
In whom are they most common?	Fair-haired individuals
What determines formation of freckles besides sun exposure?	Freckles may be a familial trait.
What is the histology of a freckle?	Increased melanin and pigment in the epidermal base cells
What are lentigines?	Small, round, dark brown macules. They can occur anywhere on the body and are generally less than 3 cm.
Are these related to freckles?	No. They have no relation to sun exposure.
What is their histology?	Increased numbers of melanocytes with dense deposits of melanin in elongated, club-shaped, epidermal rete ridges.
List 6 conditions in which lentigines are found.	Addison disease; pregnancy; lentiginosis profusa; LAMB syndrome—**L**entigines, **A**trial myxoma, **M**ucocutaneous myxomas, **B**lue nevi; leopard syndrome; Peutz-Jeghers syndrome
What are "café au lait" spots?	These are uniformly hyperpigmented macular lesions with sharp demarcation. The true hue (not always "café au lait") is determined by the natural skin tone; the deeper the color of the skin tone, the deeper the color of the spot. They may be quite large in size.

What is the histology?	Increased numbers of melanocytes and melanin in the epidermis
Are café au lait spots found in otherwise healthy children?	Yes—10% of healthy children have café au lait spots. A child in this group typically has 1–3 spots.
With what conditions may café au lait spots be associated?	McCune-Albright syndrome; neurofibromatosis (von Recklinghausen disease) (Ch 30); Russell-Silver syndrome; multiple lentigines; ataxia telangiectasia; Fanconi anemia (Ch 15, p. 176); tuberous sclerosis (Ch 30); Bloom syndrome; epidermal nevus syndrome; Chédiak-Higashi syndrome

Albinism

What is it?	A group of conditions in which there is failure or deficiency of melanin production in the skin, hair, and eyes.
What is partial albinism?	Also called piebaldism, it is characterized by sharply demarcated amelanotic patches on the forehead, anterior scalp, ventral trunk, elbows, and knees.
How is partial albinism transmitted?	As an autosomal dominant trait
How does the defective gene for partial albinism occur?	Mutation in the KIT proto-oncogene
What is the histology of the depigmented regions in partial albinism?	Absence of melanocytes and melanosomes

Waardenburg Syndrome

List 7 characteristics.	Lateral displacement of the medial canthi with dystopia canthorum, broad nasal root, heterochromic irises, congenital deafness, a white forelock, and cutaneous hypopigmentation.
What is the inheritance pattern?	Autosomal dominant with variable penetrance and expression

Vitiligo

What is it?

Acquired, sharply circumscribed depigmented macules of varying size and shape

What causes vitiligo?

Unknown, but may be due to an autoimmune mechanism. Tends to occur in areas of frequent trauma.

List 5 associated conditions.

Hypothyroidism, hyperthyroidism, adrenal insufficiency, pernicious anemia, diabetes

What is the course of vitiligo?

Spontaneous repigmentation in about 10%–20% of patients. In most patients, progression of depigmentation occurs.

What is the treatment?

Oral or topical psoralen compounds administered together with exposure to sunlight or ultraviolet (UV) light sources. Repigmentation may be partial and may take many months to occur. Topical steroids are occasionally useful. It is important to protect depigmented areas from excessive sunlight, because there is no protection provided by melanocytes.

STURGE-WEBER SYNDROME

What is it?

A condition characterized by a constellation of symptoms. The most obvious symptom is a **facial hemangioma (port wine stain)**. Seizures, hemiparesis, intracranial calcifications, and mental retardation may be components of this condition. (**Note:** Not all patients with a facial port wine stain have Sturge-Weber syndrome.)

What is the etiology?

Thought to be due to anomalous development of the vascular bed during cerebral vascularization.

What are 4 clinical manifestations, and their characteristics?

1. **Facial hemangioma** is present at birth. It may extend to the lower face, the trunk, and the mucosa of the mouth and pharynx and frequently

	occurs in the distribution of the trigeminal nerve.
	2. **Seizures,** if present, usually occur within the first year of life and become increasingly refractory to therapy.
	3. **Mental retardation** may be present; more common in patients with seizures.
	4. **Ocular manifestations**—include buphthalmos and glaucoma.

How is the diagnosis made?	1. The constellation of symptoms
	2. Radiograph of the skull—the presence of intracranial calcifications on radiograph, together with the symptoms, suggest the diagnosis.
	3. CT scan of the head—may show unilateral cortical atrophy and ipsilateral dilation of the lateral ventricle.

What are 4 components of treatment?	1. Control of seizures.
	2. Hemispherectomy or lobectomy (for intractable seizures).
	3. Laser therapy (for facial hemangioma).
	4. Monitor ocular pressure for glaucoma.

PROTEUS SYNDROME

What is it?	A disturbance of ectodermal and mesodermal growth. The etiology is unknown.

List 7 clinical manifestations.	Asymmetric overgrowth of the extremities, verrucous skin lesions, angiomas, lipomas, bone thickening, macrocephaly, excessive muscle growth

What is the treatment?	Currently there is no known treatment.

MONGOLIAN SPOTS

What are they?	Bluish areas of increased dermal melanocytosis, frequently found across the lumbosacral and gluteal regions of newborns

In which infants are they commonly found?	In infants whose natural skin has medium-to-dark pigmentation.
Are mongolian spots malignant?	No. They are thought to be benign, but may be mistaken for bruises.

CONGENITAL MELANOCYTIC NEVI

What are they?	Darkly pigmented nevi present at birth; sizes vary
Is there a risk of malignancy?	Yes. Some experts recommend removal in childhood.

TINEA VERSICOLOR

What is tinea versicolor?	A superficial fungal disease caused by *Pityrosporum orbiculare*
What are the characteristic lesions?	Round-to-oval lesions, sometimes with a fine scale, that may be either hyper- or hypopigmented

RASHES

What are 4 possible causes of diaper rash?	Irritation from urine or stool, Candidal overgrowth, allergic reaction, and bacterial infection.
What is seborrheic dermatitis?	An oily, yellow, scaly eruption, usually involving the scalp, but it may also involve cheeks, trunk, and diaper area.
What are the etiologic factors?	Unknown, but outbreaks can be associated with stress, poor hygiene, and excessive perspiration.
List 5 viral causes of a rash.	Measles (rubeola), rubella, roseola, "fifth disease," enterovirus
Describe the rash associated with:	
Measles?	Maculopapular, purplish-red rash that generally starts on the face and spreads to the extremities; it lasts 7–10 days. Koplik spots may be seen in the mouth.

With rubella?	Maculopapular rash that spreads from face to extremities; shorter in duration than the measles rash
With roseola?	Macular rash, often at the end of the febrile illness
With "fifth disease" (erythema infectiosum)?	"Slapped cheek" appearance on face; mottled or reticular rash on trunk and extremities
With enteroviruses?	Variable—may be maculopapular or macular; usually on abdomen, chest, palms, and soles
What are 2 bacterial causes of rash?	*S. pyogenes* (scarlet fever), *S. aureus* (staphylococcal scalded skin syndrome and toxic shock syndrome)
Describe the rash associated with:	
Scarlet fever?	Usually diffuse and erythematous, with a sandpaper quality. It may have darker lines in skinfold areas (Pastia's lines), and desquamate, particularly on the face.
With staphylococcal scalded skin syndrome?	Generalized, painful, and beefy red; may show blister or bullae formation.
With toxic shock syndrome?	Rash is diffuse, but usually not tender. Erythema of conjunctivae, lips, mucosa, palms, and soles may be present.

NAIL

INGROWN TOENAIL

What is it?	The side of the toenail burrows into adjoining skin, resulting in swelling, granulation tissue, erythema, and sometimes infection.
Which toe is usually affected?	The large toe
List 3 components of treatment.	1. Soak toe in warm, soapy water to clean and provide symptomatic relief. 2. Antibiotics (if infected)

3. Removal of one-third to one-half of the toenail on the affected side is ultimately needed. Removal of the entire nail with disruption of the matrix of the nail bed will keep the nail from regrowing (if desired by the patient).

How is recurrence prevented?	If the nail regrows, recurrence is common. Chances of ingrowth may be reduced by cutting nails straight across and by teasing the skin away from the nail with a cotton swab as the nail regrows.

HANGNAIL

What is it?	Growth of nail material along the lateral aspect of the nail where it joins into the skin; it is commonly deep-seated and tends to curl away from the normal nail. Discomfort occurs when this area is rubbed or caught on clothes or fabric.
How is it treated?	By pulling it out. (In some cases, freezing or providing a local anesthetic beforehand can help alleviate discomfort from the procedure.)

NAIL (SUBUNGUAL) HEMATOMA

What is it?	Blood clot collected under the nail bed secondary to trauma. It appears as a bluish collection under the nail and can be very painful.
What is the treatment?	Heat the end of a paper clip over a flame and rest it on the nail to melt the nail over the hematoma and drain it. Immediate relief is usually the rule.
What condition may exist if a lesion resembling a hematoma exists without a history of trauma?	Melanoma

PARONYCHIA

What is it?	An area of inflammation or abscess formation involving the folds of tissue at

the base (or at the lateral base) of the fingernail

What are 3 treatments?

1. Often, warm soaks induce drainage, leading to resolution.
2. Antibiotics for the surrounding cellulitis.
3. Occasionally, a small incision is needed for drainage.

FELON

What is it?

Infected collection (essentially a small abscess) in pulp of distal finger pad

List 4 signs and symptoms.

Swelling of finger pad with tenseness and sometimes erythema, extreme tenderness to touch.

What is the treatment?

1. Surgical drainage with incision in midportion of finger pad in the direction of finger.
2. Antibiotics may be needed for cellulitis.

Note: Incisions in lateral aspects of finger are to be avoided despite description of this in older sources. These incisions may damage digital nerves and vessels.

HAIR

TRICHOTILLOMANIA

What is it?

Irregular areas of incomplete hair loss due to compulsive pulling, twisting, or breaking of the hair

What causes this behavior?

In some children, this may be a benign behavior. In others, it may represent an obsessive-compulsive disorder.

What is the treatment?

If a benign habit, treatment of concurrent thumb sucking (which is usually present) may resolve the hair-damaging behavior. In children with obsessive-compulsive disorder, medical therapy with behavioral modification may be necessary.

ALOPECIA

What is it?	Partial or complete hair loss (distinguished from hypotrichosis, which is deficient hair growth)
What are the causes of true alopecia?	Inflammatory dermatoses, mechanical trauma, drugs, infection, endocrine disorders, nutritional imbalance, disturbance of the hair
List 3 causes of alopecia in children.	Alopecia areata; tinea capitis; trichotillomania
What is the treatment?	Usually alopecia will resolve when the underlying cause is treated. It is rarely primary or congenital.
What is alopecia areata?	Focal hair loss, believed to be immune-mediated
How is it treated?	Most children require no treatment. Steroids are helpful in some cases, but relapses may occur.

HYPERTRICHOSIS

What is it?	Excessive hair growth in inappropriate areas. It may be localized, generalized, permanent, or transient. The pattern of hair growth is not in a sexual distribution.
What are the etiologic factors?	It may have racial or familial forms. It is also associated with a variety of conditions, including: local trauma, malnutrition, anorexia nervosa, chronic inflammatory dermatoses, hamartomas or nevi, endocrine disorders (e.g., hypercortisolism), congenital and genetic disorders (e.g., Cornelia de Lange syndrome); a wide variety of drugs, including phenytoin, steroids, cyclosporin, minoxidil, and streptomycin

HIRSUTISM

What is it?	Excessive hair growth in appropriate areas (i.e., in a sexual pattern)

List 7 conditions or factors that are common causes.

Hyperprolactinemia, gonadal tumors (Ch 26, p. 355); endocrine insensitivity; adrenal conditions (e.g., enzyme deficiencies, neoplasms, Cushing syndrome); drugs (e.g., minoxidil, phenytoin, cyclosporin, steroids, oral contraceptives, dyazide diuretics); congenital anomalies or syndromes (e.g., trisomy 18 [Ch 30, p. 445], Cornelia de Lange syndrome, Hurler syndrome, juvenile hypothyroidism [Ch 24, p. 337); true precocious puberty (Ch 24, p. 329)

What is the treatment?

Treatment of the underlying cause

TINEA CAPITIS

What is it?

A superficial fungal infection, usually caused by *Trichophyton tonsurans* or *Microsporum canis*

List 3 ways tinea capitis is diagnosed.

1. Broken-off hair shafts may give a "black-dot" appearance (*T. tonsurans*).
2. Broken-off hair shafts may show yellow-green fluorescence with a Wood's lamp (*T. tonsurans*).
3. Both *T. tonsurans* and *M. canis* may show hyphae and spores under microscopic examination using potassium hydroxide (KOH)

In what 2 ways is it treated?

Topical antifungal agents or systemic treatment with griseofulvin as appropriate

28   Infectious Diseases

MENINGITIS

What is it?	Inflammation of the meninges
What are common clinical findings?	Fever, headache, stiff neck, changes in mental status, cerebrospinal fluid (CSF) leukocytosis
What are the 2 major classes of meningitis?	Bacterial and aseptic (usually viral)

BACTERIAL MENINGITIS

(See Chapter 10, Diseases of the Newborn, p. 97, for a discussion of neonatal bacterial meningitis.)

How does a patient with bacterial meningitis present?	Presentation is highly variable and age dependent.
Neonates and infants?	Nonspecific signs of serious illness include **tachypnea, lethargy, irritability, poor feeding, jaundice, hypoglycemia,** and **vomiting.** Child may be febrile, afebrile, or hypothermic. Later signs: **bulging fontanel, seizures,** and **poor muscle tone**
Older children?	May have more classic meningeal signs, including **Kernig** or **Brudzinski** signs (or both), **headache, photophobia, vomiting, mental status changes** (e.g., lethargy, disorientation). **Petechiae and purpura** are signs of a poor prognosis.
What are the 3 most common causative organisms from birth to 1 month of age?	Group B *streptococcus, Escherichia coli, Listeria monocytogenes*

1–3 months of age? (List 3)	Group B *streptococcus, Streptococcus pneumoniae, Haemophilus influenzae* type b
3 months to 3 years of age?	*S. pneumoniae, Neisseria meningitidis, Haemophilus influenzae* type b
Children older than 3 years of age? (List 3)	*N. meningitidis, S. pneumoniae, H. influenzae* type b
How is the diagnosis of bacterial meningitis made?	**Lumbar puncture** (LP) (See Chapter 2, Pediatric Procedures, p. 11)
List 5 tests that should be conducted on the CSF.	Gram stain, culture, cell count, glucose and protein (See Chapter 2, Pediatric Procedures, p. 12, for normal values of RBC, WBC, and protein concentration. Gram stain and CSF culture should show nothing normally. Glucose should reflect serum levels.)

List 5 CSF findings that suggest meningitis.

1. Gram stain: may show bacteria
2. Culture: will reveal specific organisms
3. Cell count: CSF leukocytosis (usually > 1000) with **predominance of polymorphonuclear neutrophil leukocytes (PMNs).** Note, however, that the presence of any PMNs in CSF is abnormal.
4. Glucose: relative **hypoglycemia** (< 60%–70% of serum glucose)
5. Protein: **elevated total protein**

List 3 issues that may cause difficulties in interpreting CSF findings.

1. "Bloody" spinal taps may confound both protein and white blood cell (WBC) levels
2. Previous treatment with antibiotics (e.g., amoxicillin for otitis) renders culture results inaccurate and may decrease WBC count.
3. Viral meningitis can have CSF profile similar to that of bacterial meningitis early in its course. A second LP may be necessary.

List 3 other findings that are suggestive of meningitis.

1. **High peripheral WBC** with left shift (caution: WBC may be low)
2. **Thrombocytopenia** with **decrease**

in hematocrit (Hct) is suggestive of disseminated intravascular coagulation (DIC) (see Chapter 15, Hematologic Disorders, p 181).

3. **Blood cultures** may be positive.

What should precede LP if high intracranial pressure (ICP) is suspected?

If elevated ICP is suspected (papilledema, focal neurologic signs), CT scan should precede LP. **Do not delay treatment in a seriously ill patient.**

What is the common treatment for bacterial meningitis?

Birth to 4 weeks of age?

Ampicillin and gentamicin.

1–3 months of age?

Ampicillin and third-generation cephalosporin, consider vancomycin if suspicious for *Streptococcus pneumoniae* meningitis.

3 months of age or older?

Third-generation cephalosporin plus vancomycin (**Note:** Determination of antibiotic sensitivities is essential. Treatment before culture should cover likely organisms in the patient's age group and clinical setting.)

What is the duration of treatment?

It depends on the patient's age, the causative organism, and the patient's response to treatment. General guidelines:
H. influenzae type b and *S. pneumoniae:* 10–14 days
N. meningitidis: 14 days
Group B *streptococcus:* 14–21 days
E. coli: 21 days
For meningitis caused by gram-negative organisms, an LP is recommended at the end of treatment to determine that the CSF is free of the organisms. This LP is often recommended for other organisms as well.

What are some other components in the management of meningitis?

1. **Fluid restriction** to two-thirds maintenance (when intravascular volume is restored) may help prevent cerebral edema.

2. **Monitor head circumference** in infants.
3. Close monitoring of **glucose, acid-base** and **volume status,** and **tissue oxygenation** is essential.

Are steroids indicated?

Steroids may decrease hearing loss in *H. influenzae* meningitis. Use varies among institutions.

List 16 complications of meningitis.

Syndrome of inappropriate diuretic hormone secretion (SIADH), cerebral edema, toxic encephalopathy, brain-stem herniation, cranial nerve palsies, deafness, seizures, subdural effusion, cerebral infarct, cortical vein thrombosis, disseminated intravascular coagulation (DIC), paresis, mental retardation, hydrocephalus, visual impairment, mental and motor delays

In what 2 groups of patients are complications most common?

1. **Newborns with gram-negative infection**
2. **Patients with pneumococcal disease** (up to 50% of patients experience complications)

What is the most common complication?

Sensorineural hearing loss (up to 20% of patients with *H. influenzae* meningitis).

What 2 bacteria cause the highest mortality rate?

S. pneumoniae and *N. meningitidis.*

ASEPTIC MENINGITIS

What are signs and symptoms of aseptic meningitis?

Similar to those of bacterial meningitis: **headache, vomiting, stiff neck, photophobia, fever, malaise, myalgia, gastrointestinal (GI) symptoms, rash, tachypnea.**

What is the clinical course?

Usually more indolent than in bacterial meningitis. Classic meningeal signs may be absent. Mental status is usually unaffected, unless encephalitis or increased ICP have developed. **It is prudent to treat as if bacterial until** culture results are available. Some viruses (e.g., herpesvirus, rabies, arbovirus) also cause encephalitis and its accompanying complications.

List 4 findings of the LP.

1. **CSF pleocytosis** is the hallmark, but usually less than in bacterial meningitis (i.e., WBC < 500).
2. **CSF lymphocytosis,** as shown by the differential; may show a higher percentage of neutrophils early in the course
3. Glucose levels are normal or elevated.
4. Protein levels are normal or elevated. **Other specific findings vary** with etiologic factors.

List 9 viral causes.

Enteroviruses (e.g., coxsackievirus, echovirus) are the most common, especially in summer and early fall. Others include **Epstein-Barr, mumps, influenza, herpesvirus, and adenoviruses,** rarely **rabies** and **arboviruses; poliovirus** in endemic areas or unimmunized populations.

How is it diagnosed?

Many viruses can be cultured from the CSF. Enteroviruses can be cultured from stool. Influenza, mumps, and adenovirus may be cultured from the nasopharynx. Serum titers (acute and convalescent) may be helpful. Herpesvirus can be difficult to verify. CT, MRI, and EEG may be useful.

How is viral meningitis treated?

Primarily supportive. Dehydration and pain sometimes necessitate hospitalization. Acyclovir is used for herpes.

What is the clinical course?

Symptoms usually last 1–3 weeks. Headache may be severe.

List 5 categories, with examples, of nonviral causes of aseptic meningitis.

Mycobacteria: *Mycobacterium tuberculosis*
Fungal: *Cryptococcus neoformans* and *Coccidioides immitis* are most

common (should be considered in immunocompromised patients)

Rickettsia: Rocky Mountain spotted fever, Q fever, typhus, and *Ehrlichia* (this should be considered when tick bite or farm animal exposure is in a child's history)

Spirochetes: leptospirosis, Lyme disease, syphilis

Parasites (very uncommon): *Naegleria fowleri* and *acanthamoeba* (amebic meningitis); *Toxoplasma gondii, cysticercosis,* and *trichinosis*

CONJUNCTIVITIS

What is it?	Inflammation of the conjunctiva
What are typical signs and symptoms of infectious conjunctivitis?	**Erythema (injection)** of sclera or inner surface of eyelids, or both; increased tearing, discharge, or both; eyelids may stick together. Pain is uncommon, although child may complain of roughness or itching.
List 3 causes of conjunctivitis.	Infection (e.g., bacteria, viruses), allergy, chemicals
Do viruses or bacteria more commonly cause conjunctivitis?	Bacteria
Which bacteria are the most common in young children?	**Non-typeable *H. influenzae*** and ***S. pneumoniae*.** *Moraxella catarrhalis, Staphylococcus aureus,* and α-*hemolytic streptococcus* are possible pathogens, but are also found in uninfected eyes.
List 2 infectious agents that particularly need to be ruled out in newborns.	*Chlamydia trachomatis, Neisseria gonorrhoeae*
Which is the most common virus isolated?	**Adenovirus**; herpesvirus and enteroviruses uncommonly cause conjunctivitis

What other condition is often associated with conjunctivitis?	**25%–33%** of patients have **otitis media;** 75% of these infections are bacterial.
How is it diagnosed?	Based on **culture;** in the newborn period, a rapid test is available for *N. gonorrhoeae* and *C. trachomatis*
How is it treated?	It will usually resolve without treatment in 7–10 days. **Topical antibiotics** include trimethoprim-sulfa-polymyxin B, erythromycin, bacitracin, gentamicin, and sulfacetamide. *S. pneumoniae* and *H. influenzae* are often resistant to aminoglycosides.
In what 2 instances are systemic antibiotics indicated?	1. When otitis media is simultaneously present (see Otitis Media, p. 403) 2. When the patient cannot tolerate topical therapy.
What is EKC?	Epidemic keratoconjunctivitis
What causes EKC?	Adenovirus type 8; EKC **is very contagious**.
List 3 symptoms.	It is associated with a **preauricular node,** and presents with **eye pain** and **photophobia**
List 4 signs and symptoms of allergic conjunctivitis.	Itching, redness, tearing, and photophobia—usually bilateral. Seasonal exacerbations and recurrent disease are common. (See Chapter 29, Allergic Diseases, p. 438.)
What is a characteristic physical finding?	Papillary hyperplasia with edema, leading to "cobblestoning" of conjunctiva.
What are 2 associated features?	1. There may be history or presence of other atopic disease 2. Child may have angioedema of eyelids
What is vernal conjunctivitis? (List 4 characteristics)	A **chronic** form of conjunctivitis, characterized by severe itching, photophobia, blurry vision, and lacrimation

What is a characteristic physical finding?	**Large papillae** on the upper eyelids

OTITIS MEDIA

What are the 3 types of otitis media?	1. Acute otitis media (AOM) 2. Otitis media with effusion (OME) 3. Chronic otitis media (COM)

AOM

What is it?	Infection of fluid in middle ear space
Why is otitis media more common in infants than in older children?	**Anatomy:** The eustachian tube drains fluid from the middle ear to the nasopharynx, and protects against reflux of nasopharyngeal pathogens. Infants have relatively horizontal eustachian tubes that become more vertical and widen as they grow. **Infections:** Babies have frequent colds, causing obstruction of the eustachian tubes. Viruses also damage the ciliated epithelium of the tube. These factors inhibit the protective function of the eustachian tube.
List 8 clinical signs of otitis media.	Prior or current upper respiratory infection (URI), fever, fussiness, sleeplessness, "pulling at ears" or ear pain, decreased hearing, vomiting, poor appetite
List 5 physical findings.	1. URI often present 2. Tympanic membrane (TM) is swollen, opaque, and discolored (red, yellow, or gray) 3. Normal TM landmarks are obscured 4. Mobility of the TM is decreased or absent on pneumatic otoscopy or tympanogram 5. Fluid may or may not be visible through the TM
What finding is the most conclusive?	**Lack of TM mobility**

List the 4 most common bacterial pathogens.

S. pneumoniae is the most common (30%–40% of cases), followed by *H. influenzae, M. catarrhalis,* and *Streptococcus pyogenes*.
S. aureus is an uncommon cause. Gram-negative enteric bacteria cause up to 15% of cases in infants < 6 weeks of age.

Viral pathogens? (List 4)

Believed to cause up to 30% of AOM cases; include respiratory syncytial virus (RSV), influenza, adenovirus, and coxsackievirus.

List 2 reasons to treat otitis media.

Treatment is thought to:
1. Prevent conductive hearing loss
2. Prevent rare complications, such as mastoiditis, meningitis, and cholesteatoma

List 5 considerations in choosing whether to treat with antibiotics.

1. Many infections are minor or viral and resolve without therapy. In some countries, AOM is rarely treated with antibiotics.
2. Nearly 100% of *M. catarrhalis,* 20% of *H. influenzae,* and 25% of *S. pneumonia* cases are beta-lactamase-producing and resistant to penicillins.
3. **Compliance:** It is not easy to give medicine to a baby. Dosing 3 or more times a day requires medication to be given at day care or at school.
4. **Cost:** New cephalosporins are effective but expensive.
5. **Resistance:** Third-generation cephalosporins have an unnecessarily wide spectrum and could contribute to emerging drug resistance.

What are the 2 usual choices of antibiotics?

Amoxicillin or erythromycin-sulfisoxazole (Pediazole)

List 3 reasons to change antibiotics.

1. **Treatment failure**—no improvement in 2–3 days on initial antibiotic with good compliance
2. **Recurrence**—another episode of AOM within 6 weeks
3. **Side effects**—diarrhea, GI upset, allergic reactions

What are some second-choice antibiotics?	1. High dose amoxicillin (80 mg/kg/day) 2. Amoxicillin (40mg/kg/day) *plus* amoxicillin/clavulanic acid 3. Cefuroxime, macrolides (erythromycin, azithromycin), cefpodoxime
What is recurrent otitis media?	Three or more episodes of AOM in 6 months, or four or more episodes in 12 months, with documented clinical resolution in between episodes
How can it be prevented?	Prophylactic antibiotic therapy with amoxicillin, sulfisoxazole, or trimethoprim-sulfamethoxazole may be effective.

OME

What is it?	Fluid (effusion) in the middle ear space without infection; it occurs alone, secondary to URI, or as a sequela of AOM
List 4 possible symptoms.	OME is often asymptomatic, but can manifest as hearing loss, "plugged ears," vertigo, or clumsiness.
What are the signs?	Fluid seen behind TM; decreased mobility of the TM
What is the clinical course?	Spontaneous resolution in majority of cases (> 50% by 3 months and 75% by 6 months); more rapid resolution following AOM (90% by 3 months)
What are complications?	1. Hearing impairment may cause abnormal language development, behavioral problems, and poor school performance. 2. OME predisposes the patient to AOM and subsequent COM
What is the treatment?	
Duration < 3 months?	Observation only; assess hearing if a condition lasts 3 months or longer.
Duration up to 6 months without hearing loss?	Antibiotics may cause more rapid resolution but are not necessary because of high rate of spontaneous resolution.

Duration of 3 months with bilateral hearing loss?	Antibiotics should be given, with close follow-up for resolution of effusion and restoration of hearing
Duration > 3 months with bilateral hearing loss?	Myringotomy with tympanostomy tube placement is indicated
Are steroids beneficial?	Benefits have not been conclusively shown, and steroids may have adverse effects. Not currently recommended.
Do decongestants or antihistamines help?	Not usually.
Is tonsillectomy or adenoidectomy helpful?	No

COM

What is it?	Inflammation of the middle ear, mastoid, or both, with otorrhea through the TM for > 3 months
List 3 complications.	Mastoiditis, labyrinthitis, cholesteatoma
What is a tympanocentesis?	Also called **myringotomy with aspiration,** it involves puncturing through the TM to collect and drain fluid from the middle ear space.
In which patients is it indicated?	Critically ill or immunocompromised patients, neonates, and patients in whom AOM is unresponsive to 2 or more full courses of antibiotics.
What are tympanostomy tubes?	Also called pressure equalization tubes **(PE tubes),** these small plastic or metal tubes are surgically placed in the TM to drain and ventilate middle ear space.
List 4 indications.	1. Recurrent AOM unresponsive to prophylactic antibiotics 2. OME with bilateral hearing impairment (> 3 months duration) 3. Severe retraction or atelectasis of TM 4. Chronic suppurative complications

List 7 complications of tympanostomy tubes.	Tympanosclerosis or atrophy, dislocation of the tube into the middle ear, cholesteatoma, extrusion of the tube, prolonged otorrhea, and complications of general anesthesia
List 6 risk factors for otitis media.	Passive smoke, day care attendance, horizontal bottle feeding, anatomic defects of oral pharynx, being a twin, experiencing first episode of otitis at less than 2 months of age

THRUSH

What is it?	Overgrowth of *Candida albicans* in oral cavity
Who gets it? (List 4 groups of children)	Infants, children on antibiotics, immunosuppressed children, and those with chronic systemic disorders
What are the clinical features?	Soft, creamy white plaques on buccal mucosa, tongue, palate, and lip commissures; lesions do not scrape off easily and leave an ulcerated red base when removed
What are the treatments?	For infants, nystatin suspension. If it fails, gentian violet may be effective. For older children not at risk for aspiration, clotrimazole topical preparation for the mouth is effective.
What are 2 prevention and control measures?	For **formula-fed infants,** nipples and pacifiers should be consistently sterilized by boiling them for 5 minutes or placing them in a sterilizer; this prevents reinfection. In **breast-fed infants,** the mother's nipples can be a source of infection. The mother should be asked about sore, red, cracked nipples; she may need treatment as well.

PHARYNGITIS/STREPTOCOCCAL PHARYNGITIS

What is pharyngitis?	Sore throat

What is the most common cause?	90% of cases are **viral.**
What is streptococcal pharyngitis?	Pharyngitis caused by group A β-hemolytic *streptococcus*
List 2 complications of streptococcal pharyngitis.	1. Acute rheumatic fever 2. Local complications (e.g., peritonsillar abscess)
List 2 ways the diagnosis is made.	Throat culture (best) or rapid antigen tests
Can streptococcal pharyngitis be diagnosed purely on clinical grounds?	Not consistently. Clinical features overlap with the more common viral causes.
List 2 ways streptococcal pharyngitis is treated.	1. Treatment of choice is penicillin, for 10 days; it may be oral or injectable. 2. Erythromycin for patients allergic to penicillin.

GINGIVOSTOMATITIS

What is it?	Inflammation of the gingiva and oral mucosa
What is the usual cause?	A primary infection with **herpes simplex virus (HSV) type 1** . HSV type 2 is a less common cause.
At what age is it commonly seen?	6 months to 3 years of age
What are typical signs and symptoms?	A prodrome of headache, fever, malaise, and local lymphadenopathy followed by erythema, swelling, and pain of gingiva and palatal mucosa. Grouped vesicles and ulcerations occur on oral mucosa. Bleeding and crusting may occur. It most frequently involves anterior gingiva and palate. Dehydration can follow when pain prevents adequate fluid intake. Secondary infection with a secondary organism may occur.
List 3 ways the diagnosis may be made.	1. It is **usually made clinically**. 2. A **Tzanck prep** of the base of the oral

lesions will show multinucleated giant cells and intranuclear inclusions.

3. Fluid from vesicles may be cultured to confirm HSV.

How can HSV gingivostomatitis be differentiated from hand-foot-mouth disease or aphthous stomatitis?

1. Hand-foot-mouth disease (**coxsackievirus**) lesions typically involve the **posterior palate and pharynx.**

2. **Aphthous stomatitis** lesions are found on **buccal, lingual, and inner lip mucosa.**

What is the clinical course?

Lesions heal spontaneously in 1–2 weeks.

Can it recur?

Reactivation of HSV, leading to recurrent infections, is common. Recurrent infections tend to be less severe with fewer and more localized lesions.

What 3 types of treatment are helpful?

1. **Pain control:** Either acetaminophen, ibuprofen, or both is usually sufficient. Diphenhydramine—antacid (Benadryl-Maalox) suspension (1:1 mix) may provide local pain relief. Viscous lidocaine can be added for children > 6 years of age.

2. **Oral hygiene:** Rinsing with chlorhexidine or glycerine-peroxide mix (for younger children) should replace tooth brushing, which may be too painful.

3. **Hydration:** Cold liquids are best tolerated. Gelatin, flavored ice-pops, and ice cream are useful. Citrus and carbonated beverages are painful to drink. Occasionally, IV fluids are needed.

When is antiviral therapy indicated?

Systemic acyclovir is indicated **only in immunocompromised patients**.

LYMPHADENITIS

What is lymphadenitis (also called adenitis)?

Swelling and inflammation of lymph nodes. It may or may not be painful depending on the etiologic factors.

List 9 common causes of lymphadenitis in children.

Reactive lymph node, staphylococcal infection, atypical mycobacterium, cat-scratch disease, mononucleosis, lymphoma, toxoplasmosis, brucellosis, tularemia

How is it managed?

Usually by treating the primary disease process.

GASTROENTERITIS

List 5 signs and symptoms of acute gastroenteritis.

Signs are variable, but may include nausea, vomiting, diarrhea, abdominal pain, excess flatulence.

What causes most cases of acute gastroenteritis?

Most cases in the US are viral.

VIRAL GASTROENTERITIS

List the 3 viruses that are most common in children.

Rotavirus, adenovirus, "Norwalk" agent

List 2 ways the viruses are spread.

Fecal-oral route, and respiratory route. Good hygiene and hand washing help reduce the risk of infection.

List 4 ways viral gastroenteritis is diagnosed.

1. Usually is a clinical diagnosis.
2. Detection of viral antigens in stool
3. Viral culture (may not be available in some hospitals)
4. Exclusion of bacterial causes by culture

How is viral gastroenteritis treated?

Usually supportive; **prevent dehydration** with IV or oral fluid and electrolyte management, depending on severity

Do most children with acute viral gastroenteritis need IV fluids?

No

What may distinguish viral from bacterial gastroenteritis?

Bacteria more commonly cause bloody diarrhea, stool leukocytes, and tenesmus. Children with **viral** gastroenteritis also may have non-GI symptoms such as cough, nasal discharge, and myalgia.

BACTERIAL GASTROENTERITIS

Name 8 bacteria that cause acute gastroenteritis.	*Salmonella, Shigella, Campylobacter jejuni, E. coli, Yersinia enterocolitica, Clostridium difficile,* food poisoning: *Clostridium perfringens* and *S. aureus* (toxin)
List 4 ways acute bacterial gastroenteritis is diagnosed.	1. Stool culture (*Salmonella, Shigella, Campylobacter, E. coli, Yersinia, C. difficile, C. perfringens*) 2. Serologic testing (*Yersinia*) 3. Toxin assay (*C. difficile*) 4. Toxin assay in food (*S. aureus*)
How is it treated?	Supportive treatment (IV or orally) for fluid and electrolyte loss. Antibiotic therapy is usually not indicated because illnesses are often self-limited. **Exception:** *Shigella* is usually treated, due to public health concerns. Extraintestinal infections (including sepsis) are indications for antibiotic treatment. Infants may be given antibiotics more readily than older children.
Why not treat the usual *Salmonella* infection?	It is usually self-limited. Treatment may prolong the "carrier state" and may not significantly alter the clinical course.
When should *Salmonella* infection be treated?	Patient is an infant or toddler (< 3 years of age); has an immune deficiency; has a systemic disease (e.g., sepsis, osteomyelitis), or has typhoid fever.
What oral rehydration regimen is recommended for gastroenteritis?	The World Health Organization (WHO) oral rehydration solution, which includes: Glucose: 90 mmol/L Sodium: 80 mmol/L Potassium: 20 mmol/L Chloride: 80 mmol/L Base (citrate): 30 mmol/L Final total osmolarity = 300 mosm/L
List 3 commercially available oral fluids that are useful.	Several are useful, including: Pedialyte, Ricelyte, Infalyte

List 4 indications for IV fluid.	Inability to drink liquids, severe vomiting, shock or impending shock, coma
Which IV fluid should be used?	It depends on the situation. Lactated Ringer's solution or normal saline for volume expansion is used in severely dehydrated patients, followed by calculated replacement of electrolytes and maintenance fluids. (See Chapter 3, Fluids and Electrolytes, p. 17, for electrolyte concentrations of GI fluids, Table 3–1.)
Should one feed a child with acute gastroenteritis?	In general, yes, but judiciously. In most children, careful feeding may promote healing and help prevent malnutrition.

URINARY TRACT INFECTION (UTI)

What does the term UTI refer to?	Usually to infection of the urethra and bladder; the term grossly encompasses ascending infections up to the kidney as well.
Are female or male children more likely to have UTIs?	In infants, males and females are affected equally. Uncircumcised male infants may have a slightly higher risk. In older children, females are affected more commonly.
What are the most common etiologic agents?	*E. coli* accounts for 70%–90% of infections. Other agents include *Klebsiella, Proteus,* and enterobacteria species.
What is the pathophysiology in infants versus children?	Infection in infants usually results from either bacteremia or migration of bacteria from the urethra. In older children, UTIs more commonly occur because of ascending bacteria from the lower urinary tract.
What is acute bacterial cystitis?	Infection of the bladder itself.
List 2 characteristics.	1. Hyperactivity of the detrusor muscle 2. Decreased functional capacity of the bladder.

**What are potential
symptoms of a UTI?**

    **In infants? (List 7
    symptoms)**

Fever, weight loss, failure to thrive,
nausea, vomiting, diarrhea, and jaundice.

    **In older children?
    (List 8 symptoms)**

Fever, urinary frequency, pain during
urination, incontinence, bed wetting,
abdominal pain, foul-smelling urine, and
hematuria.

**How is urine obtained for
analysis and culture?**

    **In infants and small
    children? (List 2 methods)**

Catheterization or **suprapubic
puncture** (See Chapter 2, Pediatric
Procedures, p. 13, for a description of the
technique for suprapubic puncture)

    In older children?

A good midstream urine specimen.

**List 4 findings that
suggest infection.**

1. Pyuria; however, infection can occur
   in the absence of pyuria. Conversely,
   pyuria can be present without
   infection.
2. Microscopic hematuria
3. An alkaline pH may suggest *Proteus*
   infection.
4. A urine culture result of 100,000
   colony-forming units/ml is diagnostic
   of infection. Occasionally, infection
   may be present with a slightly lower
   colony-forming unit count of a single
   organism.

How are UTIs treated?

Antibiotics of choice: trimethoprim-
sulfamethoxazole, nitrofurantoin, and
amoxicillin. If symptoms are not severe, it
is preferable to wait for culture results
before starting antibiotics. However, if
symptoms are bothersome, antibiotic
therapy should be started, **after** the
specimen is collected.

**If UTI is diagnosed, what
2 further workups are
required?**

1. A child with UTI should have a follow-
   up voiding cystourethrogram (VCUG)
   to assess for reflux. Reflux may
   predispose to ascending infection and

pyelonephritis. If vesicoureteral reflux (VUR) is present, prophylaxis may be needed for as long as the reflux persists. (See Chapter 21, Renal Diseases, p. 299, for a discussion of VUR.)

2. A follow-up urine culture should be obtained after treatment to confirm that the UTI is cleared. Further follow-up cultures should be done at 3-month intervals for 1–2 years.

PYELONEPHRITIS

What is it?	An infection of the renal parenchyma that is usually caused by ascending infection from the lower urinary tract.
What 2 conditions predispose a child to pyelonephritis?	Recurrent UTI and VUR
What are the clinical manifestations?	
In infants?	Signs typical of systemic infection, including fever, weight loss, failure to thrive, and irritability.
In older children?	Fever, chills, and flank or abdominal pain are typical.
List 3 laboratory tests that are valuable for diagnosis.	1. Urine culture 2. Urinalysis showing white blood cell casts 3. Peripheral WBC count may be elevated.
What imaging studies may be helpful?	1. **Ultrasound** may show hydronephrosis, a perirenal abscess, or pyonephrosis. The latter 2 conditions may require prompt drainage of purulence. 2. Renal **scanning** may confirm pyelonephritis by revealing filling defects in the renal parenchyma.
What is the treatment?	Intravenous antibiotics

What are potential complications of pyelonephritis?	Arterial hypertension, renal insufficiency, or both secondary to chronic renal damage.
List the 2 components of treatment for renal or perirenal abscesses or infections associated with obstructed urinary tract.	1. Antibiotic therapy 2. Drainage of the infected and obstructed areas using image-guided (US or CT) or surgical technique.

DACTYLITIS

What is it?	An infection of the volar fat pad of the distal portion of the finger or thumb. It is usually blistering in nature.
What are the etiologic factors?	Usually this condition occurs spontaneously. In rare cases, dactylitis may be the first manifestation of **sickle cell disease** in an infant.
List the 3 most common bacteria that cause it.	Group A β-hemolytic *streptococcus*, *S. aureus*, group B β-hemolytic *streptococcus*
What are the 2 components of treatment?	1. Incision and drainage of the blistering lesion 2. Penicillin or erythromycin therapy

SEXUALLY TRANSMITTED DISEASES (STDS)

Which age group has the highest rate of STDs?	Adolescents (Also see Chapter 14, Adolescent Medicine, p. 156)
List 8 common STDs.	1. Gonorrhea (*Neisseria gonorrhoeae*) 2. Syphilis (*Treponema pallidum*) 3. Chlamydia (*Chlamydia trachomatis*) 4. Chancroid (*Haemophilus ducreyi*) 5. Genital herpes 6. Human papillomavirus (HPV) 7. Trichomoniasis (*Trichomonas vaginalis*) 8. *Gardnerella* infection (*Gardnerella vaginalis*)
If organisms that are usually sexually transmitted are found in younger children, what should be suspected?	Child sexual abuse

GONORRHEA

What is the offending organism in gonorrhea?	*Neisseria gonorrhoeae*
What are typical symptoms?	
In males?	A purulent discharge that causes burning on urination (dysuria); occasionally infected males are asymptomatic.
In females? (List 3 symptoms)	Purulent vaginal discharge, vulvar vaginitis, dysuria (some females are asymptomatic)
What is the most common complication?	Pelvic inflammatory disease (PID)
How is the diagnosis made?	Culture of urethral or cervical discharge.
What is the treatment?	Ceftriaxone
What is the duration of treatment?	Depends on whether the disease is local or whether complications, such as PID or disseminated disease, have occurred.

SYPHILIS

What is the offending agent in syphilis?	*Treponema pallidum*
What are the symptoms of syphilis?	
Primary syphilis?	A painless **chancre** appears at the site of inoculation approximately 2–6 weeks after infection. There may be associated **adenitis**. The chancre heals spontaneously within 4–6 weeks.
Secondary syphilis?	Two to ten weeks after the chancre heals, a nonpruritic maculopapular **rash** occurs. Pustules may develop. **Condylomata** may occur around the anus and vagina. There may be an associated **flu-like illness** with lymphadenopathy. Thirty percent of people infected with secondary syphilis develop meningitis. After 1–2

months, the infection becomes latent but
may recur up to the first year.

Tertiary syphilis?

This late stage manifests with
neurologic, cardiovascular, and
granulomatous lesions.

What are diagnostic tests?

1. Demonstration of *T. pallidum* on
   darkfield microscopy as direct
   immunofluorescence on specimens
   from skin lesions, placenta, or
   umbilicus.
2. The Venereal Disease Research
   Laboratory (VDRL) and rapid plasma
   reagin (RPR) tests detect antibodies
   against a cardiolipin-cholesterol-
   lecithin complex. They are not specific
   for syphilis, but do tend to correlate
   with disease activity and are therefore
   useful in screening.
3. The fluorescent treponemal antibody
   absorption test (FTA—ABS), the
   microhemagglutination assay for
   antibodies to *T. pallidum* (MHA—
   TP), and the *T. pallidum*
   immobilization test (TPI) are tests that
   measure antibodies specific to *T.
   pallidum*. They are usually used to
   confirm findings on non-specific tests.

How is syphilis treated?

A single dose of **penicillin** is adequate
for primary, secondary, and latent
secondary disease. Treatment must be
adjusted for tertiary disease,
neurosyphilis, and congenital syphilis.

**What is the likelihood of
transmission of syphilis
from an infected mother
to her infant?**

Virtually 100%

**What is the fetal or
perinatal death rate of
infected infants?**

40%

**When should infants be
treated for syphilis?**

When there is evidence of the infection in
the mother, or when adequacy of
treatment in the mother is in question

CHLAMYDIA

Which of the *Chlamydia* species is most commonly involved in sexually transmitted infection?	*C. trachomatis*
What is another common term for *Chlamydia* infection?	Nongonococcal urethritis
What are the clinical manifestations?	These can be very similar to those of gonorrhea and include **burning** during urination as well as a urethral **discharge.** **Perihepatitis, conjunctivitis, sterility,** and **PID** are symptoms of chlamydia that has spread beyond its local site.
List 5 ways the diagnosis may be made.	1. Isolation of the organism in tissue culture from the urethra in men and from the endocervix in women and girls 2. Fluorescent antibody tests 3. Enzyme-linked immunosorbent assay (ELISA) 4. DNA probe 5. Polymerase chain reaction (PCR) assay.
How is *Chlamydia* infection treated?	Doxycycline, cefoxitin, erythromycin, and azithromycin may be adequate medications. For pregnant women, erythromycin or amoxicillin is recommended.
What symptoms may occur in infants of infected mothers?	Conjunctivitis, pneumonia, and infection of the rectum and vagina

CHANCROID

What is chancroid?	A lesion characterized by a painful, purulent, sharply delineated ulcer. There is no induration and this helps to distinguish it from a syphilis chancre. Lymphadenopathy may be associated with this condition.
What is the treatment?	Ceftriaxone

GENITAL HERPES

List the 2 viral causes in genital herpes.	HSV type 2 and HSV type 1 (may cause 10%–25% of cases)
What are clinical manifestations?	
In females?	The **vulva and vagina may have vesicles and ulcers. The cervix is the primary site of infection, and therefore the disease may be subclinical**. However, virus may still be shed, thus infecting a partner. There may be associated pain along affected nerve roots in the perineal region.
In males?	**Vesicles or ulcers occur on the penis.** The scrotum is less frequently involved. There may be associated pain along affected nerve roots in the perineal region.
What is the treatment?	There is no cure. Symptomatic and shedding phases may be shortened by the use of acyclovir.
For what other disease are women with HSV at risk?	**Cancer of the cervix;** these women should have yearly Pap smears

HUMAN PAPILLOMAVIRUS (HPV)

What is it?	This term encompasses at least 75 different types of virus that contain DNA.
What are the manifestations of sexually transmitted HPV?	Genital warts (also called condylomata acuminata)
How is the diagnosis made?	Usually by **physical examination;** however, application of **3% acetic acid** to a lesion may show a characteristic whitening that provides diagnosis.
What are some potential treatments?	Topical treatments include trichloroacetic acid, liquid nitrogen, podophyllin, and topical 5-fluorouracil. Laser therapy may be required for lesions that do not respond to medical therapy. Less common treatments include interferon and bleomycin.

What are 3 complications of infection with HPV?	Cervical dysplasia, cervical cancer, development of respiratory papillomas, which, in infants, may become malignant or may spread to a point of being uncontrollable and resulting in airway obstruction and death.

TRICHOMONAS INFECTION (TRICHOMONIASIS)

What is the offending agent in this infection?	*Trichomonas vaginalis*
What are the clinical manifestations of *Trichomonas* infection?	
In females?	There is a frothy, malodorous **vaginal discharge,** which may be accompanied by **vulvar or vaginal irritation, dysuria,** and **dyspareunia**.
In males?	Usually asymptomatic, but about 10% may experience nongonococcal urethritis.
How is the diagnosis made?	**Wet mount** examination of vaginal or urethral secretions will show the *Trichomonas*. This test is successful in about 70% of cases. Cultures may be needed to obtain a definitive diagnosis.
What is the treatment?	**Metronidazole—however, it should not be used in pregnant women. Clotrimazole** should be used in the first trimester of pregnancy if infection is suspected.

GARDNERELLA INFECTION

What is the principal manifestation of *Gardnerella* infection?	Usually a foul-smelling vaginal discharge.
How is it diagnosed?	**10% potassium hydroxide** is added to a wet preparation of the discharge. This results in the emission of a fishy odor. **Clue cells,** which are epithelial cells ringed with the rod-shaped organism, are also evident on the "wet prep."

What is the treatment?	Metronidazole, which is contraindicated in pregnant women.

PELVIC INFLAMMATORY DISEASE (PID)

What is it?	A condition that may be caused by a variety of sexually transmitted organisms that have ascended through the vaginal tract into the cervix and uterus. Subsequent migration may occur toward the tubes.
List 2 common clinical manifestations.	Lower abdominal pain, which can be severe, and often fever.
What are 2 physical findings?	1. Extreme tenderness on motion of the uterus and adnexa (i.e., the **"chandelier sign"**) 2. A **purulent discharge** from the cervical region may be present
List 3 components of diagnosis.	History, physical exam, culture of secretions Treatment is usually initiated on the basis of history and physical examination before an organism is identified.
What are common conditions in the differential diagnosis?	Appendicitis, ovarian cyst, ovarian tumor, ectopic pregnancy, UTI, inflammatory bowel disease
How is PID treated?	IV antibiotics are usually necessary and should include coverage for *N. gonorrhoeae* and *Chlamydia* species. Consideration should be given to treatment of anaerobes.
List 5 complications of PID.	Sterility, increased risk of ectopic pregnancy, chronic pain, dyspareunia, increased risk of recurring PID

COMMON VIRAL SYNDROMES

MEASLES

What is another name for measles?	Rubeola

List 6 signs and symptoms of measles.	Fever, cough, coryza, conjunctivitis, maculopapular rash, Koplik spots (enanthem)
What are 2 ways in which measles is spread?	Usually by direct contact with infectious secretions, but sometimes via airborne route
What is the incubation period?	8–12 days from exposure to onset of symptoms, and 14 days from exposure to appearance of rash
List 5 complications of measles.	Pneumonia, croup, diarrhea, encephalitis, SSPE
What is SSPE?	Subacute sclerosing panencephalitis
When can SSPE occur?	Long after the illness; average incubation period is 10.8 years after the identified measles infection.
What is the treatment for measles?	Supportive; vitamin A may be useful
Is isolation of the patient necessary?	Respiratory isolation for 4 days after onset of rash; longer for immunocompromised patients

MUMPS

What is it?	It is a systemic viral disease, most notable for **swelling of the salivary glands**. The mumps virus is a member of the **paramyxovirus** group, which includes **measles and parainfluenza.**
How is mumps spread?	Direct contact via respiratory exposure
What is the incubation period?	12–25 days, although it is usually 16–18 days
List 6 complications.	**Orchitis,** arthritis, pancreatitis, hearing loss, mastitis, renal involvement
Is isolation of the patient necessary?	Respiratory isolation for 9 days after onset of parotid swelling
What is the treatment?	Supportive

RUBELLA

What is another name for rubella?	German measles
List 2 clinical features.	1. Generalized lymphadenopathy (usually suboccipital, postauricular, cervical nodes). 2. A pink maculopapular erythematous rash appears first on the face then spreads downward.
How is rubella spread?	Direct or droplet contact with nasopharyngeal secretions
What is the incubation period?	14–21 days, but it is usually 16–18 days
Is isolation of the patient necessary?	Contact isolation for 7 days after onset of the rash
What is the treatment?	Supportive
What are potential complications?	Polyarthralgia, arthritis, thrombocytopenia, encephalitis; **the major concern is congenital rubella.**
What is congenital rubella?	Rubella infection in a fetus, acquired as a consequence of maternal infection during pregnancy
List 4 ophthalmologic complications of congenital rubella.	Cataracts, microphthalmia, glaucoma, chorioretinitis.
List 4 cardiac complications of congenital rubella.	Patent ductus arteriosus (PDA), peripheral pulmonic stenosis, atrial septal defect (ASD), ventricular septal defect (VSD)
What are other complications?	Sensorineural deafness, microcephaly, mental retardation, growth retardation, thrombocytopenia, ecchymoses/purpura (sometimes called "blueberry muffin" baby)

Is isolation of a child with congenital rubella necessary?	Contact isolation until 1 year of age, or until nasopharyngeal and urine viral cultures are consistently negative for rubella after 3 months of age.

FIFTH DISEASE

What is another name for fifth disease?	Erythema infectiosum
What is its cause?	Parvovirus B19
List 4 clinical features.	Fever, systemic illness (usually mild), a "slapped cheek" rash on the face, and a lacy or reticular rash on the extremities.
What are potential complications?	Arthralgia, arthritis, bone marrow suppression; **it may cause hydrops fetalis in the fetus of a woman infected in the first half of pregnancy**
How is it spread?	Respiratory secretions and blood
What is the incubation period?	28 days; 4–14 days on average
What is the treatment?	Supportive; immunoglobulin may be helpful in chronic infections in immunocompromised patients

ROSEOLA

What is it?	A systemic viral infection, characterized by high fever for 3–7 days, followed by a maculopapular rash; it may include respiratory or GI signs.
List 2 complications.	Febrile seizures and rarely encephalitis
What causes roseola?	Human herpesvirus type 6 and type 7
Give 2 other names for roseola.	Exanthem subitum and sixth disease
How is it spread?	Unknown—likely respiratory secretions
What is the incubation period?	5–15 days

Is isolation of an infected child necessary?	No
What is the treatment?	Supportive

VARICELLA

What is another name for varicella?	Chicken pox
List 2 clinical features	Systemic illness with fever and generalized vesicular rash
What is the cause?	Varicella-zoster virus
List 4 potential complications.	Secondary bacterial infection of skin lesions, thrombocytopenia, arthritis, pneumonia
In what 3 ways is the varicella virus spread?	Direct contact, airborne spread, contact with zoster lesions
What is the incubation period?	10–21 days, but it is usually 14–16 days
When is a child infectious?	1–4 days before lesions erupt, and for 7–10 days afterward
What is the treatment?	Supportive and symptomatic; **salicylates should be avoided.** Antiviral agents (acyclovir) can modify the course of the disease if administered early
List 2 ways chicken pox can be prevented.	1. A varicella vaccine has been developed and is recommended for universal use. 2. Varicella-zoster immune globulin (VZIG), given after exposure, can modify the course of the disease or prevent it. It is used mainly with immunocompromised patients.
What is zoster?	A painful vesicular eruption in a dermatomal distribution
What causes zoster?	Latent varicella virus that becomes active after primary systemic infection

HIV

How do children acquire HIV infection?	The vast majority of children acquire it through vertical transmission from their infected mother.
What proportion of children born to mothers with HIV infection will become infected?	About **20%–30%** of babies born to infected, untreated mothers.
When does vertical transmission of HIV infection to infants take place?	25% prepartum, 65% intrapartum, and 10% postpartum (via breast feeding)
List 3 other modes of transmission.	Contaminated blood products, sexual transmission, shared needles
Has screening of blood products affected the risk of HIV infection?	Yes—the risk from blood products has been greatly reduced, but not completely eliminated.
List the 4 major determinants of perinatal HIV transmission.	1. High maternal viral load 2. Lack of maternal anti-retroviral therapy during pregnancy 3. Vaginal delivery 4. Breast-feeding
List 3 effective measures to prevent perinatal HIV transmission from an infected mother to her infant.	1. Provide aggressive anti-retroviral therapy during pregnancy to reduce the maternal viral load. 2. Offer elective cesarean section at 38 weeks gestation. 3. Strongly discourage breast-feeding.
How effective are these measures in preventing perinatal HIV infection?	These interventions reduce the risk of perinatal transmission to < 5%.
What is the reason that HIV infection in children has not been eliminated in the US?	Failure to identify all pregnant women with HIV infection and offer them effective therapy
List 2 components of treatment that should be given to babies born to HIV-infected women.	1. Beginning at 8–12 hours after birth, these infants should receive **oral zidovudine,** continuing until 6 weeks of age.

2. Beginning at 4–6 weeks of age, these infants should receive **trimethoprim-sulfamethoxazole prophylaxis** against *Pneumocystis carinii* pneumonia.

How is perinatally acquired HIV infection diagnosed?

Polymerase chain reaction (PCR) performed at birth and at 1–2 months of age. Positive tests should be confirmed by repeat testing before a definitive diagnosis is made. Negative tests at birth and at 1–2 months of age should be repeated at 4 months of age before HIV infection is excluded.

Is testing for HIV antibody useful?

Only in children > 2 years of age. Transplacentally acquired maternal antibody to HIV can persist in children for up to 18 months after birth. Thus, antibody is not useful to definitively diagnose or exclude HIV infection in young infants.

Are newborns with HIV infection clinically ill?

Not necessarily; most are well at birth.

List 7 common clinical features of HIV infection.

Prolonged or unexplained fever, lymphadenopathy, hepatosplenomegaly, chronic diarrhea, poor weight gain, poor linear growth, parotitis

What are potential infectious complications of HIV infection in children?

1. Increased susceptibility to infection with common bacterial and viral pathogens (causing otitis media, sinusitis, pneumonia, sepsis, and meningitis)
2. Increased susceptibility to infection with opportunistic organisms (*Pneumocystis carinii, Candida albicans, Mycobacterium avium, Toxoplasma gondii,* and Cytomegalovirus)

List 4 common organ-specific complications of HIV infection.

Encephalopathy, lymphoid interstitial pneumonitis, cardiomyopathy, nephropathy

What information does measuring CD4 counts provide?	CD4 counts provide a rough measure of the **extent of destruction of the immune system by HIV.** Severe depletion of CD4 cells renders the patient susceptible to opportunistic infections. Exception: **susceptibility to *Pneumocystis carinii* pneumonia in young infants does not correlate with CD4 counts.**
How is pediatric HIV infection treated?	With a combination of anti-retroviral agents. The usual treatment consists of 2 drugs that inhibit HIV reverse transcriptase combined with a drug that inhibits HIV protease.
What is the prognosis for pediatric HIV infection?	Prior to the availability of effective therapy, the prognosis was grim, with a median survival of about 8 years. Potent anti-retroviral therapy has dramatically decreased morbidity and mortality rates. The full extent of the benefit of combination therapy is not yet known.

TUBERCULOSIS

What are 3 infecting agents for tuberculosis?	*Mycobacterium tuberculosis, Mycobacterium bovis, Mycobacterium africanum*
Which infecting agent is the most prevalent?	*M. tuberculosis*
What percent of the world's population is infected with *M. tuberculosis* ?	33%
How many people in the United States are infected with *M. tuberculosis* ?	10–20 million
Which age group has the lowest rate of tuberculosis?	5–14 years of age
How is tuberculosis transmitted?	By mucous droplets that become airborne from person to person.
Is it common for young children to infect others?	No, because often children do not have cough symptoms with tuberculosis and if

they do, the cough is not forceful enough to suspend infectious particles.

What is the primary portal of entry of tuberculosis?

The lung

What percent of patients who are infected with tuberculosis develop clinical disease?

Approximately 5%–10%; however, 40% of infected infants develop disease.

List 5 categories of children at highest risk for developing tuberculosis.

1. Children born in countries with high incidence of the disease
2. Poor and indigent children
3. Homeless children
4. Abusers of injected drugs
5. Children exposed to high-risk adults

List 4 conditions that predispose children to become symptomatic with tuberculosis once they are infected.

1. Infection with HIV
2. Immunocompromising diseases, especially malignancy
3. Immunosuppressive drug treatments
4. Age of 3 years or younger

List 2 features of the "primary complex" of tuberculosis.

1. Local infection at the portal of entry, usually the lung
2. Subsequent infection of regional lymph nodes in that area

What is the Mantoux tuberculin skin test?

This is an intradermal injection containing purified protein derivative (PPD). Usually 0.1 cc solution containing 5 tuberculin units is used for initial testing.

What defines a positive test?

1. In children with high risk of infection, an area of induration $\geq$ 5 mm
2. For other high-risk adults and children older than 4 years of age, an area of induration $\geq$ 10 mm is positive.
3. For low-risk persons, an area of induration $\geq$ 15 mm is positive.

List 5 factors that can cause a false-negative result on the tuberculin test.

Young age, malnutrition, immunosuppression, viral diseases (measles, mumps, varicella, influenza), overwhelming tuberculosis

What 2 factors can cause a false-positive response on the tuberculin test?

1. Cross-sensitization to non-tuberculous mycobacteria
2. Exposure to the bacille Calmette-Guérin (BCG) vaccine

What are some clinical manifestations of tuberculosis?

Initially, there is a lung parenchymal focus with involvement of regional lymph nodes. This may result in bronchial obstruction in small children and infants. The clinical manifestations are fairly mild, however. Infants are the most prone to showing signs and symptoms and these are usually nonproductive cough and mild dyspnea. Other generalized systemic symptoms such as fever, night sweats, anorexia, or decreased activity may occur.

List 2 radiographic findings that may be present in children with pulmonary tuberculosis.

Collapse or consolidation of a lung segment due to bronchial obstruction, signs of bacterial pneumonia

List 3 other possible pulmonary manifestations.

Pleural effusion; extension of infection to the pericardium (pericarditis); upper respiratory tract disease

What other organs may tuberculosis affect?

Any organ

What are the characteristics of central nervous system (CNS) involvement?

Meningitis with subsequent **caseous lesion** development. They affect the **brain stem** most commonly. Early symptoms resemble meningitis but may progress to coma, decerebrate posturing, and death.
CSF fluid usually shows 10–500 WBCs/mm^3, glucose level of 20–40 mg/dL, and elevated protein.

What is typical of bone involvement?

Bone involvement is usually in the **lower vertebrae**. Spondylitis (**Pott disease**) results in kyphosis.

What are manifestations of abdominal disease?

1. Abdominal lymph nodes may become infected, causing localized peritonitis or even generalized peritonitis if caseous lymph nodes rupture.
2. In the intestine, ulcers may form,

resulting in pain, diarrhea, or constipation.

What are characteristics of genitourinary disease?

Early symptoms may be subtle. However, late symptoms may include dysuria, flank or abdominal pain, and gross hematuria. Superinfection may occur. Hydronephrosis and urethral strictures may develop. In males, epididymitis or orchitis may occur.

What are symptoms of perinatal disease?

These usually occur after 2 or 3 weeks of life and include respiratory distress, fever, enlargement of the spleen or liver, poor feeding, lethargy, irritability, lymphadenopathy, abdominal distention, failure to thrive, ear drainage, and skin lesions. Chest radiograph may reveal a miliary pattern.

How is tuberculosis diagnosed?

By **isolation of the bacteria;** typically seen as **acid-fast bacteria** on staining with arylmethane. However, it may take 1–6 weeks to confirm growth in culture.

How is tuberculosis typically treated?

The most common drugs used are **isoniazid (INH)** and **rifampin**. Coverage with 2 or 3 drugs is necessary for patients with clinically active disease. This implies a large bacterial load and is meant to cover that population of bacteria that is resistant to a single drug. Patients with infection but no clinically active disease have a smaller bacterial load and may be treated with one drug.

List 2 side effects of isoniazid.

Peripheral neuritis and **hepatotoxicity**

What is the side effect of rifampin?

Hepatotoxicity

What is the typical treatment strategy for tuberculosis?

For asymptomatic infection?

Asymptomatic infection is treated with a single drug (INH) for at least 6 months.

For active disease?	A **3-drug regimen, INH, rifampin,** and **pyrazinamide,** is prescribed for 2 months and then INH and rifampin for at least another 4 months. In an area of multidrug resistant tuberculosis, treatment must be based on susceptibility patterns of isolates, usually from adult contacts.
List 3 instances in which children who do not exhibit tuberculosis disease should be treated.	1. Children with a positive PPD test should be treated with INH for 6 months. 2. INH therapy should be used for children younger than 6 years of age who have been exposed to infected adults 3. INH therapy should be used for infants born to mothers who have tuberculosis. If exposed children are PPD negative 3 months after treatment, treatment may be discontinued.
What is the BCG vaccination?	It is a vaccine for bacille Calmette-Guérin
What is its use?	It is probably best used in infants and children to reduce the risk of disseminated tuberculosis. This is especially true for infants who are at high risk of exposure due to their living environment.
Has this vaccine resulted in overall decrease in tuberculosis?	No

PERTUSSIS

What is another name for pertussis?	Whooping cough
What causes pertussis and how is it transmitted?	*Bordetella pertussis;* spread via respiratory secretions
What is the incubation period?	7–14 days

What are the 3 stages?

Catarrhal, paroxysmal, convalescent

What are characteristics of the cough?

A quick "staccato" cough, such that the child may not be able to catch his/her breath until the end of the cough. The deep breath is the "whoop." The cough is most obvious in the catarrhal stage.

What are complications of pertussis?

Pneumonia is seen, as well as CNS and GI complications, related to infection and to the consequences of violent coughing and pressure.

List 4 ways it is diagnosed.

1. Clinical suspicion with possible presence of lymphocytosis
2. Positive culture for *B. pertussis*
3. Demonstration of the organism using a fluorescent antibody test of nasopharyngeal secretions
4. PCR identification of the organism in nasopharyngeal secretions

List 3 elements of treatment.

1. Hospitalization during period of severe coughing paroxysms; the child may need suction, supplemental oxygen, nutritional support, and respiratory support
2. Antibiotic—usually erythromycin
3. Isolation until 5 days of antibiotic treatment are completed

What antibiotic prophylaxis is given, and for how long, for people exposed to pertussis?

14 days of erythromycin

Does treatment of infected persons prevent the cough?

Probably not, but those treated early may have a shorter course

How is pertussis prevented?

Vaccination

What are 2 possible complications of pertussis vaccination?

Some individuals have a febrile reaction, and there are reports of rare CNS complications. The relationship of these conditions to the vaccine is controversial.

Is protection by pertussis vaccination lifelong?

No

Is all whooping cough caused by pertussis?	No. There are viruses and other bacteria (including *Bordetella parapertussis*) that can cause a similar illness.

PARASITIC INFECTIONS AND INFESTATIONS

ROUNDWORM

What is the formal name for roundworm?	*Ascaris lumbricoides*
How big are the organisms?	Adults can be quite large (15–40 cm)
How is roundworm contracted?	Fecal-oral route (i.e., oral ingestion of eggs). The eggs hatch usually in the duodenum and the larvae penetrate the intestinal mucosa and migrate to the lungs and up the trachea, to be swallowed.
Where do the adults live?	Usually in the jejunum
What are 2 categories of symptoms of ascariasis?	1. Possible **pulmonary symptoms,** including **Loffler's pneumonia** 2. **GI signs,** including abdominal pain, loss of appetite, nausea, and vomiting.
What are 2 possible serious complications?	Intestinal obstruction and aberrant migration (to liver, eyes, brain) with inflammatory responses
How is it usually diagnosed?	By finding the eggs or the worm in stool.
What is the life span of *Ascaris* ?	Usually 2 years
List 3 treatments.	Mebendazole, pyrantel pamoate, albendazole
How can it be prevented?	Good hand washing and sanitation

VISCERAL LARVA MIGRANS

What 2 agents cause visceral larva migrans?	*Toxocara canis, T. catis*
What are they?	Dog and cat roundworms (intestinal parasites)

How do humans become infected?	Ingestion of eggs (from animal feces, perhaps in dirt)
What happens when humans ingest these eggs?	The eggs hatch in the intestines and migrate to organs (usually the liver)
What are the symptoms?	Symptoms may vary with the tissues involved. Fever, hepatomegaly, or other organ-specific findings may be present.
List 4 lab findings.	1. Eosinophilia, due to the tissue invasiveness of the parasite 2. Elevation of isohemagglutinin antibodies 3. Elevated erythrocyte sedimentation rate (ESR) 4. Positive ELISA
What is ocular larva migrans?	Eye involvement of visceral larva migrans
List 4 agents for treating visceral and ocular larva migrans.	**Diethylcarbamazine (oral), mebendazole,** or **albendazole** have been used. Dying organisms may cause an allergic or inflammatory response. **Ocular larva migrans** may also need **steroid** treatment.

PINWORMS

What is the formal name for pinworms?	*Enterobius vermicularis*
How is it transmitted?	Hand to mouth
What are the symptoms?	Perianal itching, sometimes leading to insomnia
How is it diagnosed?	Demonstration of pinworms or their eggs in the perianal region
What is the tape test?	Use of a clear adhesive tape to pick up eggs or worms from the perianal region; this pickup can be performed by the parents and the eggs or worms examined by the physician.
What is the treatment for pinworm infection?	Mebendazole

List 3 ways it can be prevented.	Practice good hygiene. Cut nails. Wash sheets, underwear, and bedclothes daily for several days to prevent reinfection.

WHIPWORM

What is the formal name for whipworm?	*Trichuris trichiura*
How is it spread?	Fecal-oral route with ingestion of infective eggs
What are potential symptoms?	The patient may be asymptomatic. Symptoms may range from abdominal pain and flatulence to rectal bleeding and prolapse, depending on the severity of the infestation.
How is it diagnosed?	Demonstration of characteristic eggs or worms in stool
What is the treatment?	Mebendazole
List 2 ways it can be prevented.	Good hygiene, sanitary disposal of human waste

HOOKWORM

What causes hookworm?	*Necator americanus* (in the United States) and *Ancylostoma duodenale*
What is the life cycle of the hookworm?	The larvae usually **burrow through the skin of the feet,** enter the bloodstream, and migrate to the lungs, where they ascend and are swallowed. They then reside in the intestines.
List 4 complications.	Irritation at the site of skin entry ("**ground itch** "), anemia, hypoproteinemia, nutritional deficiency
How is it diagnosed?	By finding ova in stools
List 2 treatments.	Mebendazole, pyrantel pamoate
List 2 ways it can be prevented.	By wearing shoes and improving sanitation

ATYPICAL MYCOBACTERIA

What are atypical mycobacteria?

Mycobacteria that are nontuberculous

How are they generally acquired?

From the environment, as opposed to person-to-person spread

List 4 categories of atypical mycobacteria.

The 4 categories are based on growth and morphology: Photochromogens, scotochromogens, nonchromogens, rapid growers

What are the most typical infectious manifestations in children?

Cervical lymphadenitis; however, children with AIDS are commonly infected systemically with *Mycobacterium avium*

Can nontuberculous mycobacteria infect other regions of the body?

Yes—particularly the skin, lungs, bones, and joints

Which mycobacterium accounts for most cases of cervical lymphadenitis?

M. avium is responsible in 80% of cases. Most other cases are caused by either *M. scrofulaceum* or *M. kansasii.*

List 2 typical symptoms of cervical lymphadenitis.

1. Enlargement of an isolated lymph node or group of nodes
2. With progressive disease, caseation may occur, resulting in drainage to the skin.

How is the definitive diagnosis made?

By isolation of the organism from a tissue sample

What is the treatment?

Surgical excision of the involved nodes

Can HIV-positive children who are infected with disseminated *M. avium* be cured of this bacterial infection?

Usually not, but multiple drug therapy may diminish the effects of the disease

29

Allergic Diseases

ATOPY

What is it?

A category of allergic reaction that implies hereditary factors. These reactions include hay fever, asthma, eczematoid dermatitis, and allergic reactions to food, drugs, and insect bites.

What is the pathophysiologic process in an atopic individual?

Selected synthesis of IgE antibodies to common environmental antigens

How is this process demonstrated in atopic individuals?

A "wheal-and-flare" reaction occurs when their skin is tested with allergenic extracts and/or elevated allergen-specific IgE antibodies in their serum.

Can nonatopic individuals form IgE antibodies?

Yes—but not to common environmental substances in the same manner that atopic individuals do

What is the definition of allergy?

A specific, acquired host reaction mediated by an immunologic mechanism, causing an undesired physiologic response.
Individuals can have allergic reactions to foods or drugs. However, a true allergy should be differentiated from an adverse reaction (commonly nausea or vomiting) that does not have a true immunologic basis. Adverse reactions without an immunologic basis are food or drug intolerances.

Are antigens and allergens the same?

Not necessarily. Allergens are antigens that provoke a specific immunologic allergic response. All allergens are antigens, although not all are good antigens. All antigens are not necessarily allergens.

List 7 laboratory values that help confirm allergic diseases.

1. Peripheral blood eosinophilia (> 500 cells/mm³)
2. Elevated serum IgE
3. Respiratory or gastrointestinal secretions containing > 10% eosinophils
4. Positive allergy skin testing (evidenced by wheals) using prick or intradermal techniques
5. Radioallergosorbent test (RAST) [allergen-specific IgE]
6. Positive food and drug challenges
7. Positive bronchial provocation tests to histamine or methacholine challenge

What are 3 treatment strategies?

Avoidance of irritant; pharmacotherapy; immunotherapy

List 8 choices in pharmacotherapy.

α-Agonists (reduce edema of mucous membranes); β-agonists (dilate airways); theophylline (treat asthma); cromolyn (smooth-muscle relaxant); topical and systemic steroids; antihistamines; anticholinergics; antileukotrienes

FOOD ALLERGIES

What are food allergies?

IgE-mediated reactions that usually occur 1–4 hours after ingestion.

List typical symptoms of food allergy.

Nausea, vomiting, diarrhea, anaphylaxis, asthma, eczema, urticaria, or angioedema.

What are nonallergic adverse food reactions?

These reactions (more common than allergic ones) can be secondary to toxic substances in food, chemical or bacterial contaminants, endogenous pharmacologic agents, or metabolic diseases in the individual.

What is the most common target organ in IgE-mediated food hypersensitivity?

The skin—may exhibit urticaria, angioedema, pruritic rash, or eczema

List 6 of the most common foods to which children are allergic.	Milk, eggs, peanuts, soybean, wheat, and fish cause over 90% of food allergy reactions.
How is food sensitivity evaluated?	**History** and **physical examination**. (Skin tests and serum RAST, which are used for measuring IgE antibodies to specific foods, are only helpful in assessing food sensitization.)
List 2 methods by which a food allergy can be confirmed.	Food challenges; elimination diets (occasionally)

ALLERGIC RHINITIS

List 4 common causes of seasonal allergies.	Outdoor inhalant allergens: tree, grass, and weed pollens (e.g., ragweed), outdoor mold spores
List 3 common causes of perennial allergies.	Indoor inhalant allergens: cat and dog dander, dust mites, molds (e.g., *Aspergillus, Penicillium*)
Whate are symptoms of allergic rhinitis?	Profuse, watery nasal discharge; itchy nose; postnasal drip; sneezing; cough. If the eyes are also involved, redness, tearing, and itching are observed (**rhinoconjunctivitis**).
What are "allergic shiners"?	Dark discoloration of the infraorbital area caused by venous stasis secondary to nasal congestion
What is the pathophysiology of allergic rhinitis?	An immediate hypersensitivity response occurs in the nasal mucosa of a sensitized individual. Specific IgE, which is stimulated by allergens, binds to mast cells. On re-exposure to the allergen, an allergen IgE-antibody reaction occurs, causing mast cell degranulation and release of mediators (e.g., **histamine, metabolites of the arachidonic acid pathway,** and **inflammatory cytokines**) which increase vascular permeability, smooth muscle contraction, mucus secretion, and pruritus.

What is the differential diagnosis?	Upper respiratory tract infection, sinusitis, nonallergic rhinitis with eosinophilia, vasomotor rhinitis, rhinitis medicamentosa

What is a Hansel stain?	An eosin methylene blue stain that shows eosinophils well. Stained cell preparations with > 10% eosinophils are highly suggestive of allergic rhinitis.

How is allergic rhinitis managed?	1. Avoidance of allergens 2. Treatment options include: antihistamines, systemic and topical decongestants, intranasal cromolyn or corticosteroids, immunotherapy

INSECT STINGS AND BITES

List 7 common stinging insects.	**Apidae family**—bumble bee, honey bee **Vespidae family**—yellow jacket, white-faced hornet, yellow hornet, wasp **Formicidae family**—fire ant All the above belong to the Hymenoptera order of insects.

List 3 classifications of reactions and the characteristics of each.	**Local:** Swelling **< 2 cm** and lasts **< 24 hours,** often with local erythema and pruritus **Large local:** Swelling **> 2 cm** and lasts up to **48–72 hours** **Systemic:** Diffuse urticaria and pruritus, laryngeal edema, bronchospasm, hypotension, abdominal cramping, nausea, and vomiting

Which classifications are involved in most typical allergic reactions?	Local or large local—most children do not have systemic reactions, and those that do occur are rarely life threatening. Of children who have life-threatening reactions, fewer than 50% have a second life-threatening event after another sting.

What are "toxic reactions"?	Nonimmunologic reactions that usually occur with multiple stings and may resemble systemic reactions

List 4 components of the long-term management of insect allergy.

Education; avoidance; kits containing epinephrine for acute treatment after a sting; immunotherapy for children who have experienced a significant systemic reaction

How effective is immunotherapy?

At least 95% effective if a maintenance dose of 100 μg venom is achieved, the amount in an average sting.

How long should injection immunotherapy be continued?

At least 3–5 years in childhood, and possibly longer for adults.

30

Genetics

DEFINITIONS

What is the difference between the terms *congenital* and *genetic*?

Congenital means appearing at birth, without regard to the cause, whereas *genetic* implies that the basis of a disease or defect, at least in part, is determined by the genetic makeup of the individual. By definition, all birth defects are congenital, but many are not genetic.

What is a malformation?

A primary defect in the formation or development of a body part or organ

What is a deformation?

A change in the shape, form, or position of a normally formed body part or organ by extrinsic or mechanical forces

What is a disruption?

A defect caused by breakdown in a previously normal body part or organ

What is a malformation syndrome?

A pattern of multiple primary malformations in an individual from a single underlying cause

What is a sequence?

A primary malformation and 1 or more secondary malformations or deformations

What is an association?

The simultaneous occurrence of 2 or more traits or abnormalities that cannot be explained by chance. The VACTERL (formerly VATER) association is the best known pediatric association.

What is an autosome?

A non-sex chromosome (i.e., a chromosome other than X or Y)

What is an autosomal condition?

A condition caused by an abnormality involving a gene on an autosome

What is a mendelian trait or condition?

A genetic condition that is inherited as a single gene trait, the occurrence and recurrence of which conform to Mendel's laws

What is an autosomal recessive trait?

A trait or condition found when the affected person has a pair of mutant genes (i.e., is homozygous) for that condition. With true autosomal recessive traits, heterozygotes are free of clinical disease.

What is an autosomal dominant trait?

A condition caused by the presence of a single mutant gene, rather than a pair of mutant genes

What is a multifactorial trait?

A trait or condition caused by the interaction of multiple genes as well as additional nongenetic factors; these traits account for many common birth defects

What is anticipation?

A phenomenon in which a genetic condition becomes more severe or has an earlier age of onset in succeeding generations. Some are associated with expansions of trinucleotide repeats.

What is mosaicism?

The presence of 2 or more genetically different cell lines in the same individual. One is usually normal.

COMMON GENETIC SYNDROMES

What is Down syndrome?

A recognizable pattern of malformations caused by the presence of extra chromosome 21 material. Also called "trisomy 21," if due to nondisjunction.

What are the features of Down syndrome?

In infants:

Hypotonia, flattened occiput (brachycephaly), redundant skin (especially on the posterior neck), flattened midface, epicanthal folds, upslanted palpebral fissures, small ears, prominent or protruding tongue, single transverse palmar creases, congenital heart disease (particularly atrioventricular canal [AVC] defect) (Ch 16)

Older children:

Same as those for infants with associated developmental delay, mental retardation, or both.

List 6 other complications.

Congenital duodenal obstruction; Hirschsprung disease (Ch 19, p. 265); hypothyroidism (congenital or acquired) (Ch 24, p. 337); congenital heart disease (Ch 16, p. 183); increased incidence of respiratory infections; increased risk of leukemia

What causes Down syndrome?

Extra material from chromosome 21, either through trisomy or a translocation. 95% of cases are caused by trisomy 21, and 5% are caused by unbalanced translocations resulting in the presence of extra chromosome 21 material or by mosaicism.

What is the most common risk factor for Down syndrome?

Advanced maternal age (older than 35 years of age at delivery)

List 6 features of trisomy 13.

Oral or facial clefts (or both), microphthalmia, postaxial polydactyly, apical scalp defects, intrauterine growth retardation, congenital heart disease

What is the prognosis for trisomy 13?

Most children die in the first year of life. Survivors are usually profoundly retarded.

List 6 features of trisomy 18.

Intrauterine growth retardation, small ears with flattened helices, small mouth, congenital heart disease, omphalocele (Ch 23, p. 320), unusual hand positioning (second and fifth fingers overlapping the third and fourth)

What is the prognosis for trisomy 18?

Most children die in the first year of life. Survivors are retarded, although some learn communication skills.

What is Turner syndrome?

Classic Turner syndrome is caused by the absence of one X chromosome in a female. About 50% of patients with the Turner syndrome phenotype have a 45,X karyotype, and about 20%–30% are mosaic. About 10%–20% have a structural rearrangement involving a deletion of part or all of the short arm of one of the two X chromosomes.

What are the features of Turner syndrome?

Girls with Turner syndrome may have short stature; delayed puberty with primary amenorrhea (caused by gonadal dysgenesis); lymphedema of the hands and feet; coarctation of the aorta (29%) (Ch 16, p. 198); kidney malformations (50%); webbed neck; shield (broad) chest; and prominent, posteriorly rotated ears

Are girls with Turner syndrome retarded?

Not usually, although they may have problems in spatial perceptual ability.

What is Klinefelter syndrome?

A syndrome seen in males who have an extra X chromosome (47,XXY)

What are the features of Klinefelter syndrome?

In young boys?

Generally few physical abnormalities.

Older patients?

Above average height, small testes, gynecomastia, fat distribution on hips and chest, below average IQ.

What is fragile X syndrome?

An X-linked condition caused by expansion of a trinucleotide repeat in the FMR1 gene

What are the features of the fragile X syndrome?

Young boys with the full mutation may have developmental delay, large ears, and a long face. Postpubertal boys usually have enlarged testes. Boys with the full mutation are usually retarded. Girls with the full mutation may also be retarded, but usually are less severely affected. They generally have few physical findings.

What is a premutation for the fragile X syndrome?

An increase in the size of the trinucleotide repeat from the normal size (usually < 50 repeats) to about 52–200 repeats. Individuals with the premutation are usually asymptomatic, but females risk having children with a full mutation.

What is Huntington disease?

A progressive autosomal dominant disorder. Onset is usually in adulthood, and characterized by progressive chorea, psychiatric problems, and dementia.

How do pediatric patients present?

Psychiatric or behavioral problems or rigidity. It is uncommon in children.

What is the cause of Huntington disease?

An expansion of a CAG nucleotide repeat in the "huntington" gene on chromosome 4

What is neurofibromatosis type 1 (von Recklinghausen disease)?

An autosomal dominant disorder characterized by hyperpigmented macules (café au lait spots) (Ch 27, p. 386) and cutaneous neurofibromata.

List 4 common findings.

Multiple (usually > 6) café au lait spots, Lisch nodules of the iris, axillary freckling, cutaneous neurofibromata

What are some complications?

Pseudoarthrosis, scoliosis, meningioma, optic glioma, seizures, learning disabilities, mental retardation, pheochromocytoma, hypertension, malignant degeneration of a neurofibroma, leukemia

What is tuberous sclerosis?

An autosomal dominant disorder characterized by hamartomas, hypopigmented skin lesions, and an increased risk of seizures and mental retardation. The kidney, heart, and eyes may also be affected by this condition.

What is the classic triad of symptoms?

Hypopigmented skin lesions, with epilepsy and mental retardation

What are 5 physical findings?

"Ash leaf" hypopigmented macules (found most commonly on the trunk), shagreen patches, adenoma sebaceum, periungual fibromas, and intracranial lesions, which are sometimes calcified

What are signs and symptoms with which pediatric patients present?

Seizures; developmental delay, mental retardation, or both; skin lesions.

Skin lesions may not be present or obvious in early infancy.

Hypopigmented skin lesions may be easier to see if viewed with a Wood's (ultraviolet) lamp.

What is the prognosis for tuberous sclerosis?

It varies. Some patients are healthy, whereas others may have severe mental retardation, seizures, or cardiac tumors.

Index

References followed by "t" denote tables